Contents

CD-ROM

- Chapter 1–28 Electronic Text

- Appendix: Table of Chemical Elements

- Glossary 1: By Word Parts

    Selected Key Prefixes, Suffixes, Word Roots, and Combining Forms Used in Medical Terms

- Glossary 2: By Meaning

    The Meanings of Selected Key Prefixes, Suffixes, Word Roots and Combining Forms Used in Medical Terms

- Index

- Workbook Answers

Preface

I hear, and I forget;
I see, and I remember;
I do, and I understand.

—An old Chinese Proverb

Today, as well as in the past, health care is one of the most complex of human endeavors. It involves all types of practitioners, differing in their education and training, and in their roles of health-care delivery.

Additionally, the quantity and variety of medical instruments, procedures, treatments, and approaches to such treatments continues to grow. At the base of it all are knowledge and understanding of fundamental biological and scientific concepts, and medical terminology. This book is designed to help you build your foundational understanding in these areas.

One of the most perplexing tasks for students beginning an education and training program in the health sciences, or individuals involved with the delivery of health care, is that of understanding and correctly using medical terms. Learning medical terminology and being able to apply specific terms can be not only challenging but fascinating as well. ***Human Biology and Medical Terminology Applications*** serves as a basic introduction and as a review and reinforcement tool. It is designed to help health professionals and students master basic medical and scientific concepts, as well as related terminology.

GOALS OF THIS BOOK

This learning system has been designed with three goals in mind:

1. To enable learners to develop the critical thinking skills necessary for understanding human biology and applying the requisite terminology;
2. To present basic subject matter in a highly interactive manner that supports learning and retention;
3. To emphasize basic facts, concepts and technical vocabulary that are critical to understanding both normal and disease processes.

SCOPE

Although ***Human Biology and Medical Terminology Applications*** presents topics ranging from simple chemistry, cells, and components of human body systems to elements of epidemiology and scientific units of measurements, it is not intended to be encyclopedic. In fact, to facilitate learning, we cover only the most important and useful basic aspects of medical terminology. In addition, descriptions of actual clinical situations and other learning devices are provided where relevant—enabling students to build their knowledge of terminology and basic concepts.

FORMAT

The unique format of this learning system is ideal for self-paced study as well as a traditional classroom experience. Students are encouraged to complete the wide variety workbook exercises contained in these pages, while referring to the full-color electronic text, which contains a rich array of visual and textual content in Adobe Acrobat (PDF) format. The illustrations used have

Human Biology and Medical Terminology Applications

George A. Wistreich, Ph. D., F(AAM), F(LSL), F(AIC), F(RSPH)

Professor of Microbiology, East Los Angeles College

PEARSON

Prentice
Hall

Upper Saddle River

Publisher: Julie Levin Alexander
Assistant to Publisher: Regina Bruno
Senior Acquisitions Editor: Mark Cohen
Associate Editor: Melissa Kerian
Editorial Assistants: Mary Ellen Ruitenberg & Jaquay Felix
Senior Marketing Manager: Nicole Benson
Marketing Assistant: Janet Ryerson
Channel Marketing Manager: Rachele Strober
Director of Production & Manufacturing: Bruce Johnson
Managing Production Editor: Patrick Walsh
Production Liaison: Danielle Newhouse
Production Editor: Michael Drew, nSight
Manufacturing Manager: Ilene Sanford
Manufacturing Buyer: Pat Brown
Design Director: Cheryl Asherman
Senior Design Coordinator: Christopher Weigand
Composition: nSight, Laserwords Pte. Ltd.
Printing & Binding: The Courier Company
Cover Printer: Phoenix Color Corp.

Notice: The author and publisher of this volume have taken care that the information and technical recommendations contained herein are based on research and expert consultation, and are accurate and compatible with the standards generally accepted at the time of publication. Nevertheless, as new information becomes available, changes in clinical and technical practices become necessary. The reader is advised to carefully consult manufacturer's instructions and information material for all supplies and equipment before use, and to consult with a healthcare professional as necessary. This advice is especially important when using new supplies or equipment for clinical purposes. The author and publisher disclaim all responsibility for any liability, loss, injury, or damage incurred as a consequence, directly or indirectly, of the use and application of any of the contents of this volume.

Photographs used with permission of the author, George A. Wistreich.

Pearson Prentice Hall™ is a trademark of Pearson Education, Inc.
Pearson® is a registered trademark of Pearson plc
Prentice Hall® is a registered trademark of Pearson Education, Inc.

Pearson Education Ltd., *London*
Pearson Education Australia Pty. Limited, *Sydney*
Pearson Education Singapore, Pte. Ltd.
Pearson Education North Asia Ltd., *Hong Kong*
Pearson Education Canada, Ltd., *Toronto*
Pearson Educación de Mexico, S.A. de C.V.
Pearson Education—Japan, *Tokyo*
Pearson Education Malaysia, Pte. Ltd.
Pearson Education, Upper Saddle River, New Jersey

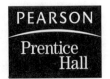

10 9 8 7 6 5 4 3 2 1

ISBN 0-13-013933-5

been carefully selected and designed to show sufficient detail for learning without students becoming bored. A number of other illustrations, including diagrams and photographs of actual disease states, and related topics, are interwoven into the electronic text chapters to effectively illustrate the subject matter.

CD-ROM: All electronic text chapters begin with a listing of competency-based objectives that clearly emphasize what learners are to accomplish. In addition all chapters introduce the specific word elements (word roots, combining forms, prefixes, and suffixes) related to the topics covered early on to aid the reader. Summarizing tables are included to emphasize what should be learned and to demonstrate approaches to organizing and applying concepts, terminology, and information.

Pronunciations for most scientific and medical terms are generally given when a term is first mentioned, as well as in various tables throughout the chapters. Knowing how to pronounce a term generally tends to lower certain barriers so that students are more likely to use and apply them.

Workbook: The workbook provides interactive exercises with clear-cut and simple-to-follow directions emphasizing the "learning by doing principle". The integration of the traditional study-guide approach with on-hands exercises have been shown to be functional motivating tools to learning. The variety and number of exercises demand learning on several levels, avoid rote memorizing, and help to keep a high level of interest.

𝒲ORKBOOK FEATURES

Those who are visually oriented will find the anatomical labeling challenge of "Vision Quizzes" in several exercises particularly challenging and beneficial to learning. Additionally, a selection of matching, multiple choice, and completion questions are designed to test and reinforce the following: student understanding and mastery of basic concepts; recognition of word elements; ability to correctly spell and pronounce medical and related terms; and enlarging a medical vocabulary.

Most chapters of the workbook contain a component titled "Increasing Your Medical Terminology Word Power", which may include actual clinical case histories, short articles. These sections provide opportunities for learners to increase their verbal skills and to expand their understanding of diseases, medical procedures, and approaches to diagnosis and treatment. Additionally "Term Search Challenges", which conclude these sections, provide a fun, option by challenging students to find specific terms hidden within a series of letters.

The correct responses for all questions are displayed on the e-text CD-ROM in the Appendices. It is important to note that the correct spelling of medical and/or scientific terms is emphasized throughout.

𝒯HE MEDICAL DICTIONARY—A COMPREHENSIVE RESOURCE

In addition to using the e-text as a resource, students are encouraged to refer to a medical dictionary during their study and throughout their careers. There are a variety of medical dictionaries from which to choose, and instructors may opt to recommend one over others. However while the approaches and presentation may vary from dictionary to dictionary, accuracy is not compromised. In general, most medical dictionaries include the following components:

- Alphabetical vocabulary: Main entries of up-to-date terms alphabetized letter by letter regardless of the spaces that occur between words.
- Definitions: Comprehensive explanations of the word of concept described.
- Pronunciations: Phonetic pronunciations of the majority of defined terms using secondary accents, and long and short vowels as indicated by marks over the vowels. Accents are shown by single (') or double (") marks to indicate emphasis on certain syllables. The marks over vowels are known as diacritics, and include the macron (ˉ) specifying the long sounds of vowels, and the breve (˘) showing the short sound. Other aspects of the pronunciations of terms can be found on pages 1-7 and 1-8 in the Chapter 1 e-text.

- Etymology: The origin and derivation of the defined term (entry) is presented in brackets following the entry. The major sources of medical terms are Latin and Greek.
- Abbreviations: Standard abbreviations for entries are included with their definitions. In addition, abbreviations may also be listed alphabetically throughout the text of some dictionaries. Abbreviations used for prescriptions and nonmedical terms may be found in Appendices.
- Synonyms: Terms having about the same meaning as the entry are listed at the end of the definition.
- Illustrations: A variety of tables and/or listings on topics such as measurement units and systems, laboratory test values, computer terms, and nutritive values of foods.

By combining the rich visual and textual information presented in the e-text, with the reinforcement provided in the workbook, and then adding the utility of a dictionary reference, students will have a complete tool set to launch their study in this exciting world of medicine.

ACKNOWLEDGMENTS

The author would also like to thank Mr. Mark Cohen, Ms. Mary Ellen Ruitenberg and other members of the editorial and production staffs of Prentice Hall, as well as Michael Drew and Robert Saley at nSight, for their untiring and imaginative efforts expended in the preparation of this workbook/e-text combination.

Thanks also to the team of reviewers for their feedback and assistance:

Julie Boles
Ithaca College
Department of Health Policy Studies
Ithaca, NY

Sue Boulden
Mount Hood Community College
Department of Medical Assisting
Gresham, OR

Recbecca Gibson
University of Akron
Department of Medical Assisting
Akron, OH

Pamela Eugene
Delgado Community College
Department of Allied Health
New Orleans, LA

Susan Buboltz
Madison Area Technical College
Department of Medical Assisting
Madison, WI

Beverly Baker
Western Iowa Technical Community College
Department of Surgery Technology
Sioux City, IA

Margaret Mazzone
Daemen College
Department of Occupational Therapy
Amherst, NY

Iris Leigh
Massachusetts Bay Community College
Department of Occupational
   Therapy Assisting
Wellesley Hills, MA

Valeria Truitt
Craven Community College
Department of Medical Office Administration
New Bern, NC

DEDICATION

To Renee, my wife, and to my sons Eddie and Phillip, whose love and encouragement have been a major part of my personal and professional life, and to my colleagues, and students, who provided the motivation and inspiration to develop an interactive approach to learn and to retain basic medical terminology and applications.

An Introduction to the Basics

"All we know is still infinitely less than still remains unknown."
—William Harvey, De Motu Cordis, Dedication

INFORMATIONAL CHALLENGE

A. Basic Word Elements

I.   Fill in the Blank

Fill in the blank with the appropriate term.

Example: A _____ appears at the beginning of another word element to change its meaning.

(The answer is ***prefix***.)

   1. A combining form consists of a _____ and a _____.
   2. A suffix is attached to the _____ of the _____
_____.
   3. A word root contains the _____ _____ of a term.
   4. A combining vowel is used to make _____ easier.
   5. A _____ may be used to specify a surgical or diagnostic test.
   6. In the term **hepatoma**, the **-oma** is a _____.
   7. In the term **osteoarthritis**, **osteo** is a _____, **arthr** is a
_____, and **-itis** is a _____.

II.   Matching 1: Medical Term Elements

Match the term component to its word element. (The same element may be used more than once.) Insert the appropriate letter in the space next to the question number.

Choices:

_____ **1.** arthr   _____ **7.** derm-   **a.** prefix
_____ **2.** cardi   _____ **8.** -ic   **b.** suffix
_____ **3.** o   _____ **9.** -itis   **c.** word root
_____ **4.** hypo-   _____ **10.** hepat-   **d.** combining form
_____ **5.** plast   _____ **11.** -oma   **e.** combining vowel
_____ **6.** cardi/o-   _____ **12.** -gram   **f.** none of the above

III.   Matching 2: Word Root Definitions

Match the word root to its meaning. (The same meaning may be used more than once.) Insert the appropriate letter in the space next to the question number.

Choices:

_____	**1.** arthr-	**a.**	liver
_____	**2.** hemat-	**b.**	joint
_____	**3.** hepat-	**c.**	heart
_____	**4.** electr-	**d.**	skin
_____	**5.** derm-	**e.**	electricity
_____	**6.** cardi-	**f.**	artery
_____	**7.** arteri-	**g.**	blood

IV.   Word Analysis 1: Word Elements

Determine a term's meaning by identifying its word elements. Separate each word element by diagonal line (/) and use the symbols indicated below to label each word element. Some answers are provided as aids.

Word Element	Symbol
word root	**wr**
combining form	**cf**
combining vowel	**cv**
prefix	**p**
suffix	**s**

	Term	Word Elements	Meaning
Example:	**endocarditis:**	**endo-** / **card** / **-itis;**	*inflammation within the*
		p wr s	*heart*

	Term	Word Elements	Meaning
1.	arthroplasty	_____	_____
2.	arthritis	_____	_____
3.	hepatoma	hepat / -oma	_____
		wr s	_____
4.	arteriosclerosis	_____	_____
5.	laryngoscope	_____	*instrument used to examine the larynx*

V.   Word Analysis 2: Combining Forms, Word Roots, Prefixes, and Suffixes

Table 1-5 lists a number of terms with their pronunciations and definitions.

   1. Analyze each term.
   2. Circle all combining forms, word roots, prefixes, and suffixes, and label them **cf, wr, p,** or **s.**
   3. Check your answers (shown in Table 1-7).

TABLE 1-5 WORD ANALYSIS 2: COMBINING FORMS, WORD ROOTS, PREFIXES, AND SUFFIXES

Term and Pronunciation	Definition
circumocular (sur'-kum-OK-ū-lar)	*around the eye*
ectocorneal (ek'-tō-KOR-nē-al)	*outside the cornea (outer layer of the eye)*
endocardiac (en'-dō-KAR-dē-ak)	*within the heart*
epimandibular (ep'-i-man-DIB-ū-lar)	*on the lower jaw*
epiotic (ep'-i-OT-ik)	*over the ear*
exocardial (eks'-ō-KAR-dē-al)	*outside the heart*
extrahepatic (eks'-tra-he-PAT-ik)	*outside the liver*
infrapatellar (in'-fra-pa-TEL-ar)	*below the patella (knee cap)*
interarticular (in'-ter-ar-TIK-ū-lar)	*between two joints*
intracellular (in'-tra-SEL-ū-lar)	*within a cell*

VI. Word Analysis 3: Combining Forms and Suffixes

Table 1-6 lists a number of terms with their pronunciations and definitions.

1. Analyze each term.
2. Circle all combining forms, word roots, prefixes, and suffixes and label them **cf**, **wr**, **p**, or **s**.
3. Check your answers (shown in Table 1-8).

TABLE 1-6 WORD ANALYSIS 3: COMBINING FORMS AND SUFFIXES

Terms and Pronunciation	Definition
arteriosclerosis (ar-te'-rē-ō-skle-RŌ-sis)	thickening or hardening of blood vessels (arteries)
cardiograph (KAR-dē-ō-graf)	instrument to measure form and force of the heart's movement
dermatopathy (der'-ma-TOP-a-thē)	any disease of the skin
hepatogastric (hep'-a-tō-GAS-trik)	pertaining to the liver and the stomach
laryngoscope (lar-IN-gō-skōp)	instrument to examine the larynx
ophthalmoscope (of-THAL-mō-skōp)	instrument to examine the interior of the eye

VII.   Vision Quiz: Combining Forms and Body Structures

Figure 1-6 shows several human body organs, which are numbered. Select the combining form that corresponds to the numbered organ or structure and write your responses next to the number.

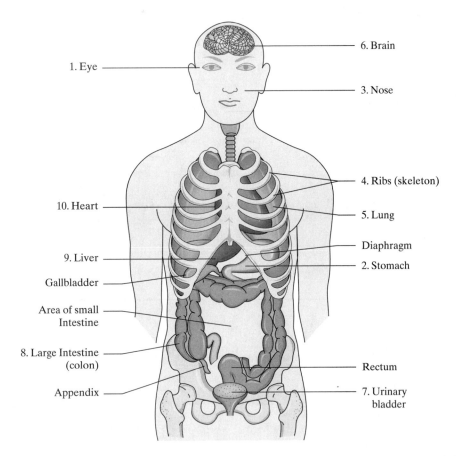

FIGURE 1-6   Vision Quiz. Several body organs are indicated in this figure. An orientation to and descriptions of body systems are provided in later chapters.

Example: The combining form appropriate for ***structure 2*** (the stomach) would be **b, gastro**.

Choices:

_____ 1.	**a.** cardio
_____ 2.	**b.** gastro
_____ 3.	**c.** hepato
_____ 4.	**d.** neuro
_____ 5.	**e.** ophthalmo
_____ 6.	**f.** pneumo
_____ 7.	**g.** skeleto
_____ 8.	**h.** uro
_____ 9.	**i.** naso
_____ 10.	**j.** colo

B. *Guides to Pronunciation*

I.   Fill in the Blank

Write the phonetic pronunciations of the terms in the spaces provided. Use a macron (‾) above vowels having the long sound.

Example: **arteriosclerosis**, ar-TER-ē-ō-skler-ō'-sis

1. prognosis _____
2. hematology _____
3. arthroscopy _____

4. endocardiac _____
5. intracellular _____
6. hemostasis _____

C. *Singular and Plural Forms*

I.   One or More?

Write "singular" or "plural" after each term or term ending.

1. cornea _____
2. lumina _____
3. abscesses _____
4. bacterium _____
5. corpus _____
6. deformities _____
7. cortices _____
8. parietes _____
9. thorax _____

10. phalanges _____
11. viscera _____
12. lumen _____
13. -ae _____
14. -on _____
15. -ses _____
16. -era _____
17. -y _____

Term Search Challenge

Locate 14 combining forms in the puzzle.

1. Write the combining form next to its definition. Then find that combining form in the puzzle and circle it.
2. Combining forms may be read from left to right, backward, up, down, or diagonally.
3. If a combining form appears more than once, circle it only once. (A combining form or a portion of it may be found inside others.)
4. Check your answers.

Clues:

1. eye _____
2. bone _____
3. larynx _____
4. electricity _____
5. joint _____
6. nerve _____
7. lung _____

8. skin _____
9. liver _____
10. artery _____
11. heart _____
12. stomach _____
13. skeleton _____
14. urine _____

Term Search Puzzle

```
O  P  H  T  H  A  L  M  O  U  R  O  N  N
E  N  R  G  A  S  T  R  O  M  A  H  R  E
L  E  R  Y  N  G  O  E  T  D  O  A  C  U
E  U  R  O  O  L  T  O  I  D  R  A  C  R
C  M  A  G  O  A  P  H  Y  E  T  F  X  O
T  O  M  S  S  L  E  R  A  R  T  E  R  I
R  T  C  O  T  I  S  I  T  M  I  S  S  I
O  T  A  P  E  H  T  T  I  A  C  A  R  D
A  O  R  I  O  G  R  A  R  T  E  R  I  O
R  R  D  R  A  M  E  L  E  O  C  T  R  U
T  C  I  T  O  C  A  R  I  T  I  S  R  R
H  G  T  A  L  A  R  Y  N  G  O  A  M  M
R  R  O  A  T  I  U  N  T  T  I  O  N  T
O  S  K  E  L  E  T  O  N  F  L  A  M  M
```

Prefixes and Their Uses

"In gaining Knowledge, you must accustom yourself to the strictest sequence . . . "
—I.P. Pavlov (1849 – 1936)

INFORMATIONAL CHALLENGE

A. General Features of Prefixes

I.   Multiple Choice

Which of the following statements are true? (Circle the correct answer/s.)

1. Most prefixes are parts of medical and scientific terms only.
2. A prefix is never used alone.
3. Prefixes usually are placed at the end of verbs, adjectives, or nouns to change their meanings.
4. In the term **antepartum** (an'-tē-PAR-tum), **ante-** is a prefix.
5. Most prefixes are parts of words in everyday language.
6. Prefixes change the meaning of terms—such as verbs, adjectives, or nouns—to which they are attached.

II.   Fill in the Blank

Fill in the blank with the appropriate word.

1. A _____ appears at the beginning of a word to change its meaning.
2. Prefixes are never used _____.
3. Most prefixes are derived from _____ and _____ sources.
4. In the term **antepartum** (an'-tē-PART-tum), **ante-** is a _____ and **–partum** is a _____.

B. Prefixes Indicating Position, Ranking, or Order of Appearance

I.   Matching: The Meaning of Prefixes

Match the prefix to its meaning. (The same meaning may be used more than once.) Insert the appropriate letter in the space next to each question number.

Choices:

_____ **1.** ante-	**a.** under	
_____ **2.** meta-	**b.** change	
_____ **3.** syn-	**c.** beyond	
_____ **4.** supra-	**d.** after	

_____ **5.** sym-	**e.** in front of
_____ **6.** sub-	**f.** above
_____ **7.** pre-	**g.** joined
_____ **8.** post-	**h.** none of the above

II.   Fill in the Blank: Prefix Applications

Fill in the blank with the appropriate word.

Choices:

a. meta-	**e.** sub-
b. pre-	**f.** post-
c. syn-	**g.** ante-
d. supra-	

Example: The **tuberculin** (tū-BER-kū-lin) skin test involves injecting test material under the skin. Such _____ **cutaneous** (ku-TA-nē-us) injections must be performed carefully so as not to draw blood.

(The answer is e., sub-.)

1. A group of signs and symptoms that accompany a disease is referred to as a(n)_____-drome.
2. The results of the laboratory test showed that the cancer spread to several body regions. This was clearly a case of cancer -_____-stasis.
3. Mrs. Jones did experience some pain and discomfort before her labor. Such _____-partum situations are not unusual.
4. Change in the appearance of a mole or any unusual bleeding may occur before the development of certain cancers. These are considered _____-cancerous symptoms.
5. The bullet lodged itself just below the collar bone or **clavicle** (KLAV-i-kul). The _____-clavian location of the bullet made it more difficult to remove.
6. Overexertion of the chest muscle during the exercise routine caused a bruising of the area just beneath the rib case. Mr. Ames was told to apply a heating pad to the _____-costal region.
7. There are genetic abnormalities that appear as a joining or fusion of two or more toes. In some cases, surgery can correct this _____-dactylism.
8. The specimen had to be taken from the area above the spine. Great care must be exercised in the removal of material from the _____-spinal location.

III.   Spell Check

Circle each incorrectly spelled term and write it correctly in the space provided.

1. antepartim   _____
2. subabdominal   _____
3. supraspinal   _____
4. metamorfosis   _____
5. preganglionic   _____

     6. symbiosis   _____

     7. postencefalitis   _____

     8. syndaktylism   _____

IV.   Word Analysis: Prefixes Indicating Position, Ranking, or Order of Appearance

Table 2-8 lists a number of terms with their pronunciations and definitions.

     1. Analyze each term.

     2. Circle all prefixes and label them **p**.

     3. Check your answers (shown in Table 2-13).

TABLE 2-8   WORD ANALYSIS: PREFIXES INDICATING POSITION, RANKING, OR ORDER OF APPEARANCE

Term and pronunciation	Definition
antecubital (an'-tē-KŪ-bi-tal)	in front of the elbow
metakinesis (met'-a-ki-NĒ-sis)	moving apart
postocular (post-OK-ū-lar)	behind the eye
preauricular (prē'-aw-RIK-ū-lar)	in front of the ear
subungual (sub-UNG-wal)	beneath the nail of a finger or toe
supracostal (soo'-pra-KOS-tal)	above the ribs
synalgia (sin-AL-jē-a)	reflex pain felt in a part distant from the site of its origin

C. Prefixes Indicating Location in Relation to Other Anatomical Parts

I.   Matching: The Meaning of Prefixes

Match the prefix to its meaning. (The same meaning may be used more than once.) Insert the appropriate letter in the space next to the question number.

Choices:

_____ **1.** endo-	**a.** outside
_____ **2.** ecto-	**b.** around
_____ **3.** epi-	**c.** below
_____ **4.** intra-	**d.** within
_____ **5.** infra-	**e.** between
_____ **6.** exo-	**f.** close to
_____ **7.** inter-	**g.** upon
_____ **8.** juxta-	**h.** middle
_____ **9.** circum-	**i.** in front of
_____**10.** peri-	**j.** across
_____**11.** trans-	**k.** behind
_____**12.** pro-	

II.   Fill in the Blank: Prefix Applications

Fill in the blank with the appropriate prefix.

Choices:

a.	infra-	**e.**	extra-
b.	medi-	**f.**	ecto-
c.	trans-	**g.**	peri-
d.	endo-	**h.**	circum-

Example: The problem was within the voice box or larynx. Such _____-laryngeal complications are not uncommon after some surgical procedures.

(The answer is d., endo-.)

1. The inflammation occurred around the eye. Treatment was simpler because of the _____-ocular site of the problem.

2. Certain viruses multiply in an area directly outside of the nucleus. Such viruses use several of the cellular structures in this _____-nuclear area for reproduction.

3. Infections within the heart may be caused by several types of microorganisms. Given the availability of an effective antibiotic and ample time, treatment of such _____-cardiac problems does not pose any difficulty.

4. The kidney machine, an instrument placed outside of the body, is used with individuals whose kidneys have completely failed. Several varieties of this _____-corporeal instrument are currently in use.

5. The x-ray showed the fracture to be just below the knee cap. Because of the _____-patellar location of the break, the entire leg was put into a cast.

6. The patient was experiencing severe pain toward the middle left side of his abdomen. This _____-al location suggested the possibility of **appendicitis** (a-pen'-di-SĪ-tis).

7. Pus formation appeared around the cornea. Its elimination from this _____-corneal area may be difficult without antibiotics.

8. Mr. Jones is not a candidate for an artificial heart. He clearly needs the transfer of a heart from a donor. The _____-plant operation should be performed as soon as an organ becomes available.

III.   Spell Check

Circle each incorrectly spelled term and write it correctly in the space provided.

1. circumokular _____
2. intraselluler _____
3. periarterial _____
4. transocular _____
5. ektositic _____
6. epidirmal _____
7. intirnasal _____
8. retrolingal _____

IV.   Word Analysis: Prefixes Indicating Location in Relation to Other Anatomical Parts

Table 2-9 lists a number of terms with their pronunciations and definitions.

   1. Analyze each term.
   2. Circle all prefixes and label them **p**.
   3. Check your answers (shown in Table 2-14).

TABLE 2-9   WORD ANALYSIS: PREFIXES INDICATING LOCATION IN RELATION TO OTHER ANATOMICAL PARTS

Term and Pronunciation	Definition
circumarticular (ser'-kum-ar-TIK-ū-lar)	around or surrounding a joint
ectocytic (ek'-tō-SĪ-tik)	outside of the cell
endoangiitis (en'-dō-an-jē-Ī-tis)	inflammation of the inner layer of blood vessels
epidermal (ep'-i-DER-mal)	outer skin layer
exoerythrocytic (ek'-sō-e-rith-rō-SI-tik)	occurring outside of red blood cells
extrahepatic(eks'-tra-hē-PAT-ik)	outside of the liver
infracostal (in'-fra-KOS-tal)	below the ribs
internasal (in'-ter-NĀ-zal)	between the nasal (nose) bones
juxtaspinal (juks'-ta-SPĪ-nal)	near the spinal column
mesobronchitis (mes'-o-bron-KĪ-tis)	inflammation of the middle layer of the **bronchi** (the two major branches of the windpipe or trachea) (TRĀ-kē-a)
periodontal (per'-ē-ō-DONT-al)	around the tooth
retrolingual (ret'-rō-LING-gwal)	behind the tongue
transaortic (trans-ā-OR-tik)	through the aorta (the main blood vessel of the arterial system)

D. *Prefixes Indicating Relationships, Rate, Origin, or Physical Condition*

I.   Matching: Prefix Meanings

Match the prefix to its meaning. (The same meaning may be used more than once.)
Insert the appropriate letter in the space next to each question number.

Choices:

_____	**1.** absent	**a.** an-
_____	**2.** unequal	**b.** ankylo-
_____	**3.** both sides	**c.** contra-
_____	**4.** painful	**d.** ambi-
_____	**5.** without	**e.** dys-
_____	**6.** fusion	**f.** con-

_____ **7.** opposite   **g.** ab-

_____ **8.** together   **h.** re-

_____ **9.** again   **i.** aniso-

II. Fill in the Blank: Applying Prefixes

Fill in the blank with the appropriate prefix.

Choices:

     a. ambi-   **e.** ab-

     b. an-   **f.** con-

     c. ankylo-   **g.** aniso-

     d. dys-   **h.** re-

Example: The patient's ability to speak was made difficult by an injury to the brain. This type of _____-phasia may result from certain virus infections.

(The answer is d., dys-.)

1. The laboratory reported a large number of red blood cells that differed from normal ones. Such _____-normal cells indicate a serious problem.

2. The use of certain drugs during pregnancy has been associated with birth defects. The _____-genital defects include the absence of limbs.

3. The tumors were found on both sides of the body. This _____-lateral involvement clearly indicated that the cancer had spread from its original site.

4. An individual with an injury to this part of the ear will be without the ability to hear. This condition of _____-acusia occurs almost immediately.

5. He does not feel any pain at all after the operation. The medication produced a state of complete _____-algesia.

6. It was quite a problem to make dentures for Mrs. Jones because of her wide upper jaw. Individuals with such unequal jaws are _____-gnathous.

7. Children with measles infections may experience a sticking together of their upper and lower eyelids. The careful application of a warm washcloth to this _____-blepharon can separate the eyelids.

8. Plastic and reconstructive surgery may be required following the separation of two or more fused fingers. This type of condition, _____-dactylia, is a congenital defect.

9. Mr. Smart's sore throat made it very difficult for him to swallow. Such _____-phagia is not uncommon with streptococcus infection.

10. Malaria is an example of a disease that periodically returns in the infected individual. The signs and symptoms of such _____-currences are usually less severe than in the original infection.

11. The white blood cells in the sample were not uniform in color. Such _____-chromatic effects are usually caused by old staining solutions.

III. Spell Check

Circle each incorrectly spelled term and write it correctly in the space provided.

     1. anallgesia   _____

     2. disgalactia   _____

    3. abrachius   _____

    4. ambelateral   _____

    5. congenital   _____

    6. disphagia   _____

    7. contralateral _____

    8. operation   _____

    9. ankylodactilia _____

IV.   Word Analysis: Prefixes Indicating Relationships, Rate, Origin, or Physical Condition

Table 2-10 lists a number of terms with their pronunciations and definitions.

    1. Analyze each term.
    2. Circle all prefixes and label them **p**.
    3. Check your answers (shown in Table 2-15).

TABLE 2-10 WORD ANALYSIS: PREFIXES INDICATING RELATIONSHIPS, RATE, ORIGIN, OR PHYSICAL CONDITION

Term and Pronunciation	Definition
abarticular (ab'-ar-TIK-ū-lar)	away or distant from a joint
anisocytosis (an-i'-sō-sī-TŌ-sis)	excessive unequal sizes of cells
ankylochilia (an'-ki-lō-KĪ-lē-a)	sticking together of upper and lower lips
dysgalactia (dis'-ga-LAK-tē-a)	defective (breast) milk secretion

E. Prefixes Indicating Direction, Source, or Rate

I.   Matching: The Meaning of Prefixes

Match the prefix to its meaning. (The same meaning may be used more than once.) Insert the appropriate letter in the space next to each question number.

                                         Choices:

_____ **1.** auto-   **a.** slow

_____ **2.** hypo-   **b.** excessive

_____ **3.** brady-   **c.** male

_____ **4.** hyper-   **d.** rapid

_____ **5.** pseudo-   **e.** less than

_____ **6.** andro-   **f.** false

_____ **7.** tachy-   **g.** self

II.   Fill in the Blank: Prefix Applications

Fill in the blank with the appropriate prefix.

Choices:

    a. brady-   **e.** andro-

    b. hyper-   **f.** pseudo-

    c. hypo-   **g.** tachy-

    d. auto-

Example: This material is not true cartilage; it merely resembles it. One can say that it is _____-cartilaginous.

(The answer is f., pseudo-.)

1. The prehistoric monster resembled a male. Its _____-id appearance was evident.
2. A woman can examine herself for breast cancer. This form of _____-diagnosis is being encouraged more.
3. The injury to his head was quite severe and caused a general slow type of body movement. This condition of _____-kinesia may also be caused by certain drugs.
4. Breathing and heart action occur independently, unlike the directed types of body function. This form of self-direction is a feature of the _____-nomic nervous system.
5. People with certain types of ulcers produce excessive amounts of acid in their gastrointestinal systems. Various drugs are available to treat such _____-acidity.
6. In blood smears of anemic patients, most red blood cells have less color than normal red blood cells. This _____-chromasia is caused by reduced amounts of hemoglobin.
7. Rapid or fast heart beating is not unusual when you are frightened. Such _____-cardia generally occurs during times of stress.
8. Laboratory and physical findings led the physician to incorrectly diagnosis inflammation of the brain. When _____-encephalitis is suspected, it is always advisable to repeat all tests.

III.   Spell Check

Circle each incorrectly spelled term and write it correctly in the space provided.

1. andropathe   _____
2. autodiagnosis   _____
3. bradicardia   _____
4. hyperlipemea   _____
5. hypoglosal   _____
6. pseudoencephalitis _____
7. tachycardia   _____
8. inflammation   _____

IV.   Word Analysis 1: Prefixes Indicating Direction, Source, or Rate

Table 2-11 lists a number of terms with their pronunciations and definitions.

TABLE 2-11   WORD ANALYSIS 1: PREFIXES INDICATING DIRECTION, SOURCE, OR RATE

Term and Pronunciation	Definition
android (AN-droyd)	resembling a male
autocytolysis (aw'-tō-sī-TOL-i-sis)	self-destruction of cells
bradycardia (brad'-ē-KAR-dē-a)	slow heart beat

(Continued)

TABLE 2-11 (CONTINUED)

Term and Pronunciation	Definition
hyperorchidism (hī'-per-OR-kid-iz-em)	excessive testicular secretion activity
hypodermic (hī'-pō-DER-mik)	under the skin
pseudoencephalitis (soo'-dō-en-sef-a-LĪ-tis)	false form of brain infection (inflammation)
tachypnea (tak'-ip-NĒ-a)	rapid breathing

1. Analyze each term.
2. Circle all prefixes and label them **p**.
3. Check your answers (shown in Table 2-16).

V.   Word Analysis 2: Prefixes, Direction, Source, or Rate

Following is a list of terms and their definitions,

1. Analyze each term.
2. Circle all word roots and combining forms and label them **wr** and **cf**, respectively.
3. Write the meaning of these word elements in the spaces provided.

	Term	Definition	Word Elements and Their Meanings
1.	hypoglossal	under the tongue	_____
2.	encephalitis	brain inflammation	_____
3.	tachycardia	rapid heart beat	_____
4.	hypodermic	under the skin	_____
5.	suprarenal	above the kidney	_____
6.	subcostal	below the ribs	_____
7.	postocular	behind the eye	_____
8.	preauricular	in front of the ear	_____
9.	subungual	under the nail	_____
10.	mesonasal	middle of the nose	_____

F. Prefixes Indicating Absence, Quantity, or Size

I.   Matching: The Meaning of Prefixes

Match the prefix to its meaning. (The same meaning may be used more than once.) Insert the appropriate letter in the space next to each question number.

Choices:

1. _____	auto-	**a.** without
2. _____	a-	**b.** twice
3. _____	macro-	**c.** half
4. _____	micro-	**d.** two
5. _____	hemi-	**e.** ten
6. _____	bi-	**f.** small
7. _____	diplo-	**g.** one
8. _____	deca-	**h.** large
9. _____	mono-	**i.** all
10. _____	milli-	**j.** one-thousandth
11. _____	poly-	**k.** many
12. _____	pan-	**l.** three
		m. four
		n. none of the above

II.   Fill in the Blank: Prefix Applications

Fill in the blank with the appropriate prefix.

Choices:

a.	poly-	**e.**	hemi-
b.	tri-	**f.**	deca-
c.	bi-	**g.**	uni-
d.	macro-		

Example: Unfortunately, one of the consequences of this genetic defect is an unusually big head. The condition of _____-cephalia is found with several disease states. (The answer is d., macro-.)

1. The drug came in ten-gram portions. Each tube had its weight indicated as _____-grams.
2. This lens has a round, raised, or convex surface on two sides. Thus it is referred to as a _____-concave lens.
3. Ms. Care experienced pain on only one side of her face. What could cause this _____-facial involvement?
4. Ms. Wilson has an abnormally large jaw. Individuals with this condition of _____-gnathia have a difficult time getting dentures that fit well.
5. Recovery from certain infections such as gonorrhea (gon'-ō-RĒ-a) may result in an arthritic (arth-RIT-ik) condition affecting many joints. Consequences such as this _____-articular disorder are not unusual.
6. One heart valve consists of three cusps. As a matter of fact, it is called the _____-cuspid.
7. Bacteria are generally one-celled. These _____-cellular forms of life are found everywhere.

III.   Spell Check

Circle each incorrectly spelled term and write it correctly in the space provided.

1. amenorhea   _____
2. biarticuler   _____

    3. hemifacial   _____
    4. semicircular   _____
    5. multicellular   _____
    6. aphasea   _____
    7. hemianalgesia   _____
    8. monodactelism   _____
    9. panarteritis   _____
    10. polygangleonic   _____

IV.   Word Analysis: Prefixes Indicating Absence, Quantity, or Size

Table 2-12 lists a number of terms with their pronunciations and definitions.

    1. Analyze each term.
    2. Circle all prefixes and label them **p.**
    3. Check your answers (shown in Table 2-17).

TABLE 2-12 WORD ANALYSIS: PREFIXES INDICATING ABSENCE, QUANTITY, OR SIZE

Term and Pronunciation	Definition
aphasia (a-FĀ-zē-a)	absence of speech
analgesia (an'-al-JĒ-zē-a)	absence of pain
bicellular (bī-SEL-ū-lar)	composed of two cells
hemianalgesia (hem'-ē-an-al-JĒ-zē-a)	lack (absence) of pain on one side (of the body)
macrocytosis (mak'-rō-sī-TŌ-sis)	larger than normal cells
microangiopathy (mī'-krō-an-jē-OP-a-thē)	pathology (disease) of small blood vessels
monodactylism (mon-ō-DAK-til-iz-em)	having one digit (finger or toe) on one hand or foot
panarteritis (pan'-ar-te-RĪ-tis)	inflammation of all parts of an artery
polyganglionic (pol'-ē-gang'-le-ŌN-ik)	involving many ganglia (nerve cell bodies)

G. Specialties in Medicine

I.   Matching: Identifying Medical Specialties

Match the specialty to its description. Insert the appropriate letter in the space next to the question number.

_____ **1.** cardiology (kar'-dē-OL-ō-jē)
_____ **2.** endocrinology (en'-dō-krin-OL-ō-jē)
_____ **3.** dermatology (der'-ma-TOL-ō-jē)
_____ **4.** otorhinolaryngology (o'-tō-rī'-nō-lā-r'-in-GOL-ō-jē)
_____ **5.** gynecology (gī'-nē-KOL-ō-jē)
_____ **6.** neurology (nū-ROL-ō-jē)

_____ **7.** obstetrics (ob-STET-riks)
_____ **8.** ophthalmology (of'-thal-MOL-ō-jē)
_____ **9.** internal medicine
_____ **10.** pediatrics (pē'-dē-AT-riks)
_____ **11.** urology (ū-ROL-ō-jē)

Choices:

   a. treatment of disorders and diseases of the nervous system
   b. care of pregnant women before, during, and after birth
   c. treatment of diseases or conditions of the eye
   d. treatment of disorders of the ear, nose, and throat
   e. treatment of diseases and injuries of internal organs and related body parts
   f. treatment of skin conditions
   g. treatment of diseases and disorders of female genital organs
   h. treatment of glands that secrete hormones
   i. treatment of urinary systems of both men and women
   j. treatment of children and adolescents.
   k. treatment of heart disorders

II.   Spell Check

Circle each incorrectly spelled term and write it correctly in the space provided.

   1. endocrinology   _____
   2. otorinolaryngology   _____
   3. guynecology   _____
   4. nurology   _____
   5. ofhtjalmology   _____
   6. pediatricks   _____
   7. cardiology   _____
   8. urology   _____

H. Increasing Your Medical Terminology Word Power

   1. Read the following case history.
   2. Prepare to answer the questions at the end of the section.
   3. Circle all unfamiliar terms with a red pencil.
   4. Underline familiar terms with a blue pencil.
   5. Use your knowledge of word elements, a medical dictionary, and the key terms to find the meanings of unfamiliar terms.

The Use of a Gastropericardial Fistula after Laparoscopic Surgery for Reflux Disease

Key Terms

adenopathy (ad'-e-NOP-a-thē)   lymph nodes exhibiting swelling and disease

atrial (Ā-trē-al)   the receiving chamber of the heart (atrium, Ā-trē-um)

fibrillation (fi'-bri-LĀ-shun)   quivering or spontaneous contraction of individual muscle fibers

fistula (FIS-tū-la)   an abnormal tubelike passage from a normal cavity or tube to a free surface or another cavity

fundoplication (fun'-dō-pī-KĀ-shun) surgical restoration to normal position of the size of the opening into the fundus of the stomach and stitching (suturing) the previously removed end of the esophagus to it

gastroesophageal (gas'-trō-e-sof'-a-JĒ-al) pertaining to the stomach and esophagus

gastroesophageal reflux a backward flow of gastric contents into the esophagus

gastropericardial (gas' trō-per-i-KAR-dē-al) stomach area near and/or around the heart

gastroscopy (gas-TRŌS-kō-pē) examination of the stomach and abdominal cavity by use of a gastroscope

infarct (in-FARKT) in this presentation, a heart attack resulting from a blood clot in the heart's arterial system.

intermittent (in'-ter-MIT-ent) occurring at intervals, coming and going

intraoperative (in'-tra-OP-er-a-tiv) occurring during surgery

laparoscopic (lap'-a-rō-SKOP-ik) abdominal surgery using an instrument called a laparoscope

paraesophageal (par'-a-e-sof'-a-JĒ-al) area around the esophagus

postprandial (post-PRAN-dē-al) following a meal

reduction (ri-DUK-shun) restoring to the normal position

reflux (RĒ-fluks) a backward flow

refractory (rē-FRAK-tō-rē) resistant to ordinary treatment

resolution (rez-ō-LŪ-shun) return to normal conditions

ulcer (UL-ser) an open sore

Introduction

Laparoscopic approaches are commonly used to treat gastroesophageal reflux disorders and diseases. Numerous studies have demonstrated the safety, effectiveness, and long-lasting benefits of these minimally invasive procedures. Intraoperative complications can occur and may be life-threatening. The physical and laboratory findings of a case in which a life-threatening gastropericardial fistula was a late complication of a laparoscopic procedure is reported here.

CASE REPORT

A 60-year-old man who was visiting Richmond, Virginia, presented to the emergency room facility in February 2001, complaining of pain in his left shoulder that spread to his neck. His medical history included the symptoms of gastroesophageal reflux that was refractory to medical therapy and prostate cancer, which had been treated with local radiation therapy three years earlier.

In October 1999, the patient had undergone a laparoscopic fundoplication, with a resolution of his reflux symptoms. The stomach was easily reduced into the abdomen from its abnormal extension near the esophagus or paraesophageal position.

On Thanksgiving Day, 1999, the patient experienced sudden and severe abdominal pains, which decreased after taking several anti-acid pills. Although he did not have additional episodes of severe pain, he experienced chronic postprandial pain. During the next four weeks he lost approximately 20 pounds and had periodic night sweats.

On December 21, 1999, the patient was admitted to the emergency room with atrial fibrillation. He was given sublingual nitroglycerin to bring the heart back to normal, and his blood pressure fell significantly, which was also corrected appropriately. The patient was found to have left supraclavicular adenopathy and an enlarged prostate gland.

He was admitted to the hospital for additional tests, corrective surgery, and treatment. Upon further testing, cardiac enzyme levels were not found to be elevated, but electrocardiographic findings suggested the presence of an old infarct. Gastroscopy showed a gastric ulcer. Biopsy specimens contained no cancer cells.

At a routine follow-up visit four months after surgery, the patient reported he was eating well and had no reflux signs or symptoms.

Questions

I.   Definitions

Give the meaning of the following prefixes.

    1. intra- _____
    2. para- _____
    3. sub- _____
    4. supra- _____
    5. post- _____
    6. peri- _____

II.   Matching: Case Report

Match the term to its meaning. Insert the appropriate letter in the space next to the question number.

Choices:

_____ **1.** intraoperative	**a.** diseased lymph nodes
_____ **2.** refractory	**b.** quivering of individual muscle fibers
_____ **3.** infarct	**c.** an abnormal tubelike passage from a normal cavity to a free surface
_____ **4.** fistula	
_____ **5.** postprandial	**d.** backward flow of gastric contents into the esophagus
_____ **6.** gastroscopy	
_____ **7.** intermittent	**e.** surgical examination of the stomach and abdominal cavity
_____ **8.** ulcer	
_____ **9.** adenopathy	**f.** blood clot, or blood vessel narrowing, leading to heart attack
____ **10.** fibrillation	
_____ **11.** gastroesophageal reflux	**g.** intervals of event coming and going
____ **12.** resolution	**h.** occurring during surgery
	i. following a meal
	j. resistant to ordinary treatment
	k. open sore
	l. return to normal

III.   Spell Check

Circle each incorrectly spelled term and write it correctly in the space provided.

    1. gastroesofageal _____
    2. laproscopik _____
    3. supraclavicular _____
    4. fistulla _____
    5. fibrillation _____
    6. atriel _____
    7. postprandial _____
    8. subliqual _____

Term Search Challenge

Locate 15 prefixes in the puzzle.

1. Write the specific prefix next to its definition. Then find that prefix in the puzzle diagram and circle it.
2. Prefixes may be read from left to right, backward, up, down, or diagonally.
3. If a prefix appears more than once, circle it only once. (A prefix may be found inside others.)
4. Check your answers.

Clues:

1. after _____
2. before _____
3. below _____
4. self _____
5. false _____
6. fast or rapid _____
7. away _____
8. both _____

9. painful _____
10. without _____
11. ten _____
12. many _____
13. outside _____
14. within _____
15. below _____

Term Search Puzzle

```
A  C  A  H  I  K  L  M  O  P  Q  E  P  S  O
M  L  B  D  P  S  E  U  D  O  O  J  O  E  T
B  R  G  H  O  A  I  L  M  U  O  U  S  M  U
I  P  Q  L  S  U  B  U  S  V  W  X  T  M  A
R  S  T  C  T  A  C  H  Y  Z  T  T  A  T  N
E  N  D  O  L  O  R  C  A  M  O  A  A  T  N
C  T  T  N  H  P  R  E  Z  O  I  V  Q  Y  K
T  R  R  T  R  I  T  S  X  L  N  S  R  H  Y
O  X  R  R  T  U  V  A  B  T  F  L  T  Y  L
Q  A  R  A  S  S  U  P  R  A  R  O  M  I  O
E  N  D  O  H  Y  P  E  R  T  A  A  W  A  P
H  D  E  C  A  N  N  A  N  L  K  Q  P  P  L
F  G  I  N  F  R  A  I  M  I  C  R  O  P  L
T  O  L  T  R  Z  Y  D  E  M  I  R  L  Y  O
A  M  B  I  M  O  P  O  N  M  D  Y  S  U  T
```

The Suffixes and Their Uses

"In gaining knowledge, you must accustom yourself to the strictest sequence. . . . "
—I.P. Pavlov (1849–1936)

INFORMATIONAL CHALLENGE

A. General Features of Suffixes

I.   Multiple Choice

Which of the following statements are true of suffixes? (Circle the correct answer/s.)

a. Most suffixes are parts of medical and scientific terms only.
b. A suffix is never used alone.
c. Suffixes are usually placed at the end of verbs, adjectives, or nouns to change their meaning.
d. In the term dermatosis (der'-ma-TŌ-sis), *-osis* is a suffix and *dermat* is a word root.
e. Most suffixes are parts of words in everyday language and make terms more specific in their meanings.
f. Suffixes change the meaning of terms such as verbs, adjectives, or nouns to which they are attached.
g. The meaning of a suffix is given first in defining an entire word.

B. Suffixes Indicating Diseases or Disorders

I.   Matching 1: Suffixes for Diseases or Disorders

Match the suffix to its meaning. (The same suffix may be used more than once.) Insert the appropriate letter in the space provided next to the question number.

Choices:

_____ **1.** -itis	**a.** softening
_____ **2.** -cele	**b.** enlargement
_____ **3.** -oma	**c.** hernia
_____ **4.** -malacia	**d.** inflammation
_____ **5.** -ectasis	**e.** fear of
_____ **6.** -megaly	**f.** tumor
_____ **7.** -emia	**g.** stretching
_____ **8.** -phobia	**h.** blood

II.   Matching 2: Suffixes for Diseases or Disorders

Match the suffix to its meaning. (The same suffix may be used more than once.)
Insert the appropriate letter in the space provided next to the question number.

Choices:

_____ **1.** -ptosis	**a.** disease or condition
_____ **2.** -rrhage	**b.** displacement
_____ **3.** -osis	**c.** flow
_____ **4.** -iasis	**d.** state of
_____ **5.** -rrhea	**e.** bleeding
_____ **6.** -rrhexis	**f.** rupture
_____ **7.** -pathy	**g.** disease

III.   Fill in the Blank: Suffix Applications

Fill in the blank with the appropriate term.

Choices:

a. -ectasis	**d.** -emia
b. -phobia	**e.** -megaly
c. -ptosis	**f.** -itis

Example: This group of viruses is known to cause an inflammation of the liver.

Cases of viral hepat-_____ occur regularly around the world.

The answer is f., -itis.

1. The infection caused the abnormal stretching of the blood vessels in Mr. Long's leg. The angi-_____ may cause a delay in his scheduled surgery.
2. This ice cream probably will raise his **blood sugar** to an abnormally high level. The high dose of sugar will cause hyperglyc-_____.
3. The strep throat is responsible for the **inflamed** tonsils. Streptococci are noted for causing tonsil-_____.
4. Her **large** facial features were caused by a hormonal abnormality. This condition, known as acro-_____ is associated with the pituitary (pi-TŪ-i-tār-ē) gland.
5. Individuals with the viral disease rabies generally have a violent **fear of water**. Apparently, the virus causes the hydro-_____ through its action on the central nervous system.
6. As a result of the accident, there was a **downward displacement** of the stomach **from its normal position**. This condition is known as gastro-_____.

IV.   Spell Check

Circle each incorrectly spelled term and write it correctly in the space provided.

1. cystoseal _____
2. angiectasis _____
3. hipergliseemea _____
4. hemorhage _____

      5. kolelitiasis   _____

      6. acromegalee   _____

      7. myelopathy   _____

      8. leucorhea   _____

      9. hepatitis   _____

V.   Word Analysis: Suffixes Indicating Diseases or Disorders

Table 3-8 lists a number of terms with their pronunciations and definitions.

      1. Analyze each term.

      2. Circle all prefixes and suffixes and label them **p** and **s**, respectively.

      3. Check your answers (shown in Table 3-13).

TABLE 3-8   WORD ANALYSIS: SUFFIXES INDICATING DISEASES OR DISORDERS

Terms and Pronunciation	Definition
dacryocele (DAK-rē-ō-sēl)	protrusion of the lacrimal (tear) sac
anemia (a-NĒ-mē-a)	lack of blood cells
cystitis (sis-TĪ-tis)	inflammation of the urinary bladder
enterolithiasis (en'-ter-ō-li-THĪ-a-sis)	formation of intestinal stones
enteromegaly (en'ter-ō-MEG-a-lē)	enlargement of the intestines
hepatoma (hep'-a-TŌ-ma)	a tumor of the liver
nephrosis (nef-RŌ-sis)	condition of kidney degeneration
enteropathy (en'-ter-OP-a-thē)	any intestinal disease
acrophobia (ak'-rō-FŌ-bē-a)	fear of high places
proctoptosis (prok'-top-TŌ-sis)	dropping down of the anus and rectum (prolapse)
gastrorrhagia (gas'-trō-RĀ-jē-a)	bleeding from the stomach
rhinorrhea (rī'-nō-RĒ-A)	watery discharge from the nose
enterorrhexis (en'-ter-ō-REKS-is)	rupture of the intestine

C. Suffixes Indicating Signs and Symptoms of Disease

I.   Matching: Suffixes for Signs and Symptoms of Disease

Match the term to its meaning. (The same meaning may be used more than once.) Insert the appropriate letter in the space provided next to the question number.

Choices:

_____ **1.** -ic	**a.** origin
_____ **2.** -algia	**b.** destruction
_____ **3.** -lysis	**c.** involuntary contractions
_____ **4.** -genic	**d.** resembling
_____ **5.** -dynia	**e.** pain
_____ **6.** -penia	**f.** decrease
_____ **7.** -spasm	**g.** none of the above

II.   Fill in the Blank: Suffix Applications

Fill in the blank with the appropriate term.

Choices:

a. -genic	**d.** -dynia
b. -algia	**e.** -spasm
c. -lysis	**f.** -penia

Example: Ms. Rose called to say that she cannot make her appointment because of the severe pain in the soles of her feet. She has a history of pod_____.

The answer is **b.**, **-algia**.

1. Being obese can cause muscle tissue **destruction**. Examination of infected laboratory animals shows such myo_____.
2. Red blood cells can be broken apart if they are placed in distilled water. The resulting hemo_____ colors the water a clear red.
3. Cold, damp conditions may cause severe nerve **pain**. This form of neur_____ tissue is quite common.
4. Certain cancers start in the skin. The dermato_____ feature can be shown by a microscopic examination.
5. Food poisoning causes painful intestinal **contractions**. Such episodes of an entero_____ can be quite disabling.
6. Prolonged use of this drug will cause a large reduction in white blood cells. The resulting leuko_____ lowers resistance.
7. The swollen liver was the result of the virus infection. This condition produced a significant amount of **pain** for the patient. Ms. Mosley's hepato_____ eventually disappeared during her recovery period. *(Do not use choice b.)*
8. Just after throwing the last ball, the catcher got a muscle **cramp**. His dactylo_____ took five minutes to pass.

III.   Spell Check

Circle each incorrectly spelled term and write its correct form in the space provided.

1. gastrodinia   _____
2. gastralgea   _____
3. osteogenic   _____
4. hemlysic   _____
5. dactylospasm   _____
6. neuralgia   _____
7. erythropenia   _____

IV.   Word Analysis: Suffixes for Signs or Symptoms Found with Disease

Table 3-9 lists a number of terms with their pronunciations and definitions.

TABLE 3-9   WORD ANALYSIS: SUFFIXES FOR SIGNS OR SYMPTOMS FOUND WITH DISEASE

Term and Pronunciation	Definition
neuralgia (nū-RAL-jē-a)	nerve pain
mastodynia (mast-ō-DIN-ē-a)	pain in the breast
carcinogenic (kar'-si-nō-JEN-ik)	producing cancer
cytolysis (sī-TOL-i-sis)	destruction of cells
erythropenia (e-rith'-rō-PĒ-nē-a)	deficiency in red blood cells
gastrospasm (GAS-trō-spaz'-em)	spasm (involuntary muscle contraction (spasm) of the stomach)

1. Analyze each term.
2. Circle all prefixes and suffixes and label them **p** and **s**, respectively.
3. Check your answers (shown in Table 3-14).

D. Suffixes Indicating Diagnostic Procedures and Measurements

I.   Matching: Suffixes Indicating Diagnostic Procedures and Measurements

Match the term to its meaning. (The same meaning may be used more than once.) Insert the appropriate letter in the space provided next to the question number.

Choices:

_____ 1. study of
_____ 2. procedure of viewing
_____ 3. instrument to examine
_____ 4. instrument to measure
_____ 5. procedure to make or study a record
_____ 6. the record of a diagnostic procedure
_____ 7. instrument to write or to record
_____ 8. procedure to measure

a. -graph
b. -scopy
c. -metry
d. -scope
e. -graphy
f. -logy
g. -meter
h. none of the above

II.   Fill in the Blank: Applying Suffixes Indicating Diagnostic Procedures and Measurements

Fill in the blank with the appropriate term.

Choices:

a. -graph
b. -scopy
c. -metry
d. -scope

e. -graphy
f. -logy
g. -gram
h. -meter

Example: The urologist is going to **examine** your bladder with the aid of this instrument called a cystoscope (SIST-ō-skōp). The cysto_____ *procedure* is not complicated.

(The answer here is b., -scopy.)

1. Since this is flu season, the lung capacity **measuring** equipment must be thoroughly cleaned between patients. However, do not use any caustic cleaner on the spiro_____.

2. The results of your test **record** from the electrocardiography (ē-lek'-trō-KAR-dē-ō'-graph-ē) department just came in. Your electrocardio_____ is normal.

3. Get a **record** of his brain waves. Send the patient to the electroencephalo_____ department for this test.

4. New **instruments** are being developed to detect cancer in the gastrointestinal tract. Modern endo_____(s) have the most up-to-date video camera attachments.

5. This child has an extremely high fever. Use the rectal thermo_____ to get a more accurate **measurement** of his temperature.

6. The specialized *study* of the psyche (SĪ-kē) together with its anatomy (an-AT-ō-mē), physiology (fiz'-ē-OL-ō-jē), and pathology is known as psychobio_____.

7. In psychology (sī-KOL-ō-jē), the **measurement** of intelligence, aptitude, behavior, and emotional reactions all belong to the specialty known as psycho_____.

8. The **procedure that will be used to visually examine** the large intestine or colon (KŌ-lon) is called colono_____.

III.   Spell Check

Circle each incorrectly spelled term and write it correctly in the space provided.

1. angiogram _____
2. sistoscopy _____
3. endoscope _____
4. spirometree _____
5. thermeter _____
6. pathology _____
7. electrocardiograph _____
8. spirometre _____
9. electrocardiographye _____

IV.   Word Analysis: Suffixes Indicating Diagnostic Procedures and Measurements

Table 3-10 lists a number of terms together with their pronunciations and definitions. Pick out the prefixes and suffixes.

1. Analyze each term.
2. Circle all prefixes and suffixes, labeling them **p** and **s**, respectively.
3. Check your answers (shown in Table 3-15).

TABLE 3-10   WORD ANALYSIS: SUFFIXES INDICATING DIAGNOSTIC PROCEDURES AND MEASUREMENTS

Term and Pronunciation	Definition
myelogram (MĪ-e-lō-gram)	record (x-ray) of spinal cord
electroencephalograph (ē-lek'-trō-en-SEF-a-lō-graf)	record of electric activity of the brain
angiography (an'-jē-OG-ra-fē)	process used to obtain a visual of blood vessels
dermatology (der'-ma-TOL-ō-jē)	study of the skin
radiometer (rā'-dē-OM-e-ter)	instrument for measurement of radiation intensity
microscope (MĪ-krō-skōp)	optical instrument used to view small objects
laparoscopy (lap-ar-OS-kō-pē)	abdominal examination process using an instrument called a laparoscope

E. Suffixes Indicating Surgical Procedures

I.   Matching 1: Suffixes Indicating Surgical Procedures Involving Incisions

Match the term to its meaning. (The same meaning may be used more than once.) Insert the appropriate letter in the space provided next to the question number.

Choices:

_____ 1. cutting	**a.** -stomy
_____ 2. puncture	**b.** -ectomy
_____ 3. incision	**c.** -cleisis
_____ 4. excision	**d.** -cenesis
_____ 5. surgical removal	**e.** -tomy
_____ 6. closing	**f.** none of these

II.   Matching 2: Suffixes Indicating Corrective Surgical Procedures

Choices:

_____ 1. binding	**a.** -clasia
_____ 2. fastening in a position	**b.** -desis
_____ 3. shaping	**c.** -plasty
_____ 4. to break	**d.** -rrhaphy
_____ 5. stitching (surgical)	**e.** -pexy
_____ 6. crushing	**f.** -tripsy
_____ 7. suturing (closing)	**g.** none of these

III.   Fill in the Blank: Applying Suffixes to Surgical Procedures

Fill in the blank with the appropriate term.

Choices:

a.	-centesis	**e.**	-clasia
b.	-ectomy	**f.**	-desis
c.	-cleisis	**g.**	-rrhaphy
d.	-tomy	**h.**	-pexy

Example: Techniques permit partial or total replacement of certain joints. The surgical procedure that involves the **excision** of a joint is called arthr_____.

(The answer here is b., -ectomy.)

1. The operation will require an incision into his chest or thorax (THŌ-raks). Thoraco_____ refers to any **incision** of the chest wall.
2. The extent of her injuries will require surgical repair to fasten or **close** the uterus. This procedure is called a hystero_____.
3. It will be necessary to remove some fluid from the cavity. Prepare the patient for the **puncture** procedure listed as para_____.
4. Surgical **removal** of the tonsils is known as tonsill_____.
5. Since the leg did not heal properly, it will have to be **broken surgically**. This calls for the osteo_____ procedure.
6. The ends of the bones should **be joined**, probably surgically. Schedule the patient for an arthro_____ procedure.
7. Surgically **fastening** a dislodged ovary is known as oophoro_____.
8. The ureter (ū-RE-ter) can be **surgically stitched** to the urinary bladder. This procedure is known as uretero_____.

IV.   Spell Check

Circle each incorrectly spelled term and write it correctly in the space provided.

1. parasentesis   _____
2. hysterocliesis   _____
3. tonsillectomy   _____
4. trachostomy   _____
5. osteoclasea   _____
6. laparoscopy   _____
7. angeography   _____
8. oophoropexy   _____
9. ureterorhaphy   _____
10. lithotripsey   _____
11. neurotomy   _____
12. angeoplasty   _____
13. phlebotomy   _____
14. colostomie   _____

V.   Word Analysis: Suffixes Indicating Surgical Procedures

Table 3-11 lists a number of terms with their pronunciations and definitions.

TABLE 3-11   WORD ANALYSIS: SUFFIXES INDICATING SURGICAL PROCEDURES

Term and Pronunciation	Definition
abdominocentesis (ab-dom'-i-nō-sen-TĒ-sis)	puncture of the abdomen
tenodesis (ten-OD-ē-sis)	binding of a tendon
laryngectomy (lar'-in-JEK-tō-mē)	excision of the larynx
nephropexy (NEF-rō-peks-ē)	fastening of a kidney
angioplasty (AN-jē-ō-plas'-tē)	shaping the structure of a vessel
herniorrhaphy (her-nē-OR-a-fē)	stitching a hernia
neurotripsy (nū-rō-TRIP-sē)	crushing a nerve
phlebotomy (fle-BOT-ō-mē)	cutting a vein
colostomy (kō-LOS-tō-mē)	opening a part of the colon

1. Analyze each term.
2. Circle all prefixes and suffixes, labeling them **p** and **s**, respectively.
3. Check your answers (shown in Table 3-16).

F. Suffixes Indicating Relationships

I.   Matching

Match the term to its meaning. (The same meaning may be used more than once.) Insert the appropriate letter in the space provided next to the question number.

Choices:

_____ **1.** pertaining to the heart
_____ **2.** pertaining to muscle
_____ **3.** pertaining to
_____ **4.** pertaining to the larynx
_____ **5.** pertaining to the breast
_____ **6.** pertaining to the nervous system
_____ **7.** pertaining to a spasm
_____ **8.** resembling fat
_____ **9.** pertaining to mucus

a. neural
b. laryngeal
c. spasmatic
d. mammary
e. -ic
f. cardiac
g. muscular
h. mucous
i. lipoid
j. none of these

II.   Fill in the Blank: Applying Suffixes

Fill in the blank with the appropriate suffix. Write the phonetic pronunciation and a brief definition of each complete term.

Example:

Word Root	Suffix	Pronunciation	Definition
alveol-	*ar*	al-VĒ-ō-lar	pertaining to air sac (of the lungs)

Choices:

a.	-ar	**e.**	-oid
b.	-ic	**f.**	-ary
c.	-eal	**g.**	-ous
d.	-al	**h.**	-tic

	Word Root	Suffix	Pronunciation	Definition
1.	gastr	_____;	_____;	_____
2.	infecti	_____;	_____;	_____
3.	mamm	_____;	_____;	_____
4.	lip	_____;	_____;	_____
5.	neur	_____;	_____;	_____
6.	skelet	_____;	_____;	_____
7.	muscul	_____;	_____;	_____
8.	spasma	_____;	_____;	_____

III.   Spell Check

Circle each incorrectly spelled term and write it correctly in the space provided.

1.	cardiak	_____
2.	larryngeal	_____
3.	adipoze	_____
4.	mukous	_____
5.	mammery	_____
6.	lipiod	_____
7.	spesmatic	_____
8.	nural	_____

IV.   Word Analysis: Suffixes Indicating Relationships

Table 3-12 lists a number of terms with their pronunciations and definitions.

TABLE 3-12   WORD ANALYSIS (SUFFIXES INDICATING RELATIONSHIPS)

Term and Pronunciation	Definition
renal (RĒ-nal)	pertaining to the kidney
tonsillar (TON-si-lar)	pertaining to a tonsil
pulmonary (PUL-mō-ne-rē)	pertaining to the lungs
colonic (kō-LON-ik)	pertaining to the colon
lacteal (LAK-tē-al)	pertaining to milk

(Continued)

TABLE 3-12   (CONTINUED)

Term and Pronunciation	Definition
epidermoid (ep'-i-DER-moyd)	pertaining to epidermis (top layers of skin)
torose or torous (TŌ-rus or TO-rus)	pertaining to a torus swelling
adenous (AD-e-nus)	pertaining to a gland
necrotic (ne-KRŌT-ik)	pertaining to death of tissue

1. Analyze each term.
2. Circle all prefixes and suffixes, labeling them **p** and **s**, respectively.
3. Check your answers (shown in Table 3-18).

G. Suffixes Indicating Diminutive Forms

I.   Definitions

Define the following terms. Write the definition in the spaces provided.

1. venula _____
2. venule _____
3. ventricle _____
4. vestibule _____
5. pustule _____
6. vesicle _____
7. papule _____
8. macula _____

II.   Spell Check

Circle each incorrectly spelled term and write it correctly in the space provided.

1. venula   _____
2. venul   _____
3. ventrikle _____
4. vestibull _____
5. pustule   _____
6. vessicle   _____
7. papule   _____

H. Increasing Your Medical Terminology Word Power

Directions:

1. Read the following case history.
2. Prepare to answer the questions at the end of the section.
3. Circle all unfamiliar terms with a red pencil.
4. Underline familiar terms with a blue pencil.
5. Use your knowledge of word elements, a medical dictionary, and the key terms to find the meanings of unfamiliar terms.

West Nile Virus Infection in New York City in 1999

Key Terms

autopsy (AW-top-sē)   examination after death to determine cause of death or disease condition.

brain stem   connects the largest part of the brain to the spinal cord.

cerebrospinal (ser'-ē-brō-SPĪ-nal) fluid a watery cushion protecting the brain and spinal cord from injury.

encephalitis (en-sef'-a-LĪ-tis)   inflammation of the brain.

epizootic (ep'-i-ZŌ-ot-ik)   any disease of animals that attack many animals in the same area.

erythematous (er'-i-THEM-a-tus)   a somewhat circular flat reddened area on the skin.

febrile (FĒ-brī-l)   pertaining to a fever.

hyperflexia (hī'-per-FLEK-sē-a)   refers to an increased flexion or bending of a joint.

lymphocytopenia (lim'-fō-sī-t'ō-PĒ-nē-a)   less than normal number of lymphocytes in the blood.

maculopapular (mak'-ū-lō-PAP-i-lar)   pertaining to a skin rash consisting of both macules and papules.

meningitis (men-in-JĪ-tis)   inflammation of the membranes covering the brain or spinal cord (meninges).

meningoencephalitis (men-in'-gō-en-sef'-a-LĪ-tis)   inflammation of the brain and its meninges.

pleocytosis (plē-'-ō-sī-TŌ-sis)   an increase in the number of lymphocytes in the cerebrospinal fluid.

Abstract

An unusual cluster of meningoencephalitis cases was reported to the New York City Department of Health in late August 1999. Most patients were over 50 years of age and presented with muscle weakness and nerve involvement. Initial investigations suggested a mosquito-borne virus disease.

Introduction

West Nile virus (WNV) was first isolated in 1937 from a blood specimen of a woman with a febrile illness in the West Nile district of Uganda. This virus is related to certain other known causes of encephalitis and is one of the world's most widely distributed viruses spread by mosquitoes. West Nile virus has caused major outbreaks of meningoencephalitis in Romania in 1996 and in Russia in 1999.

The first outbreak of the infection in humans in the United States coincided with the deaths from West Nile virus of several thousand crows and the deaths of exotic birds in two zoos located in New York City boroughs, the Bronx and Queens. This finding suggests that the virus was originally introduced into the U.S. by infected migratory or imported birds and that the infection was subsequently spread to other susceptible birds and to humans by mosquitoes. It is now apparent that WNV can infect mosquitoes, birds, and humans and those hosts, once infected with the virus—can in turn spread the disease.

Methods

Surveillance Investigation

All hospitals in New York City and neighboring areas were asked to report any suspected viral infection cases involving the central nervous system. Individuals with suspected infections were defined as those hospitalized on or after August 1, 1999, with a presumptive diagnosis of viral encephalitis indicated by fever, altered mental state, and abnormal laboratory findings such as pleocytosis. Patients with encephalitis were defined as having muscle weakness if neurologic examinations revealed flaccid paralysis, decreased strength, or hyperflexia.

Laboratory Methods

Blood and cerebrospinal fluid specimens were collected from all available suspected cases of viral encephalitis for the purposes of determining the presence of a viral agent.

Results

The results reported here focus on 59 hospitalized patients diagnosed with West Nile virus. The majority of these patients were over 50 years of age.

Laboratory Findings

Cerebrospinal fluid specimens were only available from 32 of the patients. Thirty of these showed evidence of WNV infection in the form of antibodies against the disease agent. Lymphocytopenia was a common finding.

In the four patients who died of the virus infection and on whom autopsies were performed, brain tissue was found to contain evidence of WNV.

Clinical Observations

Of the 59 patients, 37 were found to have meningoencephalitis, 17 had only meningitis, and 5 had a clinical condition characterized by fever, a mild maculopapular skin rash, and headache. Several patients had long-standing medical conditions that included diabetes, coronary artery disease, and a history of immune system deficiencies (immunosuppression). The immune system defects were the result of hormonal treatment, human immunodeficiency virus (HIV) infection, and alcoholism.

Neurologic examination of patients revealed muscle involvement documented by decreased muscle strength in 27 percent, hyperflexia in 32 percent, and flaccid paralysis in 10 percent.

Discussion

Most human West Nile virus infections are not obvious. The obvious signs and symptoms of disease are estimated to occur in about 1 of every 100 infections. The likelihood that severe neurologic illness will develop in infected individuals appears to increase with age. Underlying medical conditions may also increase the possibility of neurologic involvement and death.

From the various observations noted thus far, West Nile virus offers several potential clues that should alert health-care providers to the possibility of WNV disease. These include: (1) reports of unexpected deaths in bird and horse populations, which are likely to be early warnings preceding human infections; (2) although WNV can infect persons of all ages, the larger number of victims are over fifty years of age; (3) clinically infected persons show a pattern of muscle weakness and involvement of the nervous system, which are unusual with other types of encephalitis; and (4) patients frequently exhibit rash, and lymphocytopenia, which are unusual features of viral encephalitis.

Questions

I.   Matching 1: Suffix Identification

Match the suffix to its meaning. (The same meaning may be used more than once.)
Insert the appropriate letter in the space provided next to the question number.

Choices:

_____ **1.** -penia   **a.** inflammation
_____ **2.** -itis   **b.** deficiency
_____ **3.** -ous   **c.** pertains to
_____ **4.** -ar   **d.** abnormal condition
_____ **5.** -osis   **e.** resembles
_____ **6.** -al
_____ **7.** -tic

II.   Matching 2: Vocabulary Building

Match the term to its meaning. (The same meaning may be used more than once.)
Insert the appropriate letter in the space provided next to the question number.

Choices:

_____ **1.** hyperflexia   **a.** examination of body tissues after
_____ **2.** meningitis   death to find cause of death
_____ **3.** pleocytosis   **b.** largest part of brain connecting the
_____ **4.** brainstem   brain to the spinal cord
_____ **5.** febrile   **c.** inflammation of the brain
_____ **6.** meningoencephalitis **d.** pertaining to fever
_____ **7.** autopsy   **e.** increased flexion of a joint
_____ **8.** encephalitis   **f.** less than normal number of lym-
_____ **9.** lymphocytopenia   phocytes in the cerebrospinal fluid
                                 g. inflammation of the coverings of the
                                     brain or spinal cord
                                 h. inflammation of the brain and its
                                     meninges
                                 i. increased number of lymphocytes in
                                     the cerebrospinal fluid

III.   Spell Check

Circle each incorrectly spelled term and write it correctly in the space provided.

1. awtopsy   _____
2. febrile   _____
3. maculer   _____
4. meningitis   _____
5. encephalitis   _____
6. epizootic   _____
7. erythematos   _____
8. pleosytosis   _____

Suffix Search Challenge

Locate the 13 suffixes in the puzzle.

1. Write the suffix next to its definition. Then find that suffix in the puzzle diagram and circle it.
2. Suffixes may be read from left to right, backward, up, down, or diagonally.
3. If a suffix appears more than once, circle it only once. (A suffix may be found inside others.)
4. Check your answers.

Clues:

1. hernia or tumor _____
2. inflammation _____
3. blood _____
4. condition _____
5. to view _____
6. recording process _____
7. molding or shaping _____
8. suture or stitching _____
9. pain (list two suffixes) _____
10. resembling _____
11. excision _____
12. cutting _____

Suffix Search Puzzle

```
R  S  E  T  T  R  R  O  P  H  D  Y  N  I  A
R  N  M  A  O  M  A  T  H  P  A  R  A  C  C
H  N  I  R  H  M  L  S  I  S  X  E  H  R  R
A  M  A  L  G  I  A  F  O  G  R  A  P  H  Y
P  G  R  L  G  A  N  G  I  H  A  P  H  Y  Y
H  B  R  A  T  L  E  C  E  C  T  O  M  Y  T
Y  O  T  X  T  P  H  X  P  P  T  I  M  H  O
D  L  P  V  E  R  I  P  R  R  W  D  O  H  M
T  D  I  L  I  S  E  N  P  T  E  D  I  P  A
O  E  A  O  A  P  F  U  L  G  A  Y  L  H  A
M  B  S  M  A  S  G  R  A  V  T  X  I  R  O
Y  C  I  Y  A  S  T  R  S  T  R  E  X  R  S
E  M  S  O  C  M  T  Y  T  R  I  P  S  Y  I
I  T  I  S  S  C  O  P  Y  H  L  A  X  I  S
```

CHAPTER 4

Measurements and Dosages

"When you cannot measure it in numbers, your knowledge is of meager and unsatisfactory kind...."

—Lord Kelvin, 1883

INFORMATIONAL CHALLENGE

A. General Points to Keep in Mind and a Brief Arithmetic Review

I.   Fill in the Blank

Fill in the blank with the appropriate term.

1. Regardless of how a measurement is made, two factors always required are the _____ and the _____.
2. The two systems used to express measurements in the scientific world are the _____ and the _____.
3. As used in this chapter, a part of any quantity or unit is called a _____.
4. The value below the division line in a fraction is called the _____.
5. The value above the division line in a fraction is called the _____.
6. A decimal refers to a value of _____.
7. A _____ is a mathematical form that represents a single line of numbers described as a fraction.
8. The numbers to the left of the decimal point are _____ numbers.
9. The numbers to the right of the decimal point are _____ or _____.
10. The position of a number to the left or right of the decimal point is also known as its _____.
11. Why is it important to place a 0 (zero) before the decimal point? _____

II.   Matching: The Relationship of Whole Numbers to Decimals

Match the fraction to its equivalent decimal fractions. (The same answer may be used more than once.) Insert the appropriate letter in the space next to the question number.

Choices:

_____ **1.** one-tenth (1/10)

_____ **2.** one-thousandth (1/1,000)

_____ **3.** one-hundredth (1/100)

_____ **4.** one-millionth (1/1,000,000)

_____ **5.** one-billionth (1/1,000,000,000)

_____ **6.** one ten-thousandth (1/10,000)

_____ **7.** one hundred-thousandth (1/100,000)

_____ **8.** one ten-millionth (1/10,000,000)

a. 0.001

b. 0.01

c. 0.0001

d. 0.00001

e. 0.000001

f. 0.1

g. 0.000000001

h. 0.0000001

B. The Metric System

I.   Fill in the Blank

Fill in the blank with the appropriate term.

1. In the metric system, the basic unit of length is the _____.

2. In the metric system, the basic unit of volume is the _____.

3. In the metric system, the basic unit of mass (weight) is the _____.

4. In the metric system, the basic unit of temperature or heat is the _____.

II.   Matching 1: Prefixes and Combining Forms Associated with Measurements

Match the prefix or combining form to its meaning. Insert the appropriate letter in the space next to the question number.

Choices:

_____ **1.** giga-

_____ **2.** mega-

_____ **3.** kilo-

_____ **4.** hecto-

_____ **5.** deka-

_____ **6.** deci-

_____ **7.** centi-

_____ **8.** milli-

_____ **9.** micro-

_____ **10.** nano-

_____ **11.** pico-

a. one billion

b. one thousand

c. one-trillionth

d. one million

e. one hundred

f. one-thousandth

g. one-hundredth

h. one-tenth

i. ten

j. one-billionth

k. one millionth

l. none of the above

III.   Matching 2: Metric System Unit Symbols

Match the symbol to its prefix/meaning. Insert the appropriate letter in the space next to the question number.

Choices:

_____ **1.** p   **a.** giga-
_____ **2.** μ **b.** mega-
_____ **3.** n   **c.** kilo-
_____ **4.** m   **d.** hecto-
_____ **5.** c   **e.** deka-
_____ **6.** D   **f.** deci-
_____ **7.** H   **g.** centi-
_____ **8.** d   **h.** milli-
_____ **9.** k   **i.** micro-
                          j. nano-
                          k. pico-

IV.   Matching 3: Decimal Equivalent

Match the number to its decimal equivalent. Insert the appropriate letter in the space next to the question number.

Choices:

_____ **1.** 1 billion   **a.** 0.001
_____ **2.** one-hundredth   **b.** 0.1
_____ **3.** one-millionth   **c.** 10^{-6}
_____ **4.** one thousand   **d.** 1,000,000,000
_____ **5.** one hundred   **e.** 0.01
_____ **6.** one-thousandth   **f.** 10^{-9}
_____ **7.** one-billionth   **g.** 10^2
_____ **8.** one-trillionth   **h.** 10^3
_____ **9.** one-tenth   **i.** none of the above

V.   Spell Check

Circle each incorrectly spelled term and write it correctly in the space provided .

1. gramm   _____
2. mililiter   _____
3. microgram   _____
4. Celsius   _____
5. Fareheit   _____
6. cubik centemeter _____

C. Prescriptions and Abbreviations

I.   Fill in the Blank

Study Figure 4-7 (and Table 4-2 if necessary). Fill in the blank with the appropriate term.

1. How many times a day must the patient take this medication?

_____

2. By what route is the medication to be taken? _____

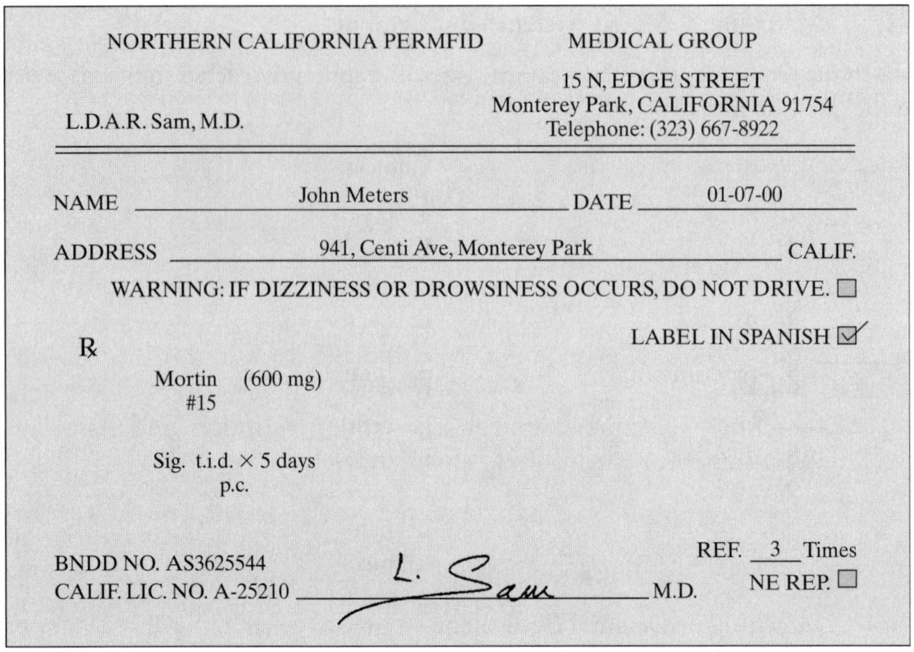

```
        NORTHERN CALIFORNIA PERMFID        MEDICAL GROUP

                                            15 N, EDGE STREET
                                        Monterey Park, CALIFORNIA 91754
         L.D.A.R. Sam, M.D.                 Telephone: (323) 667-8922


     NAME            John Meters          DATE        01-07-00

     ADDRESS        941, Centi Ave, Monterey Park            CALIF.
        WARNING: IF DIZZINESS OR DROWSINESS OCCURS, DO NOT DRIVE. ☐

       ℞                                   LABEL IN SPANISH ☑

              Mortin    (600 mg)
                #15

              Sig.  t.i.d. × 5 days
                   p.c.


     BNDD NO. AS3625544      L. Sam         REF.  3  Times
     CALIF. LIC. NO. A-25210 _____ M.D.  NE REP. ☐
```

FIGURE 4-7 A sample prescription for interpretation.

3. How long must the patient take the medication? _____
4. What is the concentration of the medication to be dispensed?
   _____
5. What does *mg* mean? _____
6. What does *sig* mean? _____

II.   Matching 1: Features of a Modern Prescription

Match the definition to its term. (The same term may be used more than once.)
Insert the appropriate letter in the space next to the question number.

                                        Choices:

_____ 1. contains the ingredients   **a.** superscription
        of the prescription
_____ 2. indicates the form in   **b.** subscription
        which the prescription is
        made   **c.** inscription
_____ 3. Rx is associated with this
        part   **d.** signature
_____ 4. contains the directions
        for the patient   **e.** none of the above
_____ 5. contains the physician's
        signature
_____ 6. contains the instructions
        for the pharmacist

III.   Matching 2: Abbreviations Used with Prescription and Associated with Time Schedules

Match the meaning to its abbreviation. Insert the appropriate letter in the space next to the question number.

Choices:

_____ **1.** immediately   **a.** ad lib
_____ **2.** as desired   **b.** q.i.d.
_____ **3.** three times/day   **c.** t.i.d.
_____ **4.** four times/day   **d.** stat
_____ **5.** two times/day   **e.** b.i.d.

IV.   Matching 3: Abbreviations Used with Prescription and Associated with Routes for Medication Administration

Match the meaning to its abbreviation. Insert the appropriate letter in the space next to the question number.

Choices:

_____ **1.** intravenously   **a.** IM
_____ **2.** intramuscularly   **b.** IV
_____ **3.** by mouth   **c.** p.o.

V.   Matching 4: Abbreviations Used with Prescription and Associated with Amounts

Match the measurement to its abbreviation. Insert the appropriate letter in the space next to the question number.

Choices:

_____ **1.** gram   **a.** U
_____ **2.** one-half   **b.** ss
_____ **3.** unit   **c.** c
_____ **4.** with   **d.** mcg or ug
_____ **5.** microgram   **e** gm

D. Increasing Your Medical Terminology Word Power 1

1. Read the following report.

2. Prepare to answer the questions at the end of the section.

3. Circle all unfamiliar terms with a red pencil.

4. Underline familiar terms with a blue pencil.

5. Use your knowledge of word elements, a medical dictionary, and the key terms to find the meaning of unfamiliar terms.

Clinical Use of Cefoxitin: A Review of Case Histories

Key Terms

abscess (AB-ses) localized collection of pus

bacteremia (bak'-ter-Ē-mē-a) bacteria in the blood

endocarditis (en'-dō-kar-DĪ-tis)   inflammation of the lining of the heart

osteomyelitis (os'-tē-ō-mī'-el-Ī-tis)   inflammation of the bone

peritonitis (per-i-tō-NĪ-tis)   inflammation of the abdominal cavity or peritoneum

pneumonia (nū-MŌ-nē-a)   inflammation of the lungs

phlebitis (fle-BĪ-tis)   inflammation of a vein

pyuria (pī-Ū-rē-a)   pus in the urine

Introduction and Overview

Cefoxitin (SĒF-ox-i-tin) is a relatively new, intravenously administered antibacterial (an'-tī-bak-TĒ-rē-al) agent. It is effective against some of the more commonly encountered disease-causing bacteria.

C ASE HISTORIES

Forty-three hospitalized patients with sixty-two clinically significant infections were treated with intravenous cefoxitin. Table 4-3 lists some of the general clinical infections treated in this study. Cefoxitin dosages ranged from 4 to 16 g/day, and the duration of therapy ranged from 3 to 43 days. Concentrations of the drug were determined before, during, and after treatment by laboratory testing of blood and other body fluid specimens.

Two patients had cefoxitin concentrations determined in both blood and abscess-fluid specimens. The first of these individuals had bacterial endocarditis. Her blood levels with a dosage of 2.0 gm of cefoxitin every 4 h were 40 μg/ml, and 125 μg/ml 1 h after the drug's administration.

The second patient was treated for pneumonia. His blood levels were 10 μg/ml 1 h before 2.0 gm of intravenous cefoxitin were injected and 26 μg/ml 1 h after the drug's administration.

TABLE 4-3   CASE HISTORY INTERPRETATIONS

Clinical Infection	Number of Patients with Condition
Abdominal abscesses (ab-DOM-i-nal AB-ses-sez)	3
Postoperative complications	1
Skin abscesses	12
Bacterial phlebitis	2
Peritonitis	2
Osteomyelitis	2
Bacterial arthritis	2
Pneumonia	2
Pyuria	1
Endocarditis	3
Bacteremia	11

Questions

I.   Fill in the blank

Fill in the blank with the appropriate term.

1. What was the antibiotic used in the treatment of patients?

_____

2. How was the antibiotic administered? _____
3. From what types of specimens were antibiotic concentrations determined? _____
4. What was the dosage of the antibiotic given per day? _____
5. Give the meaning of the following abbreviations:
   a. μg _____
   b. ml _____
6. Give the meaning of the following abbreviations:
   a. g _____
   b. h _____

II.   Matching: Disease States

Match the definition with its term. Insert the appropriate letter in the space next to the question number.

Choices:

_____ **1.** localized collection of pus
_____ **2.** bacteria in blood
_____ **3.** pus in the urine
_____ **4.** inflammation of the bone
_____ **5.** inflammation of the peritoneum
_____ **6.** inflammation of a vein
_____ **7.** inflammation of the heart

a. pyuria
b. abscess
c. bacteremia
d. endocarditis
e. peritonitis
f. phlebitis
g. osteomyelitis

III.   Spell Check

Circle each incorrectly spelled term and write it correctly in the space provided.

1. absess   _____
2. phlebitis   _____
3. bacterimia _____
4. pieuria   _____
5. peritonitis _____
6. endocarditis _____

E. Increasing Your Medical Terminology Word Power Part 2

1. Read the following report.
2. Prepare to answer the questions at the end of the section.
3. Circle all unfamiliar terms with a red pencil.
4. Underline familiar terms with a blue pencil.
5. Use your knowledge of word elements, a medical dictionary, and the key terms to find the meaning of unfamiliar terms.

A Case of Mast Cell Disease (Mastocytosis)

Key Terms

biopsy (BĪ-op-sē)   removal of a small piece of living tissue for microscopic examination

chronic (KRON-ik)   long lasting

fibrosis (fī-BRŌ-sis)   abnormal formation of fiber-containing (fibrous) tissue

hepatosplenomegaly (hep'-a-tō-splē'-no-MEG-a-lē)   enlargement of both the liver and spleen

interferon (in-ter-FĒR-on)   an anti-viral and anti-tumor agent

leukemia (loo-KĒ-mē-a)   a disease characterized by the uncontrolled growth of leukocytes and their precursors

leukopenia (loo'-kō-PĒ-nē-a)   abnormal decrease of white blood cells

macular (MAK-ū-lar)   related to discolored spots on the skin mast cells (tissue cells known for containing heparin and histamine)

mastocytosis (mas'-tō-sī-TŌ-sis)   formation of abnormal mast cells

monocytosis (mon'-ō-sī-TŌ-sis)   excessive number of monocytes in the blood

myelocyte (MĪ-el-ō-sīt)   a large red bone marrow cell from which leukocytes originate

nonpruritic (non-proo-RI-tik)   not itching

osteosclerosis (os'-tē-ō-skle-RŌ-sis)   hardening of bone with increased heaviness

platelet (PLĀT-let)   disk-shaped blood component that plays an important role in blood clotting

prednisone (PRED-ni-sōn)   a hormone with anti-inflammatory action

systemic (sis-TEM-ik)   concerning a system such as the human body

thrombocytopenia (throm'-bō-sī'-tō-PĒ-nē-a)   abnormal decrease in the number of platelets

Introduction

A 72-year-old male presented with hepatosplenomegaly and multiple macular, hyper-pigmented, nonpruritic skin lesions on his arms, legs, and trunk.

L ABORATORY FINDINGS

The patient's hemoglobin level was 9.2 **g** per **dl**, the platelet count was 110,000 per **cc**, and the white blood cell count was 34,300 per **cc** with a noticeable leukopenia. A bone marrow biopsy revealed findings consistent with the presence of chronic myelomonocytic leukemia, fibrosis, osteosclerosis, and increased numbers of mastocytes. A plasma tryptase level of 141 **μg** per **L** and the results of a skin biopsy confirmed the diagnosis of systemic mastocytosis.

T REATMENT

Treatment for the patient included 4 million to 5 million **U** of interferon-alfa given sc three times a week; prednisone 0.5 to 1.0 **mg** per **kg** of body weight/day and administered orally; and 10,000 U of epoetin twice per week given subcutaneously.

The treatment regimen resulted in a normalization of the patient's leukocyte count, a decrease in tryptase values (60 **μg** per **L**), and a stabilization of the platelet count (which was 70,000 to 120,000 platelets per **cc**).

Questions

I.   Definitions

Define the following abbreviations. Insert your answers in the spaces provided.

1. mg _____   **5.** dl _____
2. kg _____   **6.** cc _____
3. L _____   **7.** sc _____
4. U _____

II.   Matching

Match the term to its meaning. (The same meaning may be used more than once.) Insert the appropriate letter in the space next to the question number.

Choices:

_____ **1.** biopsy
_____ **2.** fibrosis
_____ **3.** hepatosplenomegaly
_____ **4.** leukopenia
_____ **5.** macular
_____ **6.** monocytosis
_____ **7.** nonpruritic
_____ **8.** osteosclerosis
_____ **9.** thrombocytopenia
_____ **10.** platelet

a. abnormal formation of fibrous tissue
b. removal of a small piece of living tissue for microscopic examination
c. an abnormal decrease of leukocytes
d. enlargement of both the liver and spleen
e. excessive number of monocytes
f. not itching
g. hardening of the bones with increased heaviness
h. abnormal decrease in the number of platelets
i. related to discolored spots on the skin
j. oval disk-shaped blood components that play an important role in blood clotting

III.   Spell Check

Circle each incorrectly spelled term and write it correctly in the space provided.

1. biopsy   _____
2. macular   _____
3. thrombocytopena   _____
4. fibrosis   _____
5. lukeemia   _____
6. osteosklerosis   _____
7. mastocytosis   _____
8. nonpuritic   _____

Term Search Challenge

Locate 18 terms and/or abbreviations in the puzzle.

1. Write the specific term next to its definition. Then find that term in the puzzle diagram and circle it.
2. Terms may be read from left to right, backward, up, down, or diagonally.
3. If a term appears more than once, circle it only once. (A term may be found inside others.)
4. Check your answers.

Clues:

1. symbol for kilo _____
2. symbol for milli _____
3. symbol for nano _____
4. prefix for one-hundredth _____
5. as desired _____
6. two times per day _____
7. three times per day _____
8. immediately _____
9. add _____
10. write on label _____
11. water _____
12. tablet _____
13. pill _____
14. capsules _____
15. gram _____
16. one-half _____
17. milliliter _____
18. unit _____

Term Search Puzzle

```
K  C  T  M  C  A  P  S  T  S
N  C  Q  U  I  H  I  I  T  A
T  T  D  D  A  F  I  M  T  Q
A  L  A  B  I  D  I  I  D  T
T  A  B  D  L  T  H  C  I  I
G  G  L  S  I  G  D  R  I  D
M  P  I  I  T  C  D  O  O  B
S  C  E  N  T  I  I  T  A  B
S  A  D  I  I  B  Q  T  I  D
U  M  D  B  P  C  S  T  A  T
```

Basic Chemistry Terminology

"The invisible in us has suddenly become visible."

—Jan Lindberg, Karolinska Institute

INFORMATIONAL CHALLENGE

A. Atoms and Elements

I.   Multiple Choice

Circle the best possible answer for each question.

1.   The study of chemical reactions in all forms of life is called _____.

   a. chemistry   **d.** physics
   b. biochemistry   **e.** biophysics
   c. biology

2.   The term "organic" refers to various substances that contain _____.

   a. hydrogen   **d.** water
   b. oxygen   **e.** carbon
   c. sulfur

3.   The smallest units of matter that enter into chemical reactions are known as _____.

   a. molecules   **d.** compounds
   b. atoms   **e.** nuclei
   c. elements

II.   Matching: Atoms and Elements

Match the term to its meaning. (The same meaning may be used more than once.) Insert the appropriate letter in the space next to the question number.

Choices:

_____ **1.** proton   **a.** positively charged particle
_____ **2.** electron   **b.** uncharged particle
_____ **3.** neutron   **c.** negatively charged particle
_____ **4.** atomic number   **d.** total number of protons and
_____ **5.** atomic weight   neutrons

_____ **6.** electron orbital
_____ **7.** isotopes
_____ **8.** electron shells
_____ **9.** an element

e. electron's pattern of movement
f. total number of protons in an atom's nucleus
g. regions of electrons at different energy levels
h. chemical atoms of an element having different numbers of neutrons
i. atoms having the same number of protons and neutrons

III.   Spell Check

Circle each incorrectly spelled term and write it correctly in the space provided.

1. element   _____
2. isotop   _____
3. electronic   _____
4. inorganik   _____
5. atomic   _____
6. molecul   _____
7. nitrojen   _____
8. sodiem   _____

B. Chemical Bonds, Molecules, and Compounds

I.   Matching: Chemical Bonds, Molecules, and Compounds

Match the term to its meaning. (The same meaning may be used more than once.) Insert the appropriate letter in the space next to the question number.

_____ **1.** bonds formed by sharing electrons
_____ **2.** negatively charged ions
_____ **3.** positively charged ions
_____ **4.** $C_6H_{12}O_6$
_____ **5.** charged chemical atom
_____ **6.** hydrogen ion
_____ **7.** two or more atoms held together by chemical bonds
_____ **8.** formula showing the kinds and numbers of chemical atoms present
_____ **9.** formula showing kinds and numbers of atoms, and numbers of electron pairs shared
_____ **10.** type of substance formed when the number of hydroxyl ions is greater than hydrogen ions
_____ **11.** type of substance formed when the number of hydrogen ions is greater than hydroxyl ions
_____ **12.** pH value of 7
_____ **13.** pH value of 9
_____ **14.** pH value of 4

Choices:

a. cations
b. covalent bonds
c. anions
d. ion
e. H^+

f. hydroxyl group
g. molecular formula
h. structural formula
i. molecule
j. base
k. acid
l. neutral condition
m. basic (alkaline) condition
n. acidic condition

C. Macromolecules

I. Definitions

Define the following prefixes.

1. sept- _____
2. pent- _____
3. hex- _____
4. tri- _____
5. di- _____
6. mono- _____
7. poly- _____
8. tetra- _____

II. Matching: Carbohydrates

Match the term to its meaning. (The same meaning may be used more than once.)
Insert the appropriate letter in the space next to the question number.

Choices:

_____ 1. subunits of large molecules
_____ 2. large molecules made up
       of smaller units
_____ 3. simple sugar
_____ 4. monosaccharides con-
       nected together
_____ 5. a six-carbon containing
       sugar
_____ 6. suffix used to indicate a
       sugar
_____ 7. a five-carbon sugar

a. pentose
b. monosaccharide
c. -ose
d. polysaccharide
e. monomers
f. hexose
g. polymer

III. Fill in the Blank

Fill in the blank with the appropriate term.

1. The two basic types of building blocks of fats are
    _____ and _____.
2. The two factors that determine the physical properties of fats
    are_____ and _____.
3. Unsaturated fatty acids contain carbon atoms joined by
    _____ bonds.

4. How many fatty acid molecules are present in the phospholipid molecule? _____

5. How does the number of fatty acid molecules in the phospholipid molecule compare with the number found in a fat molecule? _____

6. Is the number of glycerol molecules in a fat the same as that found in a phospholipid molecule? _____

IV.   Spell Check

Circle each incorrectly spelled term and write it correctly in the space provided.

1. chloroform   _____
2. faty acid   _____
3. hydrocarbon   _____
4. fosphate   _____
5. cholesterol   _____
6. waxes   _____
7. steroyd   _____
8. glycerol   _____
9. saterated   _____
10. hydrophilic   _____
11. inflamation   _____
12. phospholipid _____

V.   Fill in the Blank

Fill in the blank with the appropriate term.

1. The basic building blocks of protein are called _____.

2. The connecting link between two amino acids is called a _____.

3. The connection of two amino acids results in the formation of a _____.

4. An amino group is represented chemically as _____.

5. A carboxyl group is represented chemically as _____.

VI.   Spell Check

Circle each incorrectly spelled term and write it correctly in the space provided.

1. peptid   _____
2. carboxil   _____
3. polypeptide _____
4. ameno   _____
5. dipeptide   _____
6. enzime   _____

VII.   Fill in the Blank

Fill in the blank with the appropriate term.

1. The two types of nucleic acids are _____ and

_____.

2. What are the basic building blocks of nucleic acids called?

_____

3. List the components of the following:

    a. a nucleoside _____
    b. a nucleotide _____

4. In a DNA molecule:

    a. thymine is paired to a _____
    b. cytosine is paired to a _____

5. In a DNA molecule backbone, the deoxyribose of one nucleotide is joined to the _____ group of the next deoxyribose.

6. The nitrogen-containing bases typically contain the chemical elements _____.

VIII.   Spell Check

Circle each incorrectly spelled term and write it correctly in the space provided.

    1. riboze   _____
    2. deoxsiribose   _____
    3. nucleoside   _____
    4. uracil   _____
    5. phosphate   _____
    6. adenin   _____
    7. thymine   _____
    8. sytosine   _____
    9. quanine   _____
    10. nitrogenous   _____

D. Increasing Your Medical Terminology Word Power

1. Read the following report.
2. Prepare to answer the questions at the end of the section.
3. Circle all unfamiliar terms with a red pencil.
4. Underline familiar terms with a blue pencil.
5. Use your knowledge of word elements, a medical dictionary, and the key terms to find the meaning of unfamiliar terms.

The Universal Lipids and Associated Diseases

Key Terms

acute (a-KŪT)   having a short and relatively severe course

apolipoprotein (a'-pō-lip'-ō-PRŌ-tē-in)   nonlipid protein part of a lipoprotein

atherogenesis (ath'-er-ō-JEN-e-sis)   development of fatty degeneration of arterial walls

atherosclerosis (ath'-er-ō-skle-RŌ-sis)   hardening of the arteries caused mainly by lipid accumulation

cholesterol (kō-LES-ter-ol)   a widely distributed alcohol (sterol) in animal tissues

coronary heart disease   decreased blood flow to heart muscle resulting in an insufficient oxygen supply

deafferentation (dē-af'-er-en-TĀ-shun)   cutting the afferent (carrying nerve impulses toward the brain) nerve supply

dl or dL (DES-i-lē-ter)   a measurement of volume; 0.1 liter or 100 ml

ester (ES-ter)   a chemical compound formed by the combination of an organic acid with an alcohol (e.g., phospholipids and nucleic acids)

macrophage (MAK-rō-fāj)   protective cells of the immune system having the ability to engulf particles

mg, milligram (MIL-i-gram)   one thousandth of a gram

myocardial infarction (mī'-ō-KAR-dē-al in-FARK-shun)   blockage (occlusion) of one or more of the coronary arteries

neuronal (NŪ-rō-nal)   pertains to one or more neurons (nerve cells)

occlusion (ō-KLOO-zhun)   closure or blockage

pathogenesis (path'-ō-JEN-e-sis)   origin or development of a disease

plaque (PLAK)   a patch on an artery lining

plasma (PLAZ-ma)   liquid portion of uncoagulated blood

thrombosis (throm-BŌ-sis)   a blood clot (thrombus) in a blood vessel

triglyceride (trī-GLIS-er-īd)   combination of glycerol with three of five different fatty acids

Introduction

It is well known that atherosclerosis is the cause of coronary heart disease (**CHD**) and stroke. These conditions are the most prevalent and third most prevalent causes of death in the United States, respectively. **Lipids, lipoproteins**, and **apolipoproteins** have been linked to the pathogenesis of atherosclerosis. In addition to contributing to numerous deaths, **CHD** and **stroke** are primary causes of disability and contribute significantly to rising health costs in the U.S. **CHD** accounts for the largest proportion of heart disease.

A high concentration of *total cholesterol* (**TC**) in the blood has been found to be a major contributor to the development of **atherosclerosis** and **CHD**. About 90 million adults have cholesterol levels that put them at risk for heart disease. Most heart attacks occur in people with **CHD** and coronary artery disease (**CAD**). Both of these conditions are associated with atherosclerosis, caused by *plaque buildup* on coronary artery walls.

𝒫 ATHOGENESIS

Atherosclerotic lesions consist of fatty streaks that develop into fiber-containing plaques. Macrophages heavy with lipid deposits are typically found in such fatty areas. A buildup of plaque creates occlusions in coronary arteries and results in a decrease in or complete stoppage of the blood supply to portions of the heart. Blood clots can also cause blockages in the coronary arteries, sometimes referred to as *coronary thrombosis* or *coronary occlusion*.

Major independent risk factors believed to contribute to the development and progression of atherosclerotic vascular disease include high concentrations of plasma lipids and lipoproteins. Lipoproteins also contribute to the development of neurodegenerative diseases. In addition, changes caused by lipids have been reported to occur in Alzheimer's patients in whom neuronal loss and deafferentation are major findings.

THE ROLES OF LIPIDS, LIPOPROTEINS, AND APOLIPOPROTEINS

Lipids play both functional and structural roles in all aspects of cellular life. These include hormone precursors, aids in digestion, sources of fuel for metabolism, and energy storage. Lipids—including fatty acids, glycerol esters, and sterols—are transported to various body locations by lipoproteins such as *low-density lipoprotein* (**LDL**) and *high-density lipoprotein* (**HDL**). Closely associated with lipoproteins are protein combinations called *apolipoproteins*. The liver produces about 1.5 g of lipids daily, and another 150–300 mg of lipids are formed daily from an individual's dietary intake.

TRIGLYCERIDES

Most fatty acids form esters known as *glycerides* containing glycerol. *Triglycerides* (**TGs**) are the most common and abundant of these compounds. Numerous clinical studies have demonstrated that an elevated level of triglycerides in the blood is an important risk factor for **CHD**. Examples of factors that may contribute to elevated **TGs** in the general population include cigarette smoking, excessive alcohol consumption, high carbohydrate diets, excess weight and obesity, lack of physical activity, diseases such as Type-2 diabetes, chronic renal failure, and certain drugs such as estrogen and corticosteroids. Patients with concentrations of blood **TGs** above 150 mg per dL are considered to be at risk. The higher the concentration of **TG**, the higher the risk. In addition, pancreatitis may develop in patients having a **TG** concentration as high as 1,000 mg per dL.

CHOLESTEROL

Cholesterol has been implicated as another important key risk factor in the development of **CHD** and **atherosclerosis**. Despite its potentially harmful properties, cholesterol is essential for the formation of steroid hormones and the production of bile salts in the liver.

Lowering blood levels of cholesterol decreases risk of **CHD**, especially in the absence of other risk factors. Cholesterol concentrations greater than 240 mg per dL are considered to be a high risk.

LOW-DENSITY LIPOPROTEIN (LDL)

The main physiological function of LDL is to carry cholesterol to body cells. An LDL particle consists of a lipid center or core containing 38 percent cholesterol ester and 11 percent triglyceride. Concentrations of less than 100 mg per dL are considered optimal.

$\mathcal{H}$IGH-DENSITY LIPOPROTEIN (HDL)

HDL is involved with a major protein component in reversing cholesterol transport. Typically, an HDL molecule consists of about 50 percent protein and 50 percent lipid. Of the lipids in a HDL molecule, 30 percent are phospholipids and the remainder is cholesterol.

In general, the specific levels of HDL and LDL are based on their respective cholesterol content. Lipoprotein identification and concentration determinations are based on various physical properties and their respective apolipoprotein content.

Questions

I.   Give the Meanings

Spell out the acronyms.

      1. CHD   _____
      2. AMI   _____
      3. CAD   _____
      4. LDL   _____
      5. HDL   _____
      6. VLDL   _____
      7. TG   _____
      8. TC   _____

II.   Fill in the Blank

Fill in the blank with the appropriate term.

      1. A buildup of plaque would affect the heart's blood supply by
        _____

      2. Seven factors that may contribute to elevated TGs in the general population are _____
        _____
        _____.

      3. The value of TG concentrations within normal range is
        _____.

      4. The main physiological function of LDL is _____.
      5. The two major components of an LDL molecule are
        _____ and _____.
      6. The percent composition of the lipid in an HDL molecule is
        _____ and _____.

III.   Matching

Match the term to its meaning. (The same meaning may be used more than once.) Insert the appropriate letter in the space next to the question number.

    _____ **1.** acute
    _____ **2.** atherogenesis
    _____ **3.** apolipoprotein
    _____ **4.** atherosclerosis
    _____ **5.** myocardial infarction
    _____ **6.** neuronal
    _____ **7.** occlusion

_____ **8.** plaque
_____ **9.** thrombosis
_____ **10.** deafferentation

Choices:

    a. fatty degeneration of large arterial walls
    b. having a rapid and severe course
    c. nonlipid protein part of a lipoprotein
    d. blockage of one or more contrary arteries
    e. hardening of the arteries
    f. pertains to one or more nerve cells
    g. a patch on an artery lining
    h. closure or blockage
    i. cutting the afferent nerve supply
    j. blood clot in a blood vessel

IV.   Spell Check

Circle each incorrectly spelled term and write it correctly in the space provided.

    1. coronery   _____
    2. atherosclerosis   _____
    3. plaque   _____
    4. deaferentiation   _____
    5. cholesterel   _____
    6. oclusion   _____
    7. lypoprotiens   _____
    8. triglyceride   _____

Term Search Challenge

Locate 16 terms in the puzzle.

    1. Write the specific term next to its definition. Then find that term in the puzzle diagram and circle it.
    2. Terms may be read from left to right, backward, up, down, or diagonally.
    3. If a term appears more than once, circle it only once. (A term or abbreviation may be found inside others.)
    4. Check your answers.

Clues:

    1. The smallest unit of matter that is involved in chemical reactions.
    _____

    2. Positively charged particles in an atom's nucleus.
    _____

    3. The uncharged particle in an atom's nucleus.
    _____

    4. The listing of an element based on the number of protons in its nucleus. _____

    5. An atom with differing numbers of neutrons in its nucleus.
    _____

    6. A substance consisting of atoms having the same numbers of protons and electrons. _____

7. The total number of protons and neutrons in an atom.
_____

8. The combination of two or more atoms. _____

9. The two chemical elements always found in organic compounds.
_____, _____

10. Monosaccharides and polysaccharides are examples.
_____

11. Organic compound consisting of a molecule of glycerol and three fatty acid molecules. _____

12. The building blocks of proteins. _____

13. The abbreviation of the nucleic acid containing deoxyribose.
_____

14. The specific carbohydrate found in RNA. _____

15. The building blocks of nucleic acids. _____

Term Search Puzzle

```
N  P  O  A  T  O  M  R  V  C  W  C  H  M
U  R  H  N  O  T  I  D  A  E  E  A  Y  O
C  O  Y  D  E  L  E  M  L  E  I  R  D  L
L  T  D  L  I  P  I  D  E  N  G  B  R  E
E  O  R  E  L  E  M  E  N  T  H  O  O  C
O  N  E  U  T  R  O  N  C  A  T  N  G  U
T  G  I  S  O  T  O  P  E  T  A  Y  E  L
I  E  N  A  M  I  N  O  A  C  I  D  N  E
D  N  C  A  I  R  I  B  O  S  E  R  T  I
E  L  E  M  C  N  U  M  B  E  R  A  D  E
T  C  A  R  B  O  H  Y  D  R  A  T  E  S
```

Cellular and Tissue Organization

"The body is a state in which each cell is a citizen."

—Rudolph Virchow

A. Cellular Organization and Function

I.   Fill in the Blank

Fill in the blank with the appropriate term.

   1. Three parts that cells have in common are _____, _____, and _____.

   2. The two types of cellular organization are _____ and _____.

   3. A nucleoid is typical of _____ cells.

   4. The study of cells is known as _____.

   5. The study of tissues is called _____.

II.   Matching 1: Cellular Organization

Match the term to its meaning. Insert the appropriate letter in the space next to the question number.

Choices:

_____ **1.** nucleoid   **a.** primitive nucleus

_____ **2.** karyo   **b.** combining form for nucleus

_____ **3.** eu-   **c.** prefix meaning "true"

_____ **4.** membrane-bound internal   **d.** organelles
            cellular compartments

III.   Matching 2: Eukaryotic Cells

Match the term to its meaning. Insert the appropriate letter in the space next to the question number.

Choices:

_____ **1.** ribosomes   **a.** surrounds the nucleus

_____ **2.** microtubules   **b.** produces energy (adenosine triphosphate, or **ATP**)

_____ **3.** lysosome

_____ 4. mitochondrion
_____ 5. cell membrane
_____ 6. nuclear envelope
_____ 7. nucleus
_____ 8. Golgi apparatus

c. controls passage of materials into and out of cells

d. consists of nucleic acid and protein granules attached to endoplasmic reticulum

e. contains DNA and directs cellular activities

f. provides support internally to the cell

g. contains enzymes capable of digesting substances that enter the cell

h. site for carbohydrate synthesis and packaging of proteins for secretion

IV.   Matching 3: Prokaryotic Cells

Match the term to its meaning. Insert the appropriate letter in the space next to the question number.

Choices:

_____ 1. pilus
_____ 2. mesosome
_____ 3. cell wall
_____ 4. flagellum
_____ 5. glycocalyx
_____ 6. ribosomes
_____ 7. endospore
_____ 8. nucleoid
_____ 9. cell membrane

a. a highly heat-resistant structure

b. used for movement

c. energy production

d. provides shape to cell

e. used to transfer genetic material

f. regulates the passage of materials into and out of cells

g. provides protection against chemicals such as antibiotics

h. produces protein

i. area where DNA is localized

V.   Spell Check

Circle each incorrectly spelled term and write it correctly in the space provided.

1. prokaryotic   _____
2. silium   _____
3. membrane   _____
4. mitochondreon   _____
5. nuclolus   _____
6. rybosome   _____
7. genome   _____
8. reticulum   _____
9. pilus   _____
10. glicocalyx   _____

VI.   Vision Quiz 1: Eukaryotic Cellular Organization

Figure 6-13 shows a eukaryotic cell. Identify and write the letter of the numbered organellesin the spaces provided next to each question number.

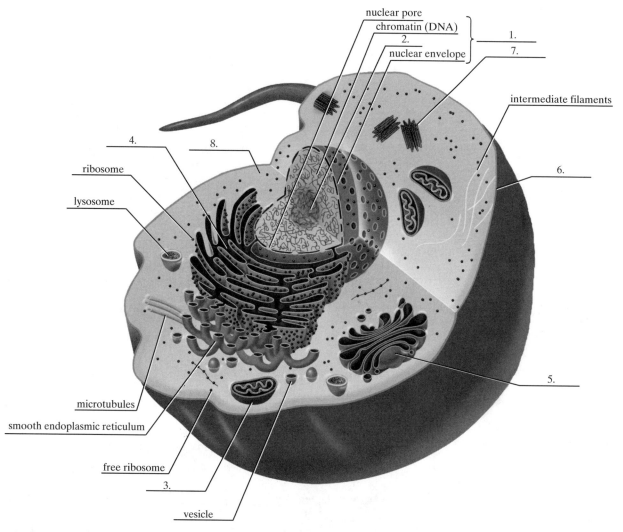

FIGURE 6-13   Vision Quiz 1: A eukaryotic cell, emphasizing its organelles.

Choices:

_____ 1.

_____ 2.

_____ 3.

_____ 4.

_____ 5.

_____ 6.

_____ 7.

_____ 8.

a. cytoplasm

b. centrioles

c. plasma (cell) membrane

d. Golgi complex

e. rough endoplasmic reticulum

f. mitochondrion

g. nucleolus

h. nucleus

VII.   Vision Quiz 2: Prokaryotic Cell

Figure 6-14 shows a prokaryotic cell. Identify and write the name of the numbered organelles in the space provided next to each question number.

Choices:

_____ 1.

_____ 2.

a. capsule

b. nucleoid

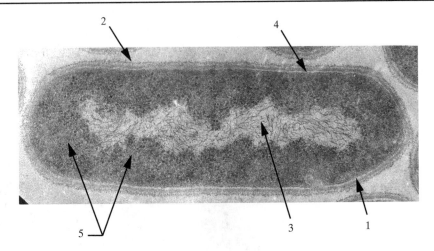

FIGURE 6-14   Vision Quiz 2: An electron micrograph.

_____ 3.   c. ribosomes
_____ 4.   d. plasma (cell membrane)
_____ 5.   e. cell wall

B. Noncellular Forms—Viruses and Prions

I.   Fill in the Blank

Fill in the blank with the appropriate word(s).

1. The nucleic acids found in virions are either
_____ or _____ but never
both.
2. Viruses depend on _____ cells and their parts for
energy and protein needs.
3. Viruses do not have the _____ typical of eukaryotic or prokaryotic cells.
4. A mature virus particle is called a _____.
5. The protein coat that surrounds the viral nucleic acid core is called a
_____.
6. The basic part of a capsid is the _____.
7. The capsid of some viruses is covered by an
_____.
8. Three shapes found among viruses are _____,
_____, and _____.

II.   Spell Check

Circle each incorrectly spelled term and write it correctly in the space provided.

1. viruses   _____
2. replication _____
3. kapsomer   _____
4. virion   _____
5. envelope   _____
6. polyhedrol _____
7. helical   _____

8. complex   _____

9. prion   _____

10. capsid   _____

III.   Vision Quiz: Bacterial Viruses

Figure 6-15 shows a bacterial virus. Identify and write the letter of the numbered structures in the spaces provided next to each question number.

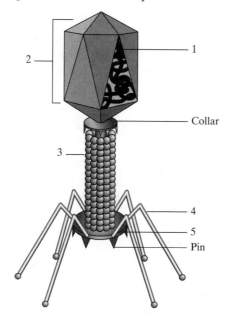

FIGURE 6-15   Vision Quiz: Bacterial viruses.

Choices:

_____ **1.**   **a.** head

_____ **2.**   **b.** tail (sheath)

_____ **3.**   **c.** nucleic acid core

_____ **4.**   **d.** base plate

_____ **5.**   **e.** tail fiber

C. Cell Division Mechanisms

I.   Matching 1: Cellular Division

Match the term to its meaning. (The same meaning may be used more than once.)
Insert the appropriate letter in the space provided next to each question number.

_____ **1.** stage between periods of mitosis

_____ **2.** active RNA and cell part synthesis

_____ **3.** DNA replication and doubling

_____ **4.** chromosome number reduction

_____ **5.** formation of special proteins involved in cell division

_____ **6.** sex cell formation process

_____ **7.** chromosome division

Choices:

     a. Gap 1

     b. Gap 2

          c. synthesis
          d. interphase
          e. meiosis
          f. mitosis

II.   Matching 2: Mitosis

Choices:

_____ **1.** mitosis stage in which chromosomes separate from each other

_____ **2.** mitotic stage in which division into two cells is complete

_____ **3.** holds chromatids together

_____ **4.** mitotic stage in which chromosomes are closely packed together within the nucleus

_____ **5.** mitotic stages in which chromosomes are in an equatorial position

_____ **6.** the stage between cycles of division

_____ **7.** half the normal number of a cell's chromosomes

_____ **8.** process of cytoplasm division

_____ **9.** the normal number of chromosomes in a cell

_____ **10.** a chromosome half

a. interphase
b. metaphase
c. anaphase
d. prophase
e. telophase
f. chromatid
g. centomere
h. diploid
i. haploid
j. cytokinesis

III.   Spell Check

Circle each incorrectly spelled term and write it correctly in the space provided.

1. myosis   _____

2. mitosis   _____

3. cromosomes   _____

4. nucleus   _____

5. nucleolis   _____

6. telaphase   _____

7. chromated   _____

8. annaphase   _____

9. centromere   _____

10. haployd   _____

IV.   Vision Quiz: Phases of Mitosis

Figure 6-16 shows a mitosis cycle. Identify and write the name of the numbered stages. Insert the appropriate letter in the space provided next to each question number.

1._____   4._____   3_____

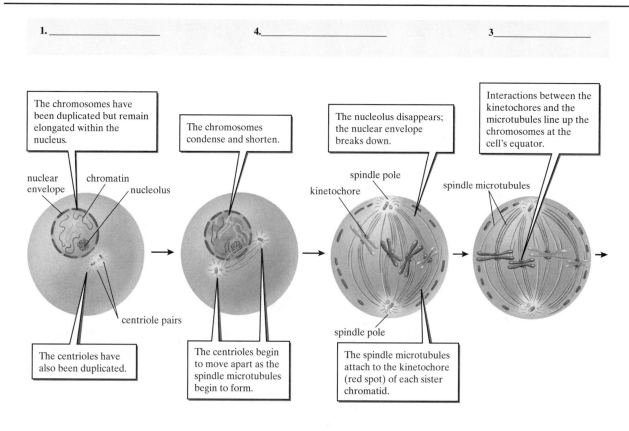

The chromosomes have been duplicated but remain elongated within the nucleus.

nuclear envelope   chromatin   nucleolus

The centrioles have also been duplicated.

centriole pairs

The chromosomes condense and shorten.

The centrioles begin to move apart as the spindle microtubules begin to form.

The nucleolus disappears; the nuclear envelope breaks down.

spindle pole
kinetochore
spindle microtubules

spindle pole

The spindle microtubules attach to the kinetochore (red spot) of each sister chromatid.

Interactions between the kinetochores and the microtubules line up the chromosomes at the cell's equator.

5._____   2._____

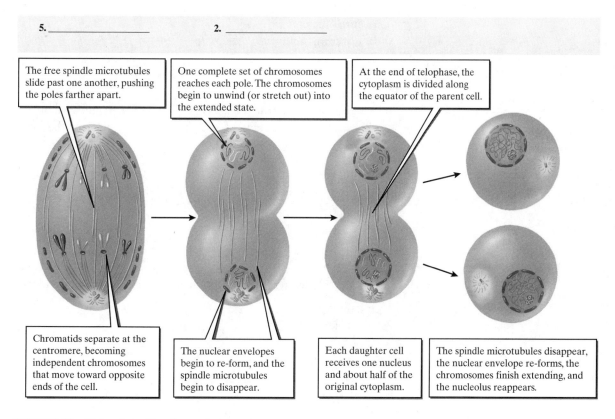

The free spindle microtubules slide past one another, pushing the poles farther apart.

Chromatids separate at the centromere, becoming independent chromosomes that move toward opposite ends of the cell.

One complete set of chromosomes reaches each pole. The chromosomes begin to unwind (or stretch out) into the extended state.

The nuclear envelopes begin to re-form, and the spindle microtubules begin to disappear.

At the end of telophase, the cytoplasm is divided along the equator of the parent cell.

Each daughter cell receives one nucleus and about half of the original cytoplasm.

The spindle microtubules disappear, the nuclear envelope re-forms, the chromosomes finish extending, and the nucleolus reappears.

FIGURE 6-16   Vision Quiz: The phases of mitosis.

Choices:

1. _____
2. _____
3. _____
4. _____
5. _____

a. anaphase
b. metaphase
c. prophase
d. interphase
e. telophase

D. Microscopes

I.   Multiple Choice

Circle the best possible answer for each question.

1. The study of the organization, structures, and functions of cells is known as _____.
   a. biochemistry
   b. cytology
   c. histology
   d. microscopy
   e. staining

2. The scientific specialty employing microscopes and stains is called

   _____.
   a. biochemistry
   b. cytology
   c. histology
   d. microscopy
   e. staining

3. Very thin slices of cells for viewing in the transmission electron microscopes are called _____.
   a. micrometers
   b. ultrathin sections
   c. dyes
   d. images
   e. sections

4. Microscopes that use ordinary visible light, magnify about 2,000 times, and show details of specimens in the range of 0.25 μm are

   _____.
   a. transmission electron microscopes
   b. scanning electron microscopes
   c. STEMs
   d. light microscopes
   e. choices *a* and *b* only

II.   Spell Check

Circle each incorrectly spelled term and write it correctly in the space provided.

1. microscope   _____
2. microskopie   _____
3. intracellular   _____
4. extracelluler   _____
5. sitology   _____
6. micrometer   _____
7. magnification   _____
8. micrografs   _____

E. Tissues and Epithelia

I.   Fill in the Blank

Fill in the blank with the appropriate term(s).

    1. In the human, similar cells arranged in layers or groups are called

    _____ .

    2. The study of tissue is known as _____ .

    3. The four basic tissue types in the human are:

    _____ , _____ ,

    _____ , and _____ .

    4. Epithelial cells arranged in single layers are referred to as being

    _____ .

    5. Epithelial cells arranged in many layers upon one another are referred
    to as being _____ .

II.   Matching

Match the term to its meaning.

Insert the appropriate letter in the space provided next to the question number.

Choices:

_____ **1.** single layer of elongated cells	**a.** simple squamous	
_____ **2.** single layer of cube-shaped cells	**b.** stratified squamous	
_____ **3.** single layer of flattened cells	**c.** stratified columnar	
_____ **4.** several layers of flattened cells	**d.** psuedostratified	
_____ **5.** several layers of elongated cells	**e.** transitional	
_____ **6.** elongated cells that appear to have a layered arrangement	**f.** simple cuboidal	
_____ **7.** cell layers specialized to undergo changes such as expression	**g.** simple columnar	

III.   Spell Check

Circle the incorrectly spelled term and write it correctly in the space provided.

    1. simple _____

    2. stratefied _____

    3. columner _____

    4. cuboidal _____

    5. transitional _____

    6. squamus _____

    7. spocrine _____

    8. pseudostratified _____

    9. holokrine _____

   10. merrocrine _____

F. Connective Tissue

I.   Fill in the Blank

Fill in the blank with the appropriate term(s).

1. Connective tissues contain the following three components:
   _____, _____, and
   _____.

2. Tissues known for their fat storage are called
   _____.

3. Three functions of connective tissue in general are
   _____, _____, and
   _____.

4. Another term for bone is _____ tissue.

5. Cells that secrete substances for bone formation are called
   _____.

6. Small cavities in a bone matrix are known as
   _____.

7. The interconnections between concentric bone lamellae and from one
   lacunae to another are called _____.

8. The three types of cartilage are _____,
   _____, and _____.

II.   Plural and Singular Forms

Write the singular form of the following terms in the spaces provided.

1. canaliculi   _____
2. lamellae   _____
3. lacunae   _____

III.   Matching 1

Match the term to its meaning. (The same meaning may be used more than once.)
Insert the appropriate letter in the space provided next to each question number.

Choices:

_____ 1. fat storage
_____ 2. protects the ends of
        bone(s) and the nose
_____ 3. supports bony skeleton
        parts
_____ 4. major component of the
        skeleton
_____ 5. phagocytosis
_____ 6. provides elasticity to blood
        vessels such as arteries
_____ 7. binds organs together

a. reticuloendothelial
b. hyaline cartilage
c. adipose tissue
d. elastic connective tissue
e. fibrocartilage
f. bone
g. loose connective tissue

IV.   Matching 2

Choices:

_____ 1. ends of bones
_____ 2. body skeleton
_____ 3. outer part of the ear

a. reticular
b. bone
c. adipose

_____ **4.** knee   **d.** elastic cartilage
_____ **5.** various organ surfaces   **e.** hyaline cartilage
                                                              f. fibrocartilage

V.   Spell Check

Circle each incorrectly spelled term and write it correctly in the space provided.

    1. adepose   _____

    2. elastik   _____

    3. cartilage   _____

    4. conective   _____

    5. fibrocartilage   _____

    6. hyalene   _____

    7. reticuloendothelial _____

    8. reticular   _____

    9. calsium   _____

    10. Haversien   _____

    11. fibrous   _____

    12. lakunae   _____

G. Muscle Tissue

I.   Fill in the Blank

Fill in the blank with the appropriate term(s).

    1. The three types of muscle tissue are _____, _____, and _____.

    2. A muscle that cannot be controlled by conscious effort is referred to as being _____.

    3. The two muscle types that cannot be controlled by conscious effort are _____ and _____.

    4. The term striated means _____.

    5. Which type of muscle tissue has intercalated disks? _____

II. Spell Check

Circle each incorrectly spelled term and write it correctly in the space provided.

    1. fibre   _____

    2. skeleton   _____

    3. sarcolema   _____

    4. interkalated   _____

    5. disk   _____

    6. volintary   _____

H. Nervous Tissue

I.   Fill in the Blank

Fill in the blank with the appropriate word(s).

    1. The two major divisions of the human nervous system are _____ and _____.

    2. Nervous tissue consists of the basic cell type known as a _____.

    3. The main parts of the basic cell type found in nervous tissue are _____, _____, and _____.

II.   Spell Check

Circle each incorrectly spelled term and write it correctly in the space provided.

    1. periferal   _____

    2. neurons   _____

    3. nervis   _____

    4. glial   _____

    5. dendrite   _____

    6. axon   _____

    7. nuroglia   _____

    8. nucelolis   _____

III.   Vision Quiz: Nervous Tissue

Figure 6-17 shows a neuron. Identify and write the name of the numbered parts.

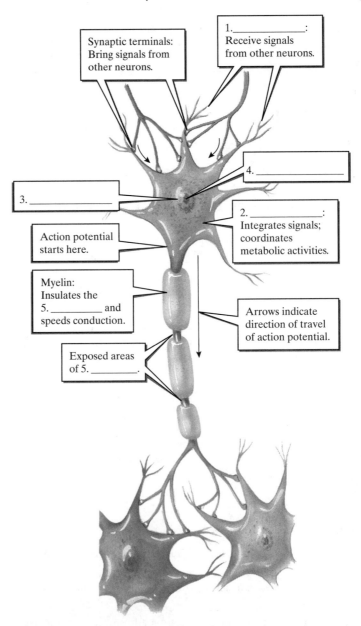

1._____:
Receive signals
from other neurons.

Synaptic terminals:
Bring signals from
other neurons.

4. _____

3. _____

2. _____:
Integrates signals;
coordinates
metabolic activities.

Action potential
starts here.

Myelin:
Insulates the
5. _____ and
speeds conduction.

Arrows indicate
direction of travel
of action potential.

Exposed areas
of 5. _____.

FIGURE 6-17   Vision Quiz: Nervous Tissue.

Choices:

_____ 1.	**a.** axon
_____ 2.	**b.** dendrites
_____ 3.	**c.** nucleus
_____ 4.	**d.** cell body
_____ 5.	**e.** nucleolus

I. Increasing Your Medical Terminology Word Power 1

1. Read the following report
2. Prepare to answer the questions at the end of the section.
3. Circle all unfamiliar terms with a red pencil.
4. Underline familiar medical terms with a blue pencil.
5. Use your knowledge of word elements, a medical dictionary, and the key terms to find the meaning of unfamiliar terms.

Calcinosis

Key Terms

calcinosis (kal'-si-NŌ-sis)   abnormal deposits of calcium in body tissues

calcium (KAL-sē-um)   a chemical element widely distributed and found naturally in various foods, such as milk products, fruits, and vegetables

dystrophic (dis-TROF-ik)   abnormal condition caused by defective nutrition

idiopathic (id'-ē-ō-PATH-ik)   diseases that can't be attributed to known causes

lesion (LĒ-shun)   injury or wound

metastatic (met'-a-STAT-ik)   spreading from one part of the body to another

systemic (sis-TEM-ik)   pertaining to the entire body rather than to one of its parts

Introduction

Calcinosis refers to the depositing of calcium within the skin or soft tissues, such as the inner linings of the cheek and lips. The abnormal condition can be classified into three types. These are (1) _dystrophic_, whereby calcium accumulates in damaged or dead tissue; (2) _metastatic_, in which normal tissue is affected by excessive amounts of either calcium or phosphorus in the blood; and (3) _idiopathic_, in which there is no recognizable cause of the condition.

C ASE HISTORY

A 65-year-old woman complaining of general discomfort in her chest and some difficulty in swallowing was taken to a local medical center. On physical examination, the patient was found to be well developed and well nourished. However, large, calcium-containing, hard, bulky masses in the skin of the chest were found. Similar lesions were also noted in the skin covering the elbows, hands, fingers, knees, and the soft tissue of the cheek. The patient indicated that some of the masses had been present for 20 years. She also complained of severe _arthritis_ (ar-THRĪ-tis) of the hands.

The personal history of the patient failed to reveal any excessive intake of milk, milk products, or vitamin D. The patient admitted to daily use of calcium tablets taken over a period of twelve years, some forty years ago. There were no signs of kidney disease and no family history of arthritis or calcinosis. Laboratory tests failed to reveal any serious underlying systemic disorder or disease process.

Questions

I.   Fill in the Blank

Fill in the blank with the appropriate term(s).

    1. The three types of calcinosis are _____, _____, and _____.

    2. Where were the lesions found on the patient? _____

    3. What condition was also found in the patient's hands? _____

II.   Spell Check

Circle each incorrectly spelled term and write it correctly in the space provided..

    1. calsinosis _____
    2. distrophik _____
    3. idiopathic _____
    4. leszun _____
    5. metastatic _____

J. Increasing Your Medical Terminology Word Power 2
A Patient with Ovarian Squamous Cell Carcinoma

Key Terms

chemotherapy (kē'-mō-THER-a-pē)   use of chemicals in the treatment of disease

histological (his-tō-LOJ-i-kal)   microscopic study of tissues

hysterectomy (his-ter-EK-tō-mē)   surgical removal of the uterus through the abdominal wall or vagina

laparatomy (lap-ar-OT-ō-mē)   surgical opening of the abdomen

multinodular (mul-tī-NŌD-ū-lar)   consisting of many small knots or small clumps of cells known as nodules

ovarian (ō-VA-re-an)   regarding the ovary

regimen (REJ-i-men)   systematic plan of activities and regulations designed to improve or keep a certain condition under control

salpingo-oophorectomy (sal-ping-gō-ō-of-ō-REK-tō-mē)   surgical removal of an ovary and fallopian (fa-LŌ-pē-an) or uterine tube

teratoma (ter-a-TŌ-ma)   congenital tumor of embryonic (developmental) tissue

tomography (tō-MOG-ra-fē)   any one of several noninvasive techniques using a special type of x-ray equipment to show an organ or tissue at a particular depth (plane)

toxicity (toks-IS-i-tē) property of being poisonous

vaginectomy (vaj-en-EK-tō-mē) surgical removal of the vagina or a portion of it

C ASE HISTORY

A 30-year-old woman was admitted to the Cancer Center for an evaluation of a pelvic (PEL-vic) mass and a vaginal tumor, which upon histological examination revealed the presence of a squamous cell carcinoma. The clinical viewpoint at this time was that the condition was unusual for a vaginal carcinoma and that the abdominal mass could be a second primary carcinoma.

Physical examination of the patient revealed a 10 × 10 × 10 cm firm mass extending to the right pelvic sidewall. Results of a laparotomy showed the presence of a 10 × 10 cm multinodular mass extending from the right ovary. Following this finding, a total abdominal hysterectomy with bilateral salpingo-oophorectomy and a partial vaginectomy were performed. Figure 6-18 shows the relationship of the ovaries, fallopian tubes, uterus, cervix, and vagina to each other. The approximate locations of the vaginal metastasis excised by the vaginectomy (area of involvement) is also shown.

Histological study of the excised tissue showed a squamous cell carcinoma of the ovary developing in an initially benign teratoma with metastasis to the vagina. The patient's postoperative course was uneventful, and she started on her first course of

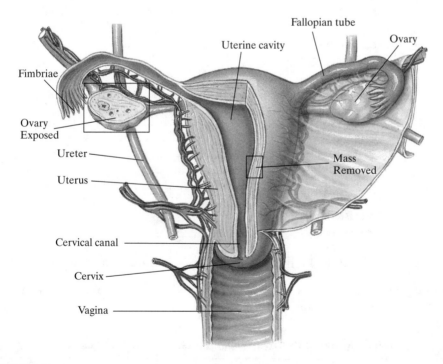

FIGURE 6-18 The relationship of the ovaries, uterine tubes, uterus, cervix, and the vagina. The approximate location of the vaginal mass removed by vaginectomy is shown. A number of additional structures also are included for general information.

chemotherapy. The patient received a specified five-course drug regimen at three-week intervals. Aside from the expected nausea and vomiting, no other indications of toxicity were noted.

Approximately nine months after the operation, a chest x-ray confirmed the presence of multiple metastatic lesions in the lungs. Because of the obvious severe progression of the disease, the patient was given external irradiation therapy in addition to the chemotherapy. Computed tomography also revealed the presence of a pelvic mass. It was hoped that the radiation treatment would help the patient. Unfortunately, little change was noted in the size of the pelvic mass, as demonstrated by further computed tomography.

Questions

I.   Matching

Match the term to its meaning. Insert the appropriate letter in the space next to each question number.

			Choices:
_____	**1.**	excision	**a.** surgical opening of the abdomen
_____	**2.**	vaginectomy	**b.** surgical removal
_____	**3.**	laparotomy	**c.** being poisonous
_____	**4.**	multinodular	**d.** excision of the vagina
_____	**5.**	toxicity	**e.** pertains to several nodules
_____	**6.**	hysterectomy	**f.** embryonically (fetal) related tumor
_____	**7.**	teratoma	**g.** surgical removal of the uterus
_____	**8.**	carcinoma	**h.** malignant tumor in epithelial tissue

II.   Spell Check

Circle each incorrectly spelled term and write it correctly in the space provided.

1. chemotherapy _____
2. histalogical _____
3. ovarien _____
4. ophorectomy _____
5. larpaotomy _____
6. bilaterel _____
7. metastetic _____
8. terratoma _____

III.   Word Analysis: Prefixes, Word Roots, Combining Forms and Suffixes

Table 6-7 lists medical terms with their pronunciations and definitions. Pick out the combining forms, word roots, prefixes, and suffixes.

TABLE 6-7   WORD ANALYSIS: PREFIXES, WORD ROOTS, COMBINING FORMS, AND SUFFIXES

Term and Pronunciation	Definition
bilateral (bī-LAT-er-al)	pertaining to both sides
carcinoma (kar'-si-NŌ-ma)	a malignant growth of epithelial tissue
chemotherapy (kē'-mō-THER-a-pē)	the treatment of a disease with drugs or chemicals

(Continued)

TABLE 6-7   (CONTINUED)

Term and Pronunciation	Definition
histological (his-tō-LOJ-i-kal)	the study of tissues
hysterectomy (his-ter-EK-tō-mē)	surgical removal of the uterus
laparotomy (lap-ar-OT-ō-mē)	surgical opening of the abdomen
oophorectomy (ō-of-ō-REK-tō-mē)	excision of an ovary
teratoma (ter-a-TŌ-ma)	congenital tumor containing primitive (embryonic) tissue
tomography (tō-MOG-ra-fē)	x-ray technique designed to show body images
vaginectomy (vaj-in-EK-tō-mē)	excision of the vagina or a part of it

1. Analyze each term in Table 6-7.
2. Circle all combining forms, word roots, prefixes, and suffixes, and label them **cf, wr, s,** and **p**, respectively.
3. Answers shown in Table 6-8.

Term Search Challenge

Locate 12 terms in the puzzle.

1. Write the specific term next to its definition. Then find that term in the puzzle diagram and circle it.
2. Terms may be read from left to right, backward, up, down, or diagonally.
3. If a term appears more than once, circle it only once. (A term or abbreviation may be found inside others.)
4. Check your answers.

Clues:

1. Functional unit of life _____
2. Type of gland that releases its product into ducts _____
3. Type of gland that directly secretes its product _____
4. The study of the structure and function of cells _____
5. Cellular organization for cells with a well-defined nucleus

   _____
6. Part of eukaryotic cell that produces ATP _____
7. Type of cell division found in human body cells _____
8. Cell with a primitive nucleus _____
9. Process by which sex cells are produced _____
10. The study of tissues and their products _____
11. General tissue group including fat and cartilage _____
12. Term for fat tissue _____

Term Search Puzzle

```
C  E  L  L  U  L  A  H  I  O  N  N  M  R  E
Y  C  M  I  T  O  S  I  S  T  C  U  I  A  L
T  H  E  R  A  C  I  S  P  L  E  U  T  A  E
O  S  I  E  N  D  O  T  N  L  N  Y  O  P  M
L  S  O  I  N  A  L  O  T  O  D  E  C  Y  E
O  Y  S  L  E  N  D  L  I  D  O  V  H  O  H
G  S  I  E  L  E  T  O  L  O  C  I  O  T  I
Y  T  S  D  O  R  P  G  V  C  R  T  N  I  S
A  E  S  R  Y  R  E  Y  I  T  I  I  D  B  T
P  R  O  K  A  R  Y  O  T  I  C  T  R  R  O
E  U  K  A  R  Y  O  T  I  C  A  A  I  H  L
L  B  C  O  N  N  E  C  T  I  V  E  O  O  O
A  D  I  P  O  S  E  D  R  A  T  E  N  R  G
E  X  O  C  R  I  N  E  R  T  E  S  R  O  Y
E  N  D  O  C  R  I  N  E  E  X  O  C  R  I
```

Organs and Systems

"Health is a state of complete physical, mental, and social well-being and not merely the absence of disease or infirmity."

—Preamble of the World Health Organization charter

INFORMATIONAL CHALLENGE

A. Organs and Organ Systems

I.   Fill in the Blank

Fill in the blank with the appropriate term(s).

1. A structure composed of two or more tissue types and grouped together to perform a specific function is a(n) _____.
2. Arrangements of several organs working together in a coordinated manner are called _____.
3. The system that coordinates circulatory functions is called the _____ system.

II.   Matching: Human Body System Components

Match the term to its meaning. (The same meaning may be used more than once.) Insert the appropriate letter in the space provided next to each question number.

Choices:

_____ 1. pituitary, thymus, and thyroid gland
_____ 2. skin, nails, and hair
_____ 3. bones and joints
_____ 4. brain, spinal cord, and nerves
_____ 5. kidney, ureters, and urinary bladder
_____ 6. nose, pharynx, trachea, and bronchi
_____ 7. mouth, intestine, and stomach
_____ 8. heart and blood vessels

a. nervous and sensory
b. urinary
c. respiratory
d. integumentary
e. skeletal
f. cardiovascular
g. gastrointestinal
h. endocrine

III.   Spell Check

Circle each incorrectly spelled term and write it correctly in the space provided.

1. stomach   _____
2. farynx   _____
3. bronki   _____
4. integumentary _____
5. trakea   _____
6. ureter   _____
7. thymose   _____
8. respiratore   _____

B. Terms Describing Organ System Parts and/or Locations

I.   Fill in the Blank: Parts or Locations of Organs or Organ Systems

Fill in the blank with the letter of the appropriate term.

1. The rounded tip or _____ of the heart points to the left and slightly downward.
2. A series of _____(s) conduct bile and other important substances into the duodenum (dū'-ō-DĒ-num), about 8–10 cm below the pyloric (pī-LOR-ik) opening of the stomach.
3. The outer surface or _____ of the cerebrum (ser-Ē-brum), the largest part of the brain, is made up of gray matter.
4. The folds found on the surface of the cerebrum are separated from one another by deep grooves or _____(s).
5. The nasal cavities or _____(s) are frequently affected during episodes of the flu.
6. This portion of the gastrointestinal _____ is obviously blocked by what appears to be a large tumor.

Choices:

a. duct
b. fissure
c. apex
d. cortex
e. tract
f. sinus

II.   Matching: Parts or Locations of Organs or Organ Systems

Match the term to its meaning. (The same meaning may be used more than once.) Insert the appropriate letter in the space provided next to each question number.

Choices:

_____ 1. an opening   a. ventricle
_____ 2. the center of an organ   b. aperture
_____ 3. an expanded or dilated   c. sinus
         part of a duct   d. corpus
_____ 4. the outer portion of an   e. apex
         organ   f. duct

_____ **5.** the part nearest the point of attachment   **g.** base

h. ampulla

_____ **6.** the tip or point of an organ   **i.** medulla

j. cortex

_____ **7.** a narrow tube   **k.** node

_____ **8.** a small bundle of tissue

_____ **9.** a body or mass

_____ **10.** a cavity

_____ **11.** a small cavity or hollow space

III.   Spell Check

Circle the term that is correctly spelled.

1. an opening is an (a) aperature, (b) apirture, (c) aperture
2. a body or mass is a (a) corpis, (b) corpus, (c) korpus
3. an expanded duct part is an (a) ampulla, (b) ampula, (c) ammpula
4. an opening in a structure is a (a) foremen (b) formann, (c) foramen
5. a groove is a (a) fissure, (b) fisure, (c) fissur
6. a small cavity is a (a) ventrikle, (b) ventricle, (c) ventricl
7. a channel is a (a) sinis, (b) signus, (c) sinus
8. a small tissue mass is a (a) knode, (b) nod, (c) node

C. *The Cavities of the Body*

I.   Fill in the Blank

Fill in the blank with the appropriate term(s).

1. The dorsal body cavity is made up of which two other cavities?
   _____ and _____
2. List the major cavities of the thoracic cavity: _____,
   _____ and _____.
3. What body structure separates the thoracic cavity from the abdominopelvic cavity? _____

II.   Matching: The Components of Body Cavities

Match the term to its meaning. (The same meaning may be used more than once.) Insert the appropriate letter in the space provided next to each question number.

Choices:

_____ **1.** brain   **a.** pelvic area

_____ **2.** trachea, aorta   **b.** abdominal cavity

_____ **3.** urinary bladder   **c.** mediastinal cavity

_____ **4.** lungs   **d.** pericardial cavity

_____ **5.** stomach, intestines   **e.** pleural cavity

_____ **6.** heart   **f.** spinal cavity

_____ **7.** nerves of the spinal cord   **g.** cranial cavity

III.   Spell Check

Circle each incorrectly spelled term and write it correctly in the space provided.

1. abdominull _____
2. dorsel _____
3. vertebral _____
4. pericardial _____
5. thorasic _____
6. pleural _____
7. viseral _____
8. pelvic _____

IV.   Vision Quiz: Body Cavities

Figure 7-7 shows the body cavities. Identify and write the name of the numbered cavity in the space provided next to the question's number.

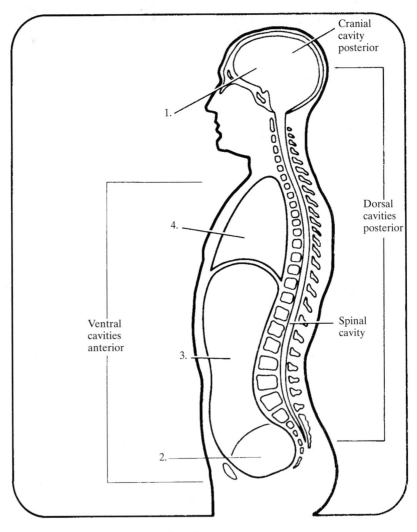

FIGURE 7-7   Vision Quiz. Body Cavities.

1. _____
2. _____
3. _____
4. _____

D. Cellular, Tissue, and Organ Responses to Injury and Disease

I.   Matching 1: Responses to Injury and Disease

Match the term to its meaning. (The same meaning may be used more than once.) Insert the appropriate letter in the space provided next to each question number.

Choices:

_____ **1.** hypertrophy
_____ **2.** atrophy
_____ **3.** hyperplasia
_____ **4.** neoplasia
_____ **5.** dysplasia
_____ **6.** metaplasia

a. abnormal tissue development
b. an increase in cell size
c. a change of a cell into another form
d. new and abnormal tissue growth
e. an increase in tissue due to cell number increases
f. decrease in cell size accompanied by reduced tissue size

II.   Matching 2: Disease-Associated Processes

Match the term to its meaning. (The same meaning may be used more than once.) Insert the appropriate letter in the space provided next to each question number.

Choices:

_____ **1.** ulcer
_____ **2.** degeneration
_____ **3.** cellulitis
_____ **4.** erythema
_____ **5.** inflammation
_____ **6.** abscess
_____ **7.** repair

a. an open sore
b. localized collection of dead tissue and leukocytes
c. spreading form of inflammation involving connective tissue
d. body process to prevent the spread of tissue injury
e. cell breakdown
f. body's attempt to replace injured cells
g. redness

III.   Matching 3: Word Elements Associated with Cellular, Tissue, and Organ Responses to Disease

Match the prefix to its meaning. Insert the appropriate letter in the space next to the question number.

Choices:

_____ **1.** cyano-
_____ **2.** erythemato-
_____ **3.** atelo-
_____ **4.** necro-
_____ **5.** path-
_____ **6.** pyreto-
_____ **7.** atroph-
_____ **8.** dys-
_____ **9.** pyo-
_____ **10.** pachy-
_____ **11.** pyro-

a. degeneration
b. heavy
c. painful
d. death
e. disease
f. incomplete
g. pus
h. heat or fire
i. blue
j. redness
k. fever

IV.   Fill in the Blank: Word Elements and Terms Used for Tissue and Organ Responses to Disease Applications

Fill in the blank with the letter of the appropriate prefix.

Choices:

   a.   atroph-
   b.   dys-
   c.   cyan-
   d.   path-
   e.   necr-
   f.   pyo-

Example: Ms. Green has a history of **painful vision**. Her _____ -*opia* has persisted for several years.

The answer here is *b.,* **dys-**.

   1.   The balloon covered her mouth and nose and caused the **dark blue appearance**. Even if oxygen is cut off for a short time, such _____ -osis will occur.
   2.   The spider bite caused a great deal of injury and resulted in tissue **death**. To limit this type of _____ -osis, surgical removal of the damaged tissue is needed.
   3.   Finding the cause of a disease is just one part of the **study of disease**. It takes years to obtain a full grasp of this medical specialty known as _____ -*ology*.
   4.   The infection was responsible for **decreases** in size or wasting away of several body organs. Such _____ -y is not remarkable.
   5.   This bacterium (bak-TĒ-rē-um), *Streptococcus pyogenes* (strep'-tō-KOK-us pī'-ō-JEN-ēz), is known to produce pus with its infections. Several such _____ -*genic* microbes are difficult to eliminate.
   6.   This is the fourth month in a row that Ms. West reported a painful menstruation episode. Her most recent x-rays show a fairly large tumor, which may be the cause of her _____ -*menorrhea*.

V.   Spell Check

Circle each incorrectly spelled term and write the correct form in the spaces provided.

   1.   atelocheila   _____
   2.   dismenorhea   _____
   3.   erythematous   _____
   4.   hiperplazia   _____
   5.   atrophe   _____
   6.   cyenosis   _____
   7.   pyonephritis   _____
   8.   piretogenous   _____
   9.   pachyglossia   _____
   10. nakrosis   _____

VI.   Word Analysis: Terms for Tissue and Organ Responses to Disease

Table 7-6 lists a number of terms with their pronunciations and definitions.

TABLE 7-6   WORD ANALYSIS: TERMS FOR TISSUE AND ORGAN RESPONSES TO DISEASE

Term and Pronunciation	Definition
atelocheilia (at'-e-lō-KĒ-lē-a)	incomplete lip development
atrophy (AT-rō-fē)	a decrease in the size of a tissue or organ; a wasting
cyanosis (sī-an-Ō-sis)	bluish discoloration of the skin
dysmenorrhea (dis'-men-ō-RĒ-a)	painful menstruation
erythematous (er'-i-THEM-a-tus)	pertaining to an area of redness over the skin
necrosis (ne-KRŌ-sis)	condition of tissue death
pachyglossia (pak-ē-GLOS-sē-a)	unusual thickness of the tongue
pathosis (path-Ō-sis)	a disease state or condition
pyonephritis (pī-ō-nef-RĪ-tis)	inflammation of the kidney with the presence of pus
pyretogenous (pī-re-TOJ-en-us)	caused by fever
pyrogenic (pī-rō-JEN-ik)	producing fever

1. Analyze each term.
2. Circle all combining forms, word roots, prefixes, and suffixes, and label them **cf**, **wr**, **p**, and **s**, respectively.
3. Check your answers (shown in Table 7-8).

E. Increasing Your Medical Terminology Word Power 1

1. Read the following report.
2. Prepare to answer the questions at the end of the section.
3. Circle all unfamiliar terms with a red pencil.
4. Underline familiar terms with a blue pencil.
5. Use your knowledge of word elements, a medical dictionary, and the key terms to find the meaning of unfamiliar terms.

Multiple System Organ Failure

Key Terms

acute respiratory distress syndrome (ARDS)   conditions associated with the ability of lungs to function normally

cholecystectomy (kō'-lē-sis-TEK-tō-mē)   removal of the gallbladder

epigastric (ep'-i-GAS-trik)   area above the pit of the stomach

hematocrit (hē-MAT-ō-krit)   laboratory test to separate the liquid portion from blood cells

hemolysis (hē-MOL-i-sis)   destruction of red blood cells

hypermetabolism (hī'-per-me-TAB-ō-liz-em)   increased rate of metabolism

hypotension   decrease in blood pressure

hypoxemia (hī-poks-Ē-mē-a)   insufficient oxygen content in the blood

laparotomy (lap-ar-OT-ō-mē)   surgical opening of the abdomen

maculopapular (mak'-ū-lō-PAP-ū-lar) rash   red or discolored patches on the skin

pathogenesis (path'-ō-JEN-e-sis)   origin and development of a disease

pathogenic (path'-ō-JEN-ik)   disease producer; refers to disease-causing capability

sepsis (SEP-sis)   microorganisms and/or their products in the bloodstream

septic shock   presence of disease-causing bacteria in the body; involves interference with blood flow to the heart and transport of oxygen to body organs

tachycardia (tak'-ē-KAR-dē-a)   abnormally rapid heart beat

tachypnea (TAK'-ip-NĒ-a)   abnormally rapid breathing

trauma (TRAW-ma)   physical injury caused by external force

ultrasonography (ul-tra-son-OG-ra-fē)   ultrasound used to produce an image of an organ or tissue

I NTRODUCTION

Multiple system organ failure (MSOF) is a relatively new diagnosis, first made in the mid-1970s in association with postoperative care. Today the condition is well recognized and frequently a fatal result of major physiologic insults, such as severe trauma, hypotension, and sepsis. MSOF is diagnosed in as many as 15 percent of the patients admitted to general critical care units. Early signs of developing MSOF are readily treated to obtain control over the cause and as a form of supportive therapy. Unfortunately, mortality ranges from 40 percent in early-phase MSOF to 90 percent or greater when three or more organs are involved. Treatment, in both early and late MSOF, is likely to be most effective when it is directed toward the central pathogenic mechanism of MSOF, namely systemic and harmful inflammation, which may lead to organ failure by direct toxic effects or by direct effects such as interference with oxygen delivery to body tissues. The many causative factors of inflammation in MSOF include those associated with the pathogenesis of sepsis.

The development of MSOF has the following four stages:

1. causative event, such as an episode of septic shock
2. period of active resuscitative (reviving) treatment, such as aggressive fluid therapy (giving large quantities of fluids)
3. a phase of hypermetabolism, during which acute respiratory distress syndrome (ARDS) may occur
4. development of liver and kidney failure

MSOF is a realistic example of situations in which patients may die of the complications of a disease rather than of the disease itself. It is a final complication of critical illness, and sepsis is usually its main cause.

The common thread that connects many cases of MSOF is sepsis. When the specific bacterial cause is known, antibiotic therapy can be specific and prompt. On the other hand, treatment may be quite broad, especially when an intra-abdominal source is suspected or the source of infection is unknown. Other than antibiotics, the key elements of MSOF therapy are restoring and maintaining oxygen transport, metabolic support, and various techniques aimed at reducing the systemic inflammation that leads to the progression of multisystem organ failure.

C ASE HISTORY

A 51-year-old male was admitted to the hospital with a one-week history of upper respiratory infection that had been treated with ampicillin. He also reported a maculopapular rash over his body and upper abdominal and epigastric pain of two days' duration. At admission the patient had fever, exhibited tachypnea, tachycardia, and hypoxemia, and showed some confusion. His chest x-ray was within normal limits. Laboratory studies included an abnormal white blood cell count. However, the hemoglobin level, hematocrit, and blood platelet count were all within normal limits. Cultures for bacterial pathogens were negative. On the third hospital day, the patient continued to show signs and symptoms of sepsis syndrome, with added evidence of hepatic and renal failure, and a decrease in blood platelet count. Abdominal ultrasonography revealed a thickened gallbladder. Exploratory laparotomy and cholecystectomy were subsequently scheduled. On the basis of findings during surgery, biopsy specimens were taken from the patient's liver and kidneys. Postoperatively, the patient experienced respiratory failure and required mechanical ventilation. When renal failure developed and persisted, the patient was started on hemodialysis. At this point, the patient was diagnosed as having sepsis syndrome with MSOF.

Questions

I.   Fill in the Blank

Fill in the blank with the appropriate term(s).

1. The antibiotic given to the patient for upper respiratory infection was
    _____.

2. What type of rash did the patient report? _____

3. Three blood tests performed were_____,
    _____, and _____.

4. Which organ(s) or system(s) failed on the third hospital day of the patient's stay?_____

5. Ultrasonography revealed _____.

6. Two surgical procedures scheduled for the patient were
    _____ and _____.

7. Three major physiologic insults known to result in MSOF are
    _____, _____,
    and _____.

II.   Matching

Match the term to its meaning. (The same meaning may be used more than once.) Insert the appropriate letter in the space next to the question number.

Choices:

_____ **1.** cholecystectomy   **a.** laboratory procedure used to sepa-
_____ **2.** epigastric   rate blood components
_____ **3.** hemolysis   **b.** destruction of red blood cells

_____ 4. hematocrit
_____ 5. hypoxemia
_____ 6. laparotomy
_____ 7. pathogenesis
_____ 8. pathogenic
_____ 9. tachycardia
_____ 10. tachypnea

c. condition caused by a lack of oxygen in blood
d. gallbladder removal
e. surgical opening of the abdomen
f. body area above the pit of the stomach
g. disease producer
h. abnormally rapid breathing
i. development and origin of a disease
j. abnormally rapid heart beat

III.   Spell Check

Circle each incorrectly spelled term and write it correctly in the space provided.

1. postopurative   _____
2. inflammation   _____
3. pathogenisis   _____
4. septic   _____
5. antibiotic   _____
6. laperotomy   _____
7. tachipnea   _____
8. platelet   _____
9. ultrasonographe   _____
10. gallbladder   _____

IV.   Word Analysis: Prefixes, Word Roots, Combining Forms, and Suffixes

Table 7-7 lists a number of terms with their pronunciations and definitions.

TABLE 7-7   WORD ANALYSIS: PREFIXES, WORD ROOTS, COMBINING FORMS, AND SUFFIXES

Term and Pronunciation	Definition
cholecystectomy (kō'-lē-sis-TEK-tō-mē)	removal of the gallbladder
epigastric (ep'-GAS-trik)	area above the pit of the stomach
hematocrit (hē-MAT-ō-krit)	laboratory test to separate the liquid portion from blood cells
hemolysis (hē-MOL-i-sis)	destruction of red blood cells
hypoxemia (hī-poks-Ē-mē-a)	insufficient oxygen content in the blood
laparotomy (lap-ar-OT-ō-mē)	surgical opening of the abdomen
pathogenesis (path'-ō-JEN-e-sis)	origin and development of a disease
pathogenic (path'-ō-JEN-ik)	disease producer
tachycardia (tak'-ē-KAR-dē-a)	abnormally rapid heart beat
tachypnea (tak'-ip-NĒ-a)	abnormally rapid breathing

1. Analyze each term.
2. Circle all combining forms, word roots, prefixes, and suffixes, and label them **cf, wr, p,** and **s,** respectively.
3. Check your answers (shown in Table 7-9).

F. Increasing Your Medical Terminology Word Power 2

1. Read the following report.
2. Prepare to answer the questions at the end of the section.
3. Circle all unfamiliar terms with a red pencil.
4. Underline familiar terms with a blue pencil.
5. Use your knowledge of word elements, a medical dictionary, and the key terms to find the meaning of unfamiliar terms.

Invasive Wound Sepsis

Key Terms

debridement (dā-brēd-MON)   removal of foreign material and dead or damaged tissue

leukocytosis (loo'-kō-sī-TŌ-sis)   increase in the number of leukocytes (white blood cells)

otitis media (ō-TĪ-tis MĒ-dē-a)   middle ear infection

pathogen (PATH-ō-jen)   disease-causing agent

periodontitis (per-ē-ō-don-TĪ-tis)   inflammation of the area around a tooth and bone

sepsis (SEP-sis)   the presence of bacteria and/or their products in the blood

sterility (ster-IL-i-tē)   free of living microorganisms

tachycardia (tak-ē-KAR-dē-a)   rapid heart beat

I NTRODUCTION

The presence of infection is determined by an imbalance between the population of pathogens and the host's defenses. Normally, a small wound is not a source of sepsis when the presence of bacteria in the blood or *septicemia* (sep-ti-SĒ-mē-a) is not accompanied by laboratory evidence of tissue invasion.

The number of pathogens on the surface of a wound can be quite high. However, the number of pathogens decreases in the upper layers until sterility is achieved. If immune system defects occur, such as a decrease in the number of normally functioning leukocytes, a life-threatening condition can develop. Treatment of wounds in these types of situations includes the surgical removal of dead or damaged tissue, called debridement, skin grafting, and the use of antibiotics.

C ASE HISTORY

A 15-year-old female was examined by her family physician and was found to have an ulcer on the anteriolateral aspect of her proximal left lower leg. There was no history of an injury to the leg. The patient's medical records showed a history of a genetic leukocyte defect that was associated with an inactive skin lesion beginning at 19 months of age, chronic otitis media, and a generalized periodontitis (per-ē-ō-don-TĪ-tis) that resulted in the removal of all her teeth by twelve years of age. The patient's father and two sisters showed the defect and a history of similar infections.

T REATMENT

The patient was given a three-month course of antibiotics. Unfortunately, treatment was unsuccessful and resulted in an enlargement of the leg ulcer. During the next three months, the follow-up treatment consisted of surgical removal of dead tissue and the use of intravenous (in-tra-VĒ-nus) antibiotics. This treatment approach also ended in failure and caused an even greater enlargement of the leg ulcer.

The patient was next admitted to the plastic surgery unit of the hospital. Following additional skin-grafting, the patient showed signs and symptoms of extreme tissue invasion. These included high fever, chills, tachycardia, and leukocytosis. Laboratory reports showed the presence of large numbers of bacteria in biopsy specimens taken from the ulcer. Additional debridement and skin grafts and the use of larger doses of antibiotics resulted in wound closure thirteen months after the initial examination of the patient.

Questions

I.   Matching: Terminology

Match the term to its meaning. Insert the appropriate letter in the space provided next to each question number.

Choices:

_____ **1.** septicemia

_____ **2.** pathogen

_____ **3.** debridement

_____ **4.** sterility

_____ **5.** otitis media

_____ **6.** tachycardia

a. middle ear infection

b. absence of living microorganisms

c. presence of pathogens and/or their products in the blood

d. rapid heart beat

e. removal of dead or impaired tissue from a wound

f. disease-causing agent

II.   Spell Check

Circle each incorrectly spelled term and write the correct form in the space provided.

1. leukocytosis _____

2. septsemia _____

3. antirolatarel _____

4. pereodontitis _____

5. intravenous _____

6. antebiotik _____

Term Search Challenge

Locate 10 terms in the puzzle.

1. Write the specific term next to its definition. Then find that term in the puzzle diagram and circle it.

2. Terms may be read from left to right, backward, up, down, or diagonally.

3. If it appears more than once, circle it only once. (A term or abbreviation may be found inside others.)

4. Check your answers.

Clues:

1. Body cavity containing the brain _____

2. Structures composed of several kinds of tissues

_____

3. General tissue group including fat and cartilage

_____

4. Body system including the skin, nails, and hair

_____

5. Body cavity containing the stomach, intestines, and pancreas

_____

6. Groups of organs working together to perform complex functions

_____

7. Body system composed of thyroid, pituitary, and related glands

_____

8. Body system that includes the heart and blood vessels

_____

9. Body cavity containing the urinary bladder and ureter

_____

10. Body cavity containing the nerves of the spinal cord

_____

Term Search Puzzle

```
C  I  R  C  U  L  A  T  I  O  N  N  E  R  V
O  C  A  R  D  I  O  V  A  S  C  U  L  A  R
S  H  O  R  A  C  I  C  P  L  E  U  R  A  L
Y  S  T  E  N  D  O  O  N  L  N  Y  M  P  H
S  S  P  I  N  A  L  R  T  O  D  E  C  Y  A
T  Y  A  L  E  N  D  G  I  D  O  V  R  O  T
E  S  K  E  L  E  T  A  L  O  C  I  A  T  I
M  T  U  D  O  R  P  N  V  C  R  T  N  I  C
S  E  A  R  Y  R  E  S  I  T  I  I  I  B  S
P  M  I  N  T  E  G  U  M  E  N  T  A  R  Y
E  S  A  B  D  O  M  I  N  A  L  A  L  M  T
L  B  C  O  N  N  E  C  T  I  V  E  T  O  O
V  L  M  E  D  I  A  S  T  I  N  U  M  D  O
I  O  E  P  I  T  H  E  L  I  A  L  L  O  R
C  O  E  N  D  O  C  R  I  N  E  O  R  O
```

The Human Body Structural Plan

"Science is not a body of knowledge, but a way of looking at the world—a creative questioning, probing, testing of all things."

—Dr. Carl Sagan, *The Dragons of Eden*

INFORMATIONAL CHALLENGE

A. Anatomical Position

I.   Fill in the Blank

Fill in the blank with the appropriate term.

1. All references to anatomical locations are based on the body position called _____.
2. The five major body regions are _____, _____, _____, _____, and _____.
3. In which body region are the eyes, nose, and mouth located? _____
4. Which major body region is also known as the chest? _____
5. Which major region includes the pubic area? _____
6. The thigh, knee, leg, and foot are parts of the region known as the _____.
7. The shoulder, forearm, and hand belong to the major body region _____.

II.   Spell Check

Circle each incorrectly spelled term and write it correctly in the space provided.

1. kranium   _____
2. posterior   _____
3. palmer   _____
4. thorex   _____
5. thoracic   _____
6. extremity   _____

III.   Vision Quiz: Anatomical Position

Figure 8-5 shows the anatomical position of the human body. Identify and write the name of the numbered body regions in the spaces provided.

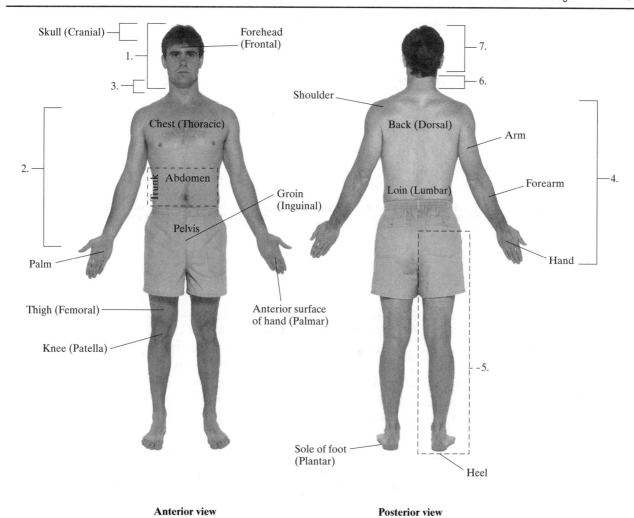

Skull (Cranial)
Forehead (Frontal)
1.
3.
Shoulder
Chest (Thoracic)
Back (Dorsal)
Arm
2.
Trunk
Abdomen
Groin (Inguinal)
Loin (Lumbar)
Forearm
4.
Pelvis
Palm
Thigh (Femoral)
Knee (Patella)
Anterior surface of hand (Palmar)
Hand
7.
6.
5.
Sole of foot (Plantar)
Heel

Anterior view   **Posterior view**

FIGURE 8-5   Vision Quiz. Anatomical Position.

1. _____   5. _____
2. _____   6. _____
3. _____   7. _____
4. _____

B. Positional and Directional Terms

I.   Fill in the Blank

Fill in the blank with the appropriate term.

1. A body lying on its abdominal surface is in the
   _____ position.
2. The front or abdominal surface of the body is referred to as the
   _____ position or direction.
3. _____ refers to a position away from the origin of
   a structure.
4. A body part located toward the tail of an animal would be in a(n)
   _____ position.
5. An object located near the surface of the body would be in a(n)
   _____ position.

6. The opposite of superior is _____.
7. The opposite of posterior is _____.
8. The opposite of dorsal is _____.
9. The opposite of deep is _____.
10. The opposite of efferent is _____.
11. The opposite of distal is _____.
12. The opposite of internal is _____.
13. The opposite of prone is _____.

II.   Matching: Terms for Position and Direction

Match the term to its meaning. (The same meaning may be used more than once.)
Insert the appropriate letter in the space provided next to the question number.

Choices:

_____ 1. away from the head
_____ 2. pertains to the center
_____ 3. lying on the back
_____ 4. located above another structure
_____ 5. conducting toward a structure
_____ 6. levels below the body surface
_____ 7. pertaining to the side
_____ 8. sole of the foot
_____ 9. the back surface
_____ 10. toward the midline

a. prone
b. lateral
c. supine
d. superior
e. central
f. afferent
g. efferent
h. deep
i. dorsal
j. medial
k. plantar
l. inferior

III.   Spell Check

Circle each incorrectly spelled term and write it correctly in the space provided.

1. afferant   _____
2. mediel   _____
3. superficial   _____
4. palmar   _____
5. proximel   _____
6. caudel   _____
7. dorsal   _____
8. distel   _____
9. prone   _____
10. soopine   _____

C. Planes of the Body

I.   Matching: Planes of the Body

Match the term to its meaning. (The same meaning may be used more than once.)
Insert the appropriate letter in the space next to the question number

_____ 1. Divides the body into equal right and left portions, and extends from anterior to posterior along the midline
_____ 2. Crosswise cut dividing the body into upper and lower portions

_____ **3.** Divides the body into anterior and posterior halves
_____ **4.** Any vertical cut or slice dividing the body into right and left portions
_____ **5.** Vertical cut next to the midsagittal plane
_____ **6.** Follows longest dimension of a body part
_____ **7.** Slanted cut across the body

Choices:

a. frontal   **e.** sagittal
b. median   **f.** transverse
c. oblique   **g.** longitudinal
d. parasagittal

II.   Spell Check

Circle each incorrectly spelled term and write it correctly in the space provided.

1. coronel   _____
2. frontel   _____
3. parasagittel _____
4. transverse   _____
5. obleque   _____
6. longitudinal _____

III.   Vision Quiz 1: Anatomical Planes (Vertical and Horizontal)

Figure 8-6A shows the vertical and horizontal planes of the human body, sagittal, frontal, and transverse. Complete this portion of this quiz by identifying the different numbered planes.

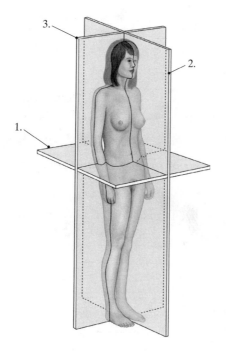

FIGURE 8-6A   Vision Quiz 1. Anatomical Planes (Vertical and Horizontal).

Write your responses in the spaces provided.

    1. _____

    2. _____

    3. _____

IV.   Vision Quiz 2: Anatomical Planes (Other Planes of Reference)

Figures 8-6B through 8-6D show the anatomical planes of the human body. Identify and write the name of the numbered body planes in the spaces provided.

    4. _____   **8.** _____

    5. _____   **9.** _____

    6. _____   **10.** _____

    7. _____   **11.** _____

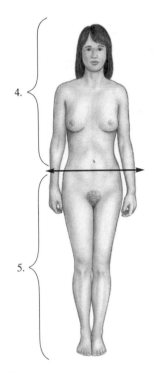

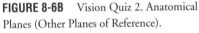

FIGURE 8-6B Vision Quiz 2. Anatomical Planes (Other Planes of Reference).

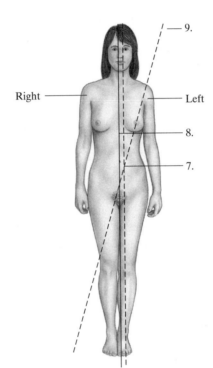

FIGURE 8-6C Vision Quiz 2. Anatomical Planes (Other Planes of Reference).

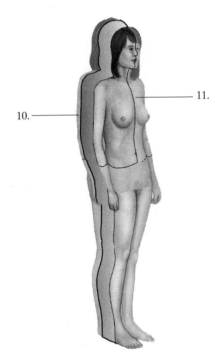

FIGURE 8-6D Vision Quiz 2. Anatomical Planes (Other Planes of Reference).

D. Anatomical Divisions of the Abdominopelvic Region

I.   Spell Check

Circle each incorrectly spelled term and write it correctly in the space provided.

    1. hypochondriak _____

    2. epigastric   _____

    3. abdominull   _____

    4. inquinal   _____

    5. asending   _____

    6. urinary   _____

    7. kolon   _____

    8. apendix   _____

E. Imaging Techniques and Approaches to Diagnosis

I.   Matching: Approaches to Disease and/or Disorder Diagnosis

Match the term to its meaning. (The same meaning may be used more than once.) Insert the appropriate letter in the space provided next to the question number

_____ **1.** The file that contains all information from a patient's medical history, physical examination, and laboratory tests is known as the _____.

_____ **2.** Striking various parts of the body during a physical examination is called _____.

_____ **3.** Feeling or touching specific body parts during a physical examination is called _____.

_____ **4.** Listening to the sounds produced by body organs during a physical examination is known as _____.

_____ **5.** Vital signs include measurements of which body functions? _____

_____ **6. TRP** stands for _____.

_____ **7. BP** stands for _____.

Choices:

a. percussion
b. palpation
c. medical or health record
d. temperature
e. auscultation

f. temperature, pulse or heart rate, respiratory rate, and blood pressure
g. temperature, respiration, pulse
h. blood pressure

II.   Spell Check

Circle each incorrectly spelled term and write it correctly in the space provided.

1. clinical   _____
2. diferenshal   _____
3. resperation   _____
4. cardinel   _____
5. percussion   _____
6. palpeytion   _____
7. auscultation   _____
8. sphygmomanometer _____

F. Increasing Your Medical Terminology Word Power 1

1. Read the following report.
2. Prepare to answer the questions at the end of the section.
3. Circle all unfamiliar terms with a red pencil.
4. Underline familiar terms with a blue pencil.
5. Use your knowledge of word elements, a medical dictionary, and the key terms to find the meaning of unfamiliar terms.

A Medical Emergency—An Unusual Hernia

Key Terms

abrasion (a-BRĀ-zhun)   scraping the surface of the skin

crepitation (krep-i-TĀ-shun)   a crackling sound

hemothorax (hē-mō-THŌ-raks)   bloody fluid in the pleural cavity

hematoma (hē-ma-TŌ-ma)   a mass of blood confined to an organ, tissue, or space

*I*NTRODUCTION

A hernia is an abnormal extension of an organ or a part of an organ through the wall of the body cavity that normally contains it. In other words, a hernia can be seen as a breaking apart of an organ or tissue. Most hernias involving the abdominal wall develop at specific regions of potential weakness. Other types of hernias include those following surgical incisions and those from blunt trauma (injury) to the internal portions of the abdomen or to the abdominal wall itself. The injury in traumatic hernias is caused by a sudden, localized force of moderate intensity that causes the splitting of muscle fibers. Since the skin is relatively elastic, it remains intact. More forceful injury may result in the penetration of the abdomen.

*C*ASE HISTORY

While driving home on a foggy night, a 29-year-old male swerved to avoid a dog and struck a lamppost. The driver was thrown forward, hitting his upper abdomen against the steering wheel. On admission to the emergency room, the patient complained of severe right upper quadrant pain spreading to the back and down the right thigh. Physical examination revealed crepitations at the base of the right lung and tenderness spreading over the right abdomen. A 10 cm oval, obvious swelling in the right upper quadrant with overlying abrasions and large, irregularly shaped hemorrhagic areas of the skin suggested a hematoma. X-ray examination revealed a hemothorax, which was subsequently treated.

Forty-eight hours after admission, the patient's vital signs were stable. Because of the RUQ swelling and complaints of pain, the skin over the hematoma was carefully opened under local anesthesia. A small bowel hernia was observed. The area was closed and repair of the injury was undertaken on the eleventh hospital day. The postoperative course was uneventful and the patient was discharged on the sixteenth hospital day. A follow-up examination four months later showed no evidence of difficulties.

Questions

I.   Fill in the Blank

Fill in the blank with the appropriate term.

   1. The location of the patient's hematoma was _____.
   2. The hemothorax was detected by _____.
   3. When did the patient's vital signs stabilize? _____.

II.   Matching

Match the term to its meaning. (The same meaning may be used more than once.) Insert the appropriate letter in the space next to the question number.

   _____ **1.** Crackling sounds heard on physical examination
   _____ **2.** Blood in the pleural cavity due to blood vessel breakage
   _____ **3.** A mass of blood confined to a tissue or space and caused by vessel breakage

Choices:

   a. hemothorax
   b. hematoma

    c. crepitation

    d. rupture

III.   Spell Check

Circle each incorrectly spelled term and write it correctly in the space provided.

    1. abraseon   _____

    2. crepitation   _____

    3. hemothorex _____

    4. hematoma   _____

    5. hernea   _____

    6. pleurel   _____

    7. quadrant   _____

    8. hemorrhagic _____

G. Increasing Your Medical Terminology Word Power 2

    1. Read the following report.

    2. Prepare to answer the questions at the end of the section.

    3. Circle all unfamiliar terms with a red pencil.

    4. Underline familiar terms with a blue pencil.

    5. Use your knowledge of word elements, a medical dictionary, and the key terms to find the meaning of unfamiliar terms.

Complications in a Severely Burned Patient

Key Terms

apnea (ap-NĒ-a)   temporary stoppage of breathing

arrest (a-REST)   stopping the motion of a part or function

coma (KŌ-ma)   condition of deep unconsciousness; the patient cannot be aroused by an external stimulus

edema (e-DĒ-ma)   local or generalized accumulation of fluid

hyperglycemia (hī'-per-glī-SĒ-mē-a)   increase in the level of blood sugar

hyperkalemic (hī'-per-kā-LĒ-mik)   excess potassium in the blood

hypernatremia (hī'-per-nā-TRĒ-mē-a)   excess sodium in the blood

kg   abbreviation for kilogram; 1,000 grams (gm) or 2.2 pounds

mL   abbreviation for milliliter; equals one-thousandth of a liter.

peritoneal dialysis (per-i-tō-NĒ-al dī-AL-i-sis)   a process that uses the lining of the peritoneal cavity to remove toxic materials and to maintain the normal composition of body fluids

resuscitation (re-sus-i-TĀ-shun)   restoring and maintaining breathing (respiratory movements)

C ASE REPORT

In the early morning of November 12, 1998, a six-month-old female, 9.3 kg infant experienced chemical burns after crawling through a large spill of concentrated laundry bleach. The length of time that the patient's skin was exposed to the bleach was not known. Upon being admitted to a local hospital the burns appeared minor and superficial and were mainly found on the abdominal quadrants.

The burns were rinsed with sterile distilled water, dried carefully, and sprayed with an anesthetic (**an-es-THET-ik**). A freshly prepared paste of sodium bicarbonate (**SŌ-dē-um bī-KAR-bō-nāt**) was then applied to the extent of the chemical burns on the anterior portions of the trunk and certain parts of the face that were also involved. Further examination showed the burns to be both superficial and deep and involving at least 22 percent of the body surface.

Treatment also included the intravenous administration of 5 percent glucose (**GLŪ-cose**) in distilled water to maintain an adequate urinary output. The output later increased to 25 to 30 ml per hour.

About 40 hours after being admitted, the patient experienced seizures and periodic apnea. Because of continuing seizures and other difficulties, the patient was transferred to the County Medical Center at 1:45 P.M. on November 14, 1998. On admission the patient exhibited occasional twitching movements, an elevated body temperature of 40°C, and an elevated breathing rate. At 3:00 P.M. peritoneal dialysis was started to correct both the hypernatremia and edema. At approximately 4:00 A.M. on November 15, during the 13 hours of dialysis, respiratory and circulatory arrest occurred. The patient was resuscitated (**re-SUS-i-tā-ted**) and placed on a mechanical respirator. The dialysis was discontinued, after which the patient slipped into a deep coma. The patient never regained consciousness and was pronounced dead at 10:45 A.M. on November 15, 1998.

Questions

I.   Fill in the Blank

Fill in the blank with the appropriate term.

    1. What was the causative material in the case? _____

    2. Upon being admitted, where were the burns initially found?

        _____

    3. What material was administered to maintain urinary output of the patient? _____

    4. What procedure was used to correct the conditions of hypernatremia and edema? _____

II.   Matching

Match the term to its meaning. (The same meaning may be used more than once.) Insert the appropriate letter in the space next to the question number.

Choices:

_____ **1.** coma		**a.** temporary stoppage of breathing
_____ **2.** hypernatremia		**b.** excess sodium in the blood
_____ **3.** hyperkalemic		**c.** abbreviation for kilogram
_____ **4.** hyperglycemia		**d.** abbreviation for milliliter
_____ **5.** apnea		**e.** localized accumulation of fluid
_____ **6.** edema		**f.** excess potassium in the blood
_____ **7.** kg		**g.** increase in blood sugar level
_____ **8.** ml		**h.** abnormal unconsciousness in a patient

III.   Spell Check

Circle the incorrectly spelled term and write it correctly in the space provided.

    1. koma   _____

    2. apnea   _____

    3. hyperglycemia _____

    4. milliliter   _____

    5. anesthetik   _____

    6. peritoneal   _____

    7. sucros   _____

    8. resusitation   _____

Term Search Challenge

Locate 12 terms in the puzzle.

    1. Write the specific term next to its definition. Then find that term in the puzzle and circle it.

    2. Terms may be read from left to right, backward, up, down, or diagonally.

    3. If it appears more than once, circle it only once. (A term or abbreviation may be found inside others.)

    4. Check your answers.

Clues:

    1. Abbreviation for right upper quadrant of the abdomen _____

    2. Term pertaining to the side _____

    3. Term for lying on the belly _____

    4. Term for lying on the back _____

    5. Abdominal region of the navel _____

    6. Abbreviation for computerized axial tomography _____

    7. Directional term for beneath the surface _____

    8. Directional term for towards the back _____

    9. Directional term for carrying away from an organ _____

    10. Term for near the surface _____ .

    11. Term for plane cutting diagonally across _____

    12. Term for vertical plane that divides the body into right and left portions

    _____

Term Search Puzzle

P	H	Y	P	O	C	H	O	N	D	R	I	A	C	D
O	Y	P	R	O	N	E	P	B	S	T	E	R	I	S
S	P	S	E	U	M	B	I	L	I	C	A	L	O	A
T	O	U	S	P	E	L	S	O	C	I	E	A	R	G
E	G	P	P	L	V	O	U	L	B	C	Q	A	I	I
R	A	E	I	D	O	P	P	A	L	L	U	N	T	T
I	S	R	T	S	L	D	I	T	E	E	I	S	E	T
O	T	F	O	A	L	P	N	E	M	A	A	Q	U	A
R	R	I	R	U	Q	R	E	R	P	R	S	P	U	L
V	I	C	Y	C	L	E	P	A	E	T	T	E	N	E
I	C	I	A	A	U	S	S	L	T	A	I	I	L	I
C	A	A	T	L	P	U	T	Q	U	T	C	O	C	N
A	D	L	E	F	F	E	R	E	N	T	S	R	A	L
L	U	M	D	E	E	P	E	R	E	N	T	A	T	A

An Introduction to Disease

"They can strike anywhere, anytime. On a cruise ship, in the corner restaurant, in the grass just outside the back door. And anyone can be a carrier...."

—Michael D. Lemonick, *Time Magazine*, Sept. 12, 1994

INFORMATIONAL CHALLENGE

A. *Types of Diseases and Causes*

I.   Fill in the Blank

Fill in the blank with the appropriate term.

1. Any disturbance or disruption of a body structure or function is referred to as a(n) _____.

2. List three things a medical model attempts to do: _____, _____, and _____.

3. A disease that can spread from person to person is referred to as _____.

II.   Matching 1: General Terminology

Match the term to its meaning. (The same meaning may be used more than once.) Insert the appropriate letter in the space next to the question number.

Choices:

_____ **1.** etiology	**a.** process associated with a disease's development
_____ **2.** pathology	**b.** cause of a disease
_____ **3.** prognosis	**c.** predicting the outcome of a disease or condition
_____ **4.** pathogenesis	**d.** study of the nature and cause of a disease
_____ **5.** sequelae	**e.** unknown cause of a disease or disorder
_____ **6.** idiopathic	**f.** after-effects

III.   Matching 2: Classification of Diseases According to Causes and Related Factors

Match the term to its meaning. (The same meaning may be used more than once.) Insert the appropriate letter in the space next to the question number.

Choices:

_____ **1.** idiopathic
_____ **2.** immunologic
_____ **3.** congenital
_____ **4.** genetic
_____ **5.** noncommunicable
_____ **6.** nosocomial
_____ **7.** communicable
_____ **8.** heart attack
_____ **9.** malnutrition
_____ **10.** metabolic

a. disease appearing at birth
b. disease having a hereditary basis
c. disease of unknown origin
d. disease resulting from a defect in the immune system
e. hospital-acquired disease
f. disease or condition that cannot be spread from person to person
g. disease that can be spread from person to person
h. disease or disorder caused by a hormonal deficiency
i. disease caused by an insufficient amount of a food component such as minerals or vitamins
j. degenerative disease

IV.   Spell Check

Circle each incorrectly spelled term and write it correctly in the space provided.

1. conjenital   _____
2. ideopathic   _____
3. measles   _____
4. imunity   _____
5. strok   _____
6. infectious   _____
7. iatrogenic   _____
8. nosocomial   _____
9. seguellee   _____
10. sychogenic   _____

B. Features of Epidemiology

I.   Fill in the Blank

Fill in the blank with the appropriate term.

1. The specialist who gathers statistics concerning the prevalence of frequency of disease is a(n) _____.
2. A series of epidemics is a(n) _____.
3. The abbreviation DRG means _____.
4. List the five items needed to assign a specific patient's case to a DRG:

_____, _____, _____,

_____, _____

II.   Matching: Epidemiological Terminology

Match the term to its meaning. (The same meaning may be used more than once.)
Insert the appropriate letter in the space next to the question number.

Choices:

_____ 1. mortality rate
_____ 2. endemic
_____ 3. sporadic
_____ 4. morbidity rate
_____ 5. pandemic
_____ 6. epidemic

a. the number of new cases of a disease per 100,000 in a population or unit of population per year
b. a disease occurring in an irregular pattern
c. a disease constantly present within a population but involving few persons
d. the number of persons that die as a result of a specific disease in a specific time period
e. a sudden increase in the number of cases of a disease
f. a series of epidemics

III.   Spell Check

Circle each incorrectly spelled term and write it correctly in the space provided.

1. statistiks   _____
2. epideemeologist   _____
3. prevalance   _____
4. rubeolla   _____
5. insidence   _____
6. categories   _____

C. The Bacteria: Shapes, Staining Reactions, and Growth Requirements

I.   Fill in the Blank

Fill in the blank with the appropriate term.

1. The study of bacteria is called _____.
2. List the three basic shapes found among bacteria: _____, _____, _____.
3. Preparations used to grow bacteria are known as _____.
4. Two staining procedures used for detection and identification are _____, _____.

II.   Matching 1: Bacterial Morphology and Arrangements

Match the term to its meaning. (The same meaning may be used more than once.) Insert the appropriate letter in the space next to the question number.

Choices:

_____ 1. diplococcus
_____ 2. streptobacillus
_____ 3. staphylococcus
_____ 4. tetrad
_____ 5. streptococcus
_____ 6. spirochete
_____ 7. vibrio
_____ 8. sarcinae

a. grapelike clusters of cocci
b. rods in chains
c. cocci in pairs
d. compressed spiral
e. cocci in a chain
f. boxlike arrangement of four cocci
g. short curved form
h. boxlike arrangement of eight cocci

III.   Matching 2: Oxygen Requirements

Match the term to its meaning. (The same meaning may be used more than once.)
Insert the appropriate letter in the space next to the question number.

Choices:

_____ **1.** grows only in absence of oxygen
_____ **2.** grows only in presence of oxygen
_____ **3.** grows under aerobic or anaerobic
         conditions
_____ **4.** requires less oxygen than found
         in ordinary conditions

a. aerobe
b. microaerophilic
c. anaerobe
d. facultative anaerobe

IV.   Spell Check

Circle each incorrectly spelled term and write it correctly in the space provided.

1. sifilis   _____
2. preon   _____
3. antibiotic   _____
4. cocci   _____
5. spirilum   _____
6. spirochete   _____
7. tetrad   _____
8. tuberkulosis   _____
9. airobe   _____
10. microairophilic _____
11. staflococcus   _____
12. vibreo   _____

V.   Vision Quiz: Morphological Arrangements of Bacteria

Figure 9-14 shows the morphological arrangements found among bacteria. Identify
and write the appropriate terms in the spaces provided.

1. _____   **6.** _____
2. _____   **7.** _____
3. _____   **8.** _____
4. _____   **9.** _____
5. _____   **10.** _____

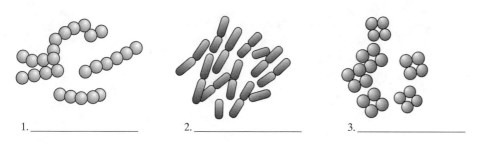

1. _____   2. _____   3. _____

FIGURE 9-14   Vision Quiz. Morphological Arrangements of Bacteria.

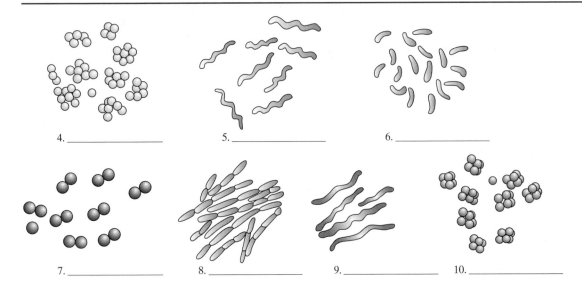

4. _____   5. _____   6. _____

7. _____   8. _____   9. _____   10. _____

FIGURE 9-14   (Continued)

D. Fungi, Protozoa, Viruses, Viroids, and Prions

I.   Fill in the Blank

Fill in the blank with the appropriate term.

1. The study of fungi is called   _____.
2. The study of viruses is called   _____.
3. The study of protozoa is called _____.
4. List two infectious disease agents smaller than a virus: _____ and _____.
5. List three human diseases caused by prions: _____, _____, and _____.

II.   Matching 1: Fungi and Protozoa

Match the term to its meaning. (The same meaning may be used more than once.) Insert the appropriate letter in the space next to the question number.

Choices:

_____ **1.** mycelium
_____ **2.** reproductive unit of a fungus
_____ **3.** yeast
_____ **4.** threadlike filaments of cellular strands
_____ **5.** active feeding stage of protozoa
_____ **6.** reproductive unit of protozoa

a. unicellular fungus
b. hyphae
c. trophozoite
d. fungal colony
e. spore
f. cyst

III. Matching 2: Viruses, Viroids, and Prions

Match the term to its meaning. (The same meaning may be used more than once.)
Insert the appropriate letter in the space next to the question number.

                                    Choices:

_____ **1.** capsid   **a.** individual virus particles
_____ **2.** viroid   **b.** consists of pure protein
_____ **3.** envelope   **c.** protein covering of viral nucleic acid
_____ **4.** virion   **d.** part that covers capsid
_____ **5.** prion   **e.** consists of only nucleic acid

IV. Spell Check/Multiple Choice

Circle each correctly spelled term. The meaning of each term is given as an aid.

1. the structural unit of a mold: hypha, hyfa, hyftha
2. the fungal colony: miselium, micelium, mycelium
3. the study of fungi: micology, mycoleje, mycology
4. whip-like structures used for movement: flagela, flajela, flagella
5. protozoon active feeding stage: tofozoite, trophozoite, tropozoite
6. protozoon reproductive stage: sist, syst, cyst
7. a protozoan gastrointestinal infection: amoebic dysentery, amoebic dizentery, amoebic dysentarry
8. the protein covering of a virus: kapsid, capsid, casid

E. Helminths and Infectious Diseases

I. Fill in the Blank

Fill in the blank with the appropriate term.

1. Two general types of medically important flatworms are _____ and _____.
2. List the three general parts of a tapeworm. _____, _____, and _____.
3. A worm having both male and female reproductive organs is referred to as being _____.
4. The parts of a scolex can include _____ and _____.
5. Another term for a worm's egg is _____.

II. Matching: Helminth Terms

Match the term to its meaning. (The same meaning may be used more than once.)
Insert the appropriate letter in the space next to the question number.

                                    Choices:

_____ **1.** ovum   **a.** tapeworm head
_____ **2.** proglottid   **b.** tapeworm
_____ **3.** cestode   **c.** egg

_____ **4.** scolex	**d.** fluke (a form of flatworm)
_____ **5.** trematode	**e.** roundworm
_____ **6.** nematode	**f.** tapeworm body segment
_____ **7.** suckers and hooklets	

III.   Spell Check

Circle each incorrectly spelled term and write it correctly in the space provided.

1. helminth   _____
2. hermafroditisim _____
3. sestode   _____
4. ova   _____
5. skolex   _____
6. proglotid   _____

F. Disease Transmission

I.   Fill in the Blank

Fill in the blank with the appropriate term.

1. A contaminated inanimate object is called a(n) _____.
2. List three different types of arthropod known to transmit disease agents: _____, _____, and _____.
3. Hospital-acquired infections are called _____.
4. Sources of disease agents in nature are referred to as _____.
5. Two main factors known to help pathogens establish a disease process are _____ and _____.

II.   Spell Check

Circle each incorrectly spelled term and write it correctly in the space provided.

1. formites   _____
2. transmision   _____
3. arthropid   _____
4. resrevoir   _____
5. toksin   _____
6. carrier   _____
7. enzyme   _____
8. nosomial   _____
9. rabies   _____
10. tick   _____

G. Word Elements Used with Microbes and Disease

I.   Matching 1: Word Element Applications

Complete the term with the appropriate word element.

1. His condition worsened because bacteria invaded the circulatory system. Mr. Gen has _bacter_____.

2. Ms. Foss found an amazing cream for her fungus infection. The label indicated it would stop the growth of fungi. In other words it was *fungi*_____.

3. This newly discovered microorganism resembles bacteria. It is a _____*oid*.

4. Bacteria that appear as spherical forms in chains are called _____*cocci*.

5. A pus-forming microbe is referred to as being _____ *genic*.

6. A disease resulting from a poisonous substance represents a _____ *pathic* condition.

7. The new drug was found to be capable of destroying the flu virus. It is *viri*_____ in most situations if used as directed.

Choices:

- **a.** -cidal
- **b.** bacteri-
- **c.** strepto-
- **d.** -emia
- **e.** -static
- **f.** pyo-
- **g.** toxico-

II.   Matching 2: Prefixes and Suffixes Used with Microorganisms and Diseases

Match the term to its meaning. (The same meaning may be used more than once.) Insert the appropriate letter in the space next to the question number.

Choices:

_____ **1.** -cidal	**a.**	pertains to killing
_____ **2.** -iasis	**b.**	blood condition
_____ **3.** -emia	**c.**	spherical
_____ **4.** micro-	**d.**	pertains to stopping
_____ **5.** -static	**e.**	small
_____ **6.** -coccus	**f.**	abnormal condition
_____ **7.** -sis	**g.**	condition or state of

III.   Matching 3: Word Roots and/or Combining Forms Used with Microorganisms and Diseases Part 1

Match the term to its meaning. (The same meaning may be used more than once.) Insert the appropriate letter in the space next to the question number.

Choices:

_____ **1.** tox/o	**a.**	shape
_____ **2.** morph/o	**b.**	infection
_____ **3.** py/o	**c.**	poison
_____ **4.** pyr/o	**d.**	pus
_____ **5.** seps/o	**e.**	fever

IV.   Matching 4: Word Roots and/or Combining Forms Used with Microorganisms and Diseases Part 2

Match the term to its meaning. (The same meaning may be used more than once.) Insert the appropriate letter in the space next to the question number.

		Choices:
_____ **1.** ov/o		**a.** clusters
_____ **2.** myc/o		**b.** fungus
_____ **3.** vir		**c.** worm
_____ **4.** staphyl/o		**d.** egg
_____ **5.** strept/o		**e.** virus
_____ **6.** helmin		**f.** twisted chain
_____ **7.** bi/o		**g.** life

V.   Spell Check

Circle each incorrectly spelled term and write it correctly in the space provided.

1. micrococus   _____
2. bacterisidal   _____
3. stafflocorcus   _____
4. ambiasis   _____
5. bactereemia   _____
6. fungistatic   _____
7. bacterioyd   _____
8. morphology   _____
9. pyrojenic   _____
10. toxicopathy   _____
11. pyogenic   _____
12. mykoid   _____

VI.   Word Analysis: Prefixes, Word Roots, Combining Forms, and Suffixes

Table 9-5 lists a number of terms with their pronunciations and definitions.

TABLE 9-5   WORD ANALYSIS: PREFIXES, WORD ROOTS, COMBINING FORMS, AND SUFFIXES

Term and Pronunciation	Definition
micrococcus (mī-krō-KOK-us)	small spherical cell
bactericidal (bak-ter-i-SĪ-dal)	destructive to or destroying bacteria
staphylococcus (staf-il-ō-KOK-us)	spherical cells in a cluster
bacteremia (bak-ter-Ē-mē-a)	bacteria in the blood
amoebiasis (am-ē-BĪ-a-sis)	an intestinal disease caused by amoeba
bacteriosis (bak-tē-rē-Ō-sis)	any disease caused by bacteria
fungistatic (FUN-ji-stat-ik)	pertaining to stopping the growth of fungi

(Continued)

TABLE 9-5   (CONTINUED)

Term and Pronunciation	Definition
bacterioid (bak-TĒR-ē-oyd)	resembling bacteria
morphology (mor-FOL-ō-jē)	study of shape and structure
mycoid (MĪ-koyd)	fungus-like
pyogenic (pī-ō-JEN-ik)	pus-producing
pyrogenic (pī-rō-JEN-ik)	fever-producing
streptococcus (strep-tō-KOK-us)	spherical cells in a chain
toxicopathy (toks-i-KOP-a-thē)	any disease caused by a poison
toxic (TOKS-ik)	pertaining to or caused by a poison

1. Analyze each term.
2. Circle all combining forms, word roots, prefixes, and suffixes and label them **cf**, **wr**, **p**, and **s**, respectively.
3. Check your answers (shown in Table 9-6).

H. Increasing Your Medical Terminology Word Power 1

1. Read the following report.
2. Prepare to answer the questions at the end of the section.
3. Circle all unfamiliar terms with a red pencil.
4. Underline familiar terms with a blue pencil.
5. Use your knowledge of word elements, a medical dictionary, and the key terms to find the meaning of unfamiliar terms.

Lyme (LĪM) Disease

Key Terms

acrodermatitis (ak-rō-der-ma-TĪ-tis)   inflammation of the skin on the extremities (arms and legs)

arthritis (ar-THRĪ-tis)   inflammation of a joint

erosion (e-RŌ-shun)   eating away of tissue

meningitis (men-in-JĪ-tis)   inflammation of a nerve or nerves

radiculoneuritis (ra-dik-ū-lō-nū-RĪ-tis)   inflammation of spinal nerve roots

spirochete (SPĪ-rō-kēt)   corkscrew-shaped bacterium

tick (tik)   blood-sucking insect having a hard, external surface and segmented body (consisting of several sections)

torticollis (tor-ti'-KOL-is)   stiff neck

Introduction

Approximately 22 years ago, a puzzling and seemingly new multiorgan syndrome identified in Lyme, Connecticut, was put on the medical map as Lyme disease. Since then, early reports of the infectious disease have been traced back to 19th century Europe. Lyme disease has plagued Europeans for nearly one hundred years, but before the U.S. epidemics no one had linked the unrelated range of symptoms to a single cause, namely a spirochete.

L YME (LĪM) DISEASE

Lyme disease is caused b the spirochete *Borrelia burgdorferi* (bor-RĒ-lē-a, berg-DOR-fer-ī) that is spread by the bites of small ticks. The disease-transmitting ticks are so small that their bites are often not noticed. Humans in 45 states as well as Europe, Asia, and Australia have thus far been infected. In 1984, the cases of Lyme disease outnumbered those of Rocky Mountain spotted fever (another bacterial disease), and Lyme became the most common tick-borne disease in the United States.

C LINICAL COURSES

Lyme disease follows three stages: *an acute stage*, *a second stage*, and *a late stage*, in which destructive arthritis, neurologic disease, or *acrodermatitis* may occur. The first stage typically includes a circular rash that can reach several centimeters in diameter as the disease progresses. The rash appears two days to a few weeks after the bite at the site of injury. Joint stiffness, headache, and torticollis also occur in the first stage. In the second stage, meningitis, cranial *neuritis* (nū-RĪ-tis), and radiculoneuritis typically appear. In the third stage, arthritis and neurologic symptoms become chronic.

T REATMENT

Without treatment, the spirochetes multiply and the disease worsens. Approximately 20 percent of untreated victims develop acute neurologic and cardiac symptoms and problems. About one-half experience arthritis, most commonly in the knees. The symptoms of arthritis last for several weeks to months, then lessen somewhat and eventually recur. If Lyme disease is not recognized early, it poses difficulties in diagnosis and treatment. Antibiotics help during all stages of the disease, but are most effective when given early.

P REVENTION

In 1988, a Lyme disease vaccine was approved for use by the Food and Drug Administration (FDA). It appears, however, to be only 70 to 80 percent effective.

Questions

I.   Matching: Lyme Disease Signs, Symptoms, and Related Factors

Match the term to its meaning. (The same meaning may be used more than once.) Insert the appropriate letter in the space next to the question number.

Choices:

_____ **1.** spirochete
_____ **2.** erosion
_____ **3.** arthritis
_____ **4.** neuritis
_____ **5.** radiculoneuritis
_____ **6.** acrodermatitis
_____ **7.** meningitis
_____ **8.** torticollis

a. inflammation of spinal cord membranes
b. stiff neck
c. corkscrew-shaped bacterium
d. inflammation of skin on the legs or arms
e. eating away of tissue
f. spinal nerve root inflammation
g. nerve inflammation
h. joint inflammation

II.   Spell Check

Circle each incorrectly spelled term and write it correctly in the space provided.

1. acrodermatis _____
2. meningidis _____
3. nuritis _____
4. tik _____
5. lime disease _____
6. spirokete _____
7. cardiac _____
8. inflamation _____
9. torticollis _____
10. neurologic _____

I. Increasing Your Medical Terminology Word Power 2

1. Read the following report.
2. Prepare to answer the questions at the end of the section.
3. Circle all unfamiliar terms with a red pencil.
4. Underline familiar terms with a blue pencil.
5. Use your knowledge of word elements, a medical dictionary, and the key terms to find the meaning of unfamiliar terms.

A Case of Eczema Vaccinatum

Key Terms

b.i.d. twice daily

confluent (KON-floo-ent) running together, as in situations when pustules combine

contraindication (kon'-tra-in-di-KĀ-shun) not using a form of treatment that is otherwise considered appropriate for a particular condition

dermatitis (der'-ma-TĪ-tis) skin inflammation

eczema (EK-ze-ma)   skin inflammation accompanied by a variety of eruptions such as blisters, redness, and crusts

eczema vaccinatum (EK-ze-ma VAK-sin-at-um)   cutaneous inflammatory condition with formation of a variety of skin lesions; occurs as a complication of vaccination or because of contact with a recently vaccinated individual

immunoglobulin (im-ū-nō-GLOB-ū-lin)   protective proteins produced by the body's immune system

intermittent (in-ter-MIT-ent)   periodic

prophylactic (prō-feh-LAK-tik)   protective measure

pruritis (proo-RĪ-tus)   severe itching

pustule (PUS-tūl)   small skin blister filled with lymph or pus

smallpox (SMAWL-pox)   contagious, fever-producing viral infection; prevented by immunization with vaccinia (vak-SIN-ē-a)

t.i.d.   three times a day

umbilicated (um-BIL-i-kā-ted)   refers to a central depressed point

vaccinia (vak-SIN-ē-a)   cowpox virus; used to immunize against smallpox

vesicle (VES-i-kl)   small sac or blister filled with fluid

ℬ ACKGROUND

The last documented case of the viral disease smallpox occurred in 1977. The apparent eradication of this disease resulted in the World Health Organization recommendation in May 1980 to stop routine smallpox vaccination. However, because of the potential threat of smallpox being used as a biological warfare weapon, the United States Army continues to vaccinate active-duty soldiers with vaccinia virus after testing for human immunodeficiency virus (HIV) infection. Several contraindications for vaccination exist. These include immunodeficiency, atopic dermatitis, pregnancy, and primary vaccination during acute febrile illness. Some adverse vaccination consequences can also develop.

Overview

Eczema vaccinatum is a potentially fatal complication that occurs in persons with eczema and other forms of dermatitis. The condition usually occurs in children under the age of five years. Typical signs and symptoms of eczema vaccinatum include fever, toxicity (toks-IS-i-tē), and a widespread eruption of vesicular and pustular lesions. At first these lesions are superficial and papular, but they progress to vesicular and finally to pustular forms. Crusting develops by the seventh day of illness, with crust shedding occurring within two weeks. In the majority of cases full recovery occurs and skin lesions heal without scarring. However, death may result when extensive involvement of the internal organs develops or if inflammation of the brain or encephalitis complicates the situation.

𝒞 ASE REPORT

On August 25, 2000, a nineteen-month-old female was taken to the emergency room of a local medical hospital. The patient had a fever of 101°F to 102°F and exhibited a "chickenpox-like rash." The child was referred to the dermatology clinic for a physical examination and laboratory tests.

Physical examination showed multiple early papulovesicular lesions, and in some body areas the lesions progressed to an umbilicated pox stage. Confluent lesions were found in the ears, nape of the neck, mid-abdomen, elbows, and knees. Crusting of the isolated lesions was present, suggesting a secondary bacterial infection.

The patient's treatment included Alpha-Keri baths t.i.d. for her pruritis and antibiotics b.i.d. for the secondary bacterial infection. Laboratory cultures yielded the bacterium *Enterococcus faecalis* (en'-ter-ō-KOK-us fē'-KAL-us), which was found to be sensitive to the antibiotics ampicillin (amp'-i-SIL-in) and gentamicin (jen'-ta-MĪ-sin).

Questions

I.   Matching: Eczema Vaccinatum Signs and Treatment

Match the term to its meaning. (The same meaning may be used more than once.) Insert the appropriate letter in the space next to the question number.

Choices:

_____ **1.** the property of being poisonous	**a.** eczema
_____ **2.** severe itching	**b.** superficial
_____ **3.** having a central depression	**c.** pruritis
_____ **4.** skin inflammation	**d.** pustule
_____ **5.** skin inflammation with eruptions such as blisters	**e.** prophylactic
_____ **6.** confined to the surface	**f.** toxicity
_____ **7.** a protective measure	**g.** dermatitis
_____ **8.** small skin lesion filled with pus	**h.** umbilicated
_____ **9.** t.i.d.	**i.** vesicle
_____ **10.** b.i.d.	**j.** twice daily
_____ **11.** blister filled with fluid	**k.** three times daily
_____ **12.** periodic	**l.** intermittent

II.   Spell Check

Circle each incorrectly spelled term and write it correctly in the space provided.

1. exzema _____
2. papul _____
3. prophylactic _____
4. puritus _____
5. pustule _____
6. vesickle _____
7. umbilicated _____
8. vacinia _____
9. toxicity _____
10. inflammation _____

J. Increasing Your Medical Terminology Word Power 3

1. Read the following report.
2. Prepare to answer the questions at the end of the section.

3. Circle all unfamiliar terms with a red pencil.

4. Underline familiar terms with a blue pencil.

5. Use your knowledge of word elements, a medical dictionary, and the key terms to find the meaning of unfamiliar terms.

Necrotizing Fasciitis

Key Terms

anesthesia (an'-es-THĒ-zē-a)   partial or complete loss of feeling with or without a loss of consciousness

crepitation (krep-i-TĀ-shun)   crackling sound

histology (his-TOL-ō-jē)   microscopic study of tissues

mortality rate   number of deaths per unit of population

necrosis (nē-KRŌ-sis)   dead tissue surrounded by healthy tissue

perirectal (per'-i-REK-tal)   extending around the rectum

postoperative   period following surgery

prognosis (prog-NŌ-sis)   prediction of the outcome of a disease and an estimate of the possibility for recovery

rectum (REK-tum)   lower part of the large intestine

superficial fascia (soo'-per-FISH-al FASH-ē-a)   fibrous covering that supports and separates muscle

tissue (TISH-ū)   group of similar cells that act together in performing a particular function

ulcer (UL-ser)   open sore

Introduction

The disease state of *necrotizing* (NĒ-krō-tī-zing) *fasciitis* (FASH-i-ī-tis) is a relatively rare, rapidly acting, soft-tissue infection. The superficial fascia are primarily involved. The infection often extends to the surrounding tissues and leads to their destruction. The necrotizing process is generally quite rapid and eventually involves the skin. The prognosis of necrotizing fasciitis depends to a large extent on the promptness of an accurate diagnosis and appropriate treatment. Effective treatment mainly consists of surgical *debridement* (dē-brēd-MON) of all necrotic tissue and the administration of antibiotics. Necrotizing fasciitis occurs postoperatively after minor injury or due to inadequate care of perirectal abscesses or skin ulcers.

S TUDY

A review was conducted of 15 cases of necrotizing fasciitis that occurred over a ten-year period. The review involved all medical records, surgical summaries, *biopsy* (BĪ-op-sē) and *autopsy* (AW-top-sē) reports, and histologic slides used for diagnosis. The histologic findings included necrosis of superficial fascia, the presence of microorganisms within the destroyed fascia, and an absence of muscle involvement.

    The patients in the study were compared with respect to age, underlying disease, specific signs and symptoms, antibiotic administration, and supportive care. The presenting signs of several patients were nonspecific and included *edema* (e-DĒ-ma) or tissue swelling, *erythema* (redness), skin necrosis, skin ulcerations, blisters, local loss of feeling (*anesthesia*, an-as-THĒ-zē-a), occasional crepitation from involved areas, and a slight fever. The average age of the patient was 54.1 years with a range from 18 to 83. In the majority of cases, the initiating cause was a minor cut. Diagnosis was based on histologic examination and isolation of several microorganisms associated with skin and related tissue infections. The mortality rate was 45.4 percent.

This study clearly showed that the diagnosis of necrotizing fasciitis early in the development of the disease is difficult. It is also quite obvious from this study that rapid, life-saving surgical debridement of the necrotic tissue requires early recognition and diagnosis of necrotizing fasciitis and its differentiation from other diseases.

Questions

I.   Matching: Necrotizing Fasciitis Signs

Match the term to its meaning. (The same meaning may be used more than once.) Insert the appropriate letter in the space next to the question number.

Choices:

_____	**1.** debridement	**a.** excessive amount of fluid in tissue
_____	**2.** fascia	**b.** connective tissue layer covering muscles
_____	**3.** crepitation	**c.** fascia inflammation
_____	**4.** superficial	**d.** tissue that is dead or dying
_____	**5.** necrotic	**e.** crackling sound
_____	**6.** fasciitis	**f.** surgical removal of dead tissue
_____	**7.** edema	**g.** limited to the surface

II.   Spell Check

Circle each incorrectly spelled term and write it correctly in the space provided.

1. ulser   _____
2. nekrosis   _____
3. crepitation _____
4. progknowsis _____
5. perirectal   _____
6. autopsy   _____

Term Search Challenge

Locate 12 terms in the puzzle.

1. Write the specific term next to its definition. Then find that term in the puzzle diagram and circle it.
2. Terms may be read from left to right, backward, up, down, or diagonally.
3. If a term appears more than once, circle it only once. (A term may be found inside others.)
4. Check your answers.

Clues:

1. The spherical form of bacteria (singular form) _____
2. The abbreviation for diagnosed-related groups (plural) _____
3. The term that refers to predicting the outcome of a disease _____

4. The study of the cause of a disease process _____
5. The process associated with a disease's development _____
6. The study of the nature and cause of disease _____
7. A disease appearing at time of birth _____
8. A disease resulting from procedures administered by health care personnel _____
9. Another term for the body's resistance against disease _____
10. The microscopic forms of life found in the body, *micro-* _____
11. A disease of unknown cause _____
12. The term for a hospital-acquired infection _____

Term Search Puzzle

```
G  E  N  I  T  A  L  N  O  S  I
E  T  I  O  L  C  O  G  Y  O  D
P  R  O  G  N  O  S  I  S  C  I
I  D  G  O  Z  C  P  A  T  O  O
S  I  S  E  G  C  O  T  H  M  P
B  I  O  T  A  U  L  R  M  I  A
D  I  D  R  G  S  T  O  O  A  T
P  A  T  H  O  L  O  G  Y  L  H
F  G  I  G  E  N  E  S  I  S  I
E  T  I  O  L  O  G  Y  P  Q  C
I  M  M  U  N  I  T  Y  Y  G  T
```

Oncogenesis and Cancers

"But some say that cancer is so called because it adheres to any parts which it seizes upon in an obstinate manner like the crab."

—Paul of Aegina on Medicine (7th Century)

INFORMATIONAL CHALLENGE

A. Normal and Cancerous Processes and Classification of Cancers

I.　Fill in the Blank

Fill in the blank with the appropriate term.

1. The development or formation of tumors is referred to as onco-_____.

2. The medical specialty concerned with tumors is called onco-_____.

3. The three broadly recognized groups of cancers are _____, _____, and _____.

4. Neoplasms of lymphoid tissue are called _____.

5. The group of cancers originating in leukocytes is referred to as _____.

6. Tumors of pigment-producing cells are called _____.

7. A benign, pigmented skin lesion is known as a(n) _____.

8. The combining form *adeno* refers to a(n) _____.

9. A tissue-invasive and destructive tumor would be an example of a(n) _____ tumor.

II.　Matching: Tumor Types

Match the term to its meaning. (The same meaning may be used more than once.) Insert the appropriate letter in the space next to the question number.

Choices:

_____ 1. melanoma
_____ 2. teratoma
_____ 3. lymphoma
_____ 4. nevus
_____ 5. retinoblastoma
_____ 6. benign tumor

a. lymphoid tissue neoplasm
b. mixed tissue tumor
c. associated with pigment-producing cell
d. Hodgkin's disease
e. embryonic tumor
f. noninvasive tumor

III.   Spell Check

Circle each incorrectly spelled term and write it correctly in the space provided.

1. oncogenesis   _____
2. leukemia   _____
3. benine   _____
4. nephroblastoma   _____
5. kneeoplasm   _____
6. differentiation _____
7. myosarcoma   _____
8. Hogdkin's   _____

B. Word Elements Used in Association with Neoplasms

I.   Matching 1: Combining Forms Used in Association with Neoplasms

Match the term to its meaning. (The same meaning may be used more than once.) Insert the appropriate letter in the space next to the question number.

Choices:

_____ 1. radi/o   a. tumor
_____ 2. onc/o   b. cancerous
_____ 3. scirrh/o   c. chemical
_____ 4. chem/o   d. rays
_____ 5. tox/o   e. small growths
_____ 6. aden/o   f. hard
_____ 7. carcin/o   g. cold
_____ 8. cry/o   h. poison
_____ 9. polyp/o   i. gland

II.   Matching 2: Combining Forms, Suffixes, and Prefixes Used in Association with Neoplasms

Match the term to its meaning. (The same meaning may be used more than once.) Insert the appropriate letter in the space next to the question number.

Choices:

_____ 1. -plasia   a. lymph
_____ 2. papill/o   b. formation
_____ 3. ple/o   c. many
_____ 4. cyst/o   d. nipple-like
_____ 5. lymph/o   e. closed sac
_____ 6. blast/o   f. immature
_____ 7. neo-   g. new
_____ 8. -plasm   h. middle
_____ 9. medull/o

III. Spell Check

Circle each incorrectly spelled term and write it correctly in the space provided.

1. anaplasia   _____
2. chemotherapey   _____
3. sistosarcoma   _____
4. dysplasia   _____
5. mutajen   _____
6. adeknowma   _____
7. radiotaxemia   _____
8. carcinolysis   _____

IV. Word Analysis: Combining Forms and Word Roots

Table 10-11 lists a number of terms with their pronunciations and definitions.

TABLE 10-11 WORD ANALYSIS: COMBINING FORMS AND WORD ROOTS

Term and Pronunciation	Brief Description
anaplasia (an-a-PLĀ-zē-a)	loss of typical cellular structure and function (reverting to a more primitive cell type)
metaplasia (met-a-PLĀ-zē-a)	a reversible process in which one type of specialized cell is substituted for another resulting in a change in formation or development
neopathy (nē-OP-a-thē)	a new disease
cystosarcoma (sis-tō-sar-KŌ-ma)	connective tissue tumor containing cysts
dysplasia (dis-PLĀ-zē-a)	abnormal development of tissue
neoplasm (NĒ-ō-plaz-em)	new (generally abnormal) tissue formation
adenoma (ad-e-NŌ-ma)	a gland tumor
blastoma (blas-TŌ-ma)	a tumor or neoplasm consisting of immature cells
carcinolysis (kar'-si-NOL-i-sis)	destruction of cancer cells
chemotherapy (kē'-mō-THER-a-pē)	chemical treatment
cryogenic (KRĪ-ō-jen'-ik)	pertains to a substance that produces low temperatures
cystoid (SIS-toyd)	resembling a closed sac

(Continued)

TABLE 10-11   (CONTINUED)

Term and Pronunciation	Brief Description
medullary (MED-ū-lar'-ē)	pertaining to the middle or inner portion
mutagen (MŪ-ta-jen)	any agent that causes permanent genetic changes
oncologist (ong-KOL-ō-jist)	tumor specialist
papillary (PAP-i-lar-ē)	nipple-like
pleomorphic (plē-ō-MOR-fik)	having many forms
polypectomy (pol-i-PEK-tō-mē)	surgical removal of small growths
radiotoxemia (rā'-dē-ō-tok-SĒ-mē-a)	blood poisoning effect produced by x-ray exposure
scirrhoma (skir-Ō-ma)	a hard (cancerous) tumor
teratoid (TER-a-toyd)	resembling a malformed fetus or monster
toxic (TOKS-ik)	pertaining to a poisonous condition or state

1. Analyze each term.
2. Circle all combining forms, word roots, prefixes, and suffixes and label them **cf**, **wr**, **p**, and **s**, respectively.
3. Check your answers (shown in Table 10-12).

C. Staging and Grading Systems and Pathological Descriptive Terminology

I.   Fill in the Blank

Fill in the blank with the appropriate term.

1. Give the meaning of TNM in this type of staging system: T = _____, N = _____, and M = _____.
2. Give the designation in the TNM staging system used to indicate a *carcinoma in situ*: _____
3. What is the basis of staging in the TNM system? _____
4. What is the purpose of the Papanicolaou smear? _____
5. The basic document used to record information pertinent to cancers by a tumor registry is called a(n) _____.
6. List the three general types of tumor registries: _____, _____, and _____.

II.   Matching 1: Pathological Terms for Gross Features of Tumors

Match the term to its meaning. (The same meaning may be used more than once.) Insert the appropriate letter in the space next to the question number.

Choices:

_____ 1. fungating
_____ 2. polypoid
_____ 3. multicentric
_____ 4. verrucous
_____ 5. sessile
_____ 6. encapsulated

a. occurring at several sites in the same type of tissue
b. wartlike growth
c. having no stem
d. a growth pattern similar to a fungus
e. contained in a covering
f. tumor with a stem

III.   Matching 2: Pathological Terms for Microscopic Features of Tumors

Match the term to its meaning. (The same meaning may be used more than once.)
Insert the appropriate letter in the space next to the question number

Choices:

_____ 1. *carcinoma in situ*
_____ 2. infiltrative
_____ 3. mucinous
_____ 4. undifferentiated
_____ 5. hyperplasia
_____ 6. dysplasia
_____ 7. nodular
_____ 8. *in vivo*

a. abnormal development of tissue
b. excessive production of normal cells in an organ
c. containing mucus
d. pertains to tightly packed small cell clusters
e. in a living system
f. loss of cellular specialization
g. confined to one site
h. extending beyond normal tissue borders

IV.   Spell Check

Circle each incorrectly spelled term and write it correctly in the space provided.

1. inflamatory   _____
2. enkapsulaed   _____
3. scirhouis   _____
4. necrotic   _____
5. papilloma   _____
6. alveolar   _____
7. verrucous   _____
8. disseminated   _____

D. Carcinogens, Carcinogenesis, and Cancer Treatment and Detection

I.   Fill in the Blank

Fill in the blank with the appropriate term.

1. The development of a cancerous process is called _____.
2. Tissues that are stimulated to increase their number are said to have undergone _____-plasia.
3. A chemical initiating a cancerous process is referred to as a(n) _____.
4. The process that changes normal cells into malignant ones is called _____.

5. Substances known for their ability to bring about permanent genetic changes are called _____.

6. The use of chemicals in the treatment of disease is called

_____.

II.   Matching 1: General Terminology

Match the term to its meaning. (The same meaning may be used more than once.) Insert the appropriate letter in the space next to the question number.

Choices:

_____ **1.** immunotherapy
_____ **2.** tumorostatic
_____ **3.** tumoricidal
_____ **4.** mutation
_____ **5.** tumorigenesis
_____ **6.** chemicals, radiation, viruses
_____ **7.** rapid growth, production of fetal proteins, reversion to immature cells, and failure to differentiate

a. known cancer-producing agents
b. properties of cells that undergo malignant transformation
c. permanent genetic change
d. chemical that kills tumor cells
e. form of treatment that stimulates the immune system to react to a cancerous process
f. chemical agent that stops tumor growth
g. term for tumor production

III.   Matching 2: General Approaches to Cancer Treatment

Match the term to its meaning. (The same meaning may be used more than once.) Insert the appropriate letter in the space next to the question number.

Choices:

_____ **1.** irradiation
_____ **2.** radiosensitizers
_____ **3.** modality
_____ **4.** used in immunotherapy
_____ **5.** ionizing radiation
_____ **6.** lymphocyte-activated killer cells

a. method
b. drugs that increase tumor sensitivity to x-rays
c. therapeutic application of x-rays
d. bacillus of Calmette and Guérin
e. white blood cells activated by interleukin-2
f. energy given off by radioactive atoms and x-rays

IV.   Matching 3: Laboratory Test and Clinical Procedures Used in Cancer Detection

Match the term to its meaning. (The same meaning may be used more than once.) Insert the appropriate letter in the space next to the question number.

Choices:

_____ **1.** carcinoembryonic antigen test
_____ **2.** estrogen receptor assay
_____ **3.** human chorionic gonadotropin test

a. measures specific hormone receptor sites
b. measures enzyme levels related to liver injury
c. test for cervical cancer

_____ **4.** glutamic-pyruvic transaminase test

_____ **5.** Pap smear

_____ **6.** scans

_____ **7.** prostate-specific antigen test or assay

d. tumor-associated blood test for gastrointestinal cancer

e. test for testicular cancer

f. test for prostate cancer

V.   Matching 4: Surgical Procedures Used in Cancer Therapy and Detection

Match the term to its meaning. (The same meaning may be used more than once.) Insert the appropriate letter in the space next to the question number.

Choices:

_____ **1.** aspiration

_____ **2.** electrocoagulation

_____ **3.** enucleation

_____ **4.** laparotomy

_____ **5.** cryosurgery

_____ **6.** peritoneoscopy

_____ **7.** microscopically controlled surgery

_____ **8.** resection

_____ **9.** needle biopsy

a. procedure to remove an entire mass

b. use of cold to destroy tissue

c. suction procedure

d. use of high-frequency electric current to clot tissue

e. procedure used to examine peritoneal cavity

f. microscopic procedure to precisely determine entire margin of cancer

g. procedure for partial excision of body structures

h. use of a special needle and suction to remove specimens for cytological examination

VI.   Matching 5: Features of Chemotherapeutic Agents

Match the term to its meaning. (The same meaning may be used more than once.) Insert the appropriate letter in the space next to the question number.

_____ **1.** steroid hormones

_____ **2.** alkylating agents

_____ **3.** antimetabolites

_____ **4.** antibiotics

_____ **5.** alkaloids

Choices:

a. primarily prevents normal DNA formation

b. slows tumor growths and interrupts formation of selected hormones

c. chemicals that resemble those required by cells for normal functioning

d. drugs that interfere with protein, DNA, or RNA formation in infectious diseases

e. chemicals derived from plants and used in combination with other chemotherapeutic agents

VII.   Spell Check

Circle each incorrectly spelled term and write it correctly in the space provided.

1. carcinojenesis   _____

2. radiocurable   _____

3. excavation   _____

4. enuclaetion _____

5. criosurgery _____

6. peretoneoscopy _____

7. alkaling _____

8. sturoid _____

E. Medical Vocabulary Building

I.   Matching

Match the term to its meaning. (The same meaning may be used more than once.)
Insert the appropriate letter in the space next to the question number.

_____ **1.** glioblastoma

_____ **2.** immunotherapy

_____ **3.** medulloblastoma

_____ **4.** mucositis

_____ **5.** rhabdomyosarcoma

_____ **6.** thymoma

_____ **7.** dedifferentiation

_____ **8.** exacerbation

_____ **9.** immunosuppression

_____ **10.** violaceous

Choices:

a. treatment of disease with immunological materials

b. malignant tumor of the brain, usually of the cerebral hemispheres

c. oral mucosa inflammation, usually caused by radiation exposure

d. malignant tumor of the fourth ventricle and cerebellum

e. thymus gland tumor

f. malignant tumor originating in striated muscle tissue

g. process whereby normal cells lose their specialization and turn malignant

h. having a violet color

i. process of preventing immune responses

j. increasing the severity of disease signs and symptoms

II.   Spell Check

Circle each incorrectly spelled term and write it correctly in the space provided.

1. immunosupresion _____

2. gloiblastoma _____

3. mucocitis _____

4. exaserbation _____

5. medulloblastoma _____

6. rhabdomyosarcoma _____

F. Abbreviations

I.   Matching 1: Abbreviations Associated with Neoplasms and Related Conditions

Match the term to its meaning. (The same meaning may be used more than once.)
Insert the appropriate letter in the space next to the question number.

Choices:

_____ **1.** DNA   **a.** *carcinoma in situ*
_____ **2.** bx   **b.** alpha-fetoprotein
_____ **3.** chem.   **c.** American Cancer Society
_____ **4.** DFI   **d.** biopsy
_____ **5.** ACS   **e.** deoxyribonucleic acid
_____ **6.** CIS   **f.** excision
_____ **7.** AFP   **g.** chemotherapy
_____ **8.** ER   **h.** estrogen receptor
_____ **9.** st   **i.** disease-free interval
_____ **10.** exc.   **j.** stage

II.   Matching 2: Abbreviations Associated with Neoplasms and Related Conditions

Match the term to its meaning. (The same meaning may be used more than once.) Insert the appropriate letter in the space next to the question number.

Choices:

_____ **1.** TNM   **a.** Papanicolaou's test
_____ **2.** NERD   **b.** no evidence of recurrence
_____ **3.** RAtx   **c.** protocol
_____ **4.** NER   **d.** metastases
_____ **5.** Pap smear   **e.** tumor, node, metastases
_____ **6.** Ga   **f.** gallium
_____ **7.** prot.   **g.** radiation therapy
_____ **8.** TAA   **h.** no evidence of recurrent disease
_____ **9.** NPDL   **i.** tumor-associated antigen
_____ **10.** mets   **j.** nodular, poorly differentiated lymphocytes

G. *Increasing Your Medical Terminology Word Power 1*

1. Read the following report.
2. Prepare to answer the questions at the end of the section.
3. Circle all unfamiliar terms with a red pencil.
4. Underline all familiar terms with a blue pencil.
5. Use your knowledge of word elements, a medical dictionary, and the key terms to find the meaning of unfamiliar terms.

Ovarian Squamous Cell Carcinoma Derived from a Dermoid Cyst

Key Terms

chemotherapy (kē'-mō-THER-a-pē)   the use of chemicals in the treatment of disease

cm (centimeter)   one-hundredth of a meter

histological (his'-tō-LOG-i-kal)   microscopic study of tissues

hysterectomy (his-ter-EK-tō-mē)   surgical removal of the uterus through the abdominal wall or vagina (va-JĪ-na)

laparotomy (lap-ar-OT-ō-mē)   surgical opening of the abdomen

ovarian (ō-VA-rē-an)   pertaining to the ovary

regimen (REJ-i-men)   a systemic plan of activities and regulations designed to improve or keep a certain condition under control

salpingo-oophorectomy (sal-ping'-gō-ō'-ōf-ō-REK-tō-mē)   surgical removal of an ovary and fallopian (fa-LŌ-pē-an) tube

toxicity (toks-IS-i-tē)   the property of being poisonous

vaginectomy (vaj-in-EK-tō-mē)   surgical removal of the vagina or a portion of it

Introduction

A 30-year-old female was admitted to the Cancer Center for an evaluation of a pelvic mass and a vaginal tumor, which upon histological examination revealed the presence of a squamous cell carcinoma. The clinical viewpoint at this time was that the condition was unusual for a vaginal carcinoma and that the abdominal mass could be a second primary ovarian carcinoma.

C ASE REPORT

Physical examination of the patient revealed a 10 × 10 × 10 cm firm mass extending to the right pelvic sidewall. Results of a laparotomy showed the presence of a 10 × 10 cm multinodular mass extending from the right ovary. Following this finding, a total abdominal *hysterectomy* with bilateral salpingo-oophorectomy and a partial *vaginectomy* were performed.

Histological study of the excised tissue showed a squamous cell carcinoma of the ovary developing in an initially benign teratoma and a metastasis to the vagina. The patient's postoperative course was uneventful, and she was started on her first course of chemotherapy. The patient received a specified five-course drug regimen at three-week intervals. Aside from the expected nausea and vomiting, no other indications of toxicity were noted.

Approximately six months after the operation, a chest x-ray confirmed the presence of multiple metastatic lesions in the lungs. Because of the obvious severe progression of the disease, the patient was given external irradiation therapy in addition to the previously administered chemotherapeutic regimen. Computerized tomography also revealed the presence of a pelvic mass. It was hoped that the radiation treatment would benefit the patient. Unfortunately, little change was noted in the dimensions of the pelvic mass as assessed by further computerized tomography.

Questions

I.   Fill in the Blank

Fill in the blank with the appropriate term.

1. What did the laparotomy show? _____

2. Following the results of the laparotomy what three specific operations were performed on the patient? _____,
_____, and _____

3. What were the findings of the chest x-ray six months after the laparotomy? _____

_____

4. What treatments were given to the patient? _____

_____

II.   Matching

Match the term to its meaning. (The same meaning may be used more than once.) Insert the appropriate letter in the space next to the question number.

Choices:

_____ **1.** excision
_____ **2.** vaginectomy
_____ **3.** laparotomy
_____ **4.** multinodular
_____ **5.** toxicity
_____ **6.** hysterectomy
_____ **7.** teratoma
_____ **8.** carcinoma

a. surgical opening of the abdomen
b. surgical removal
c. being poisonous
d. excision of the vagina
e. having many nodules
f. embryonically related tumor
g. surgical removal of the uterus
h. malignant tumor in epithelial tissue

III.   Spell Check

Circle each incorrectly spelled term and write it correctly in the space provided.

1. pelvic   _____
2. sqamous   _____
3. multinodular   _____
4. metastatic   _____
5. bylateral   _____
6. fallopaen   _____
7. ovarien   _____
8. vajinectomy   _____
9. laparotomy   _____
10. toxicity   _____

H. Increasing Your Medical Terminology Word Power 2

1. Read the following report.
2. Prepare to answer the questions at the end of the section.
3. **Circle** all unfamiliar terms with a red pencil.
4. **Underline** familiar terms with a blue pencil.
5. Use your knowledge of word elements, a medical dictionary, and the key terms to find the meaning of unfamiliar terms.

Renal-Cell Carcinoma Extension into the Inferior Vena Cava and Right Atrium

Key Terms

angiography (an'-jē-OG-ra-fē)   procedure to obtain an x-ray of blood vessels after ingestion of radiopaque substance

atrium (Ā-trē-um)   a chamber (here the reference is to the heart chamber)

cm   one-hundredth of a meter

diabetes mellitus (dī'-a-BĒ-tēz, mel-i-TUS)   a carbohydrate metabolism disorder; type I is insulin dependent, and type II is non-insulin-dependent

diastole (dī-AS-tō-lē)   normal period in heart cycle during which the heart dilates and the cavities (chambers) of the heart fill with the blood

dyspnea (disp-NĒ-a)   labored breathing

echocardiography (ek'-ō-kar'-dē-OG-ra-fē)   using ultrasound to see internal heart structures

inferior vena cava (VĒ-na CĀ-va)   main vein draining the lower portion of the body

nephrectomy (neh-FREK-tō-mē)   surgical removal of a kidney

prolapse (prō-LAPS)   a falling or dropping down of an organ or internal body structure

pulmonic (pul-MON-ik)   pertaining to the lungs

regurgitation (rē-gur'-ji-TĀ-shun)   a backward flowing

renal (RĒ-nal)   pertaining to the kidney

transesophageal (trans'-ē-sof'-a-JĒ-al)   across the esophagus

transthoracic (trans'-thō-RAS-ik)   across the thorax

ventricle (VEN-tri-kl)   a lower heart chamber

C ASE HISTORY

An obese 80-year-old female with a history of hypertension and type II diabetes mellitus experienced dyspnea on the climbing of stairs in her home. The patient also had an obvious swelling of her legs for two to three months earlier.

C LINICAL FINDINGS

Transthoracic echocardiography revealed a right atrial mass with an obvious extension into the inferior vena cava. Further follow-up with computerized tomography of the patient's chest and abdomen showed that this mass originated in the left kidney. The results of coronary angiography and bone scanning were normal.

A radical left nephrectomy and excision of the right atrial mass were performed. Interoperative transesophageal echocardiography revealed a mass in the right atrium that prolapsed into the right ventricle during diastole. In addition moderate regurgitation, and a normal aorta and pulmonary artery were noted.

P ATHOLOGY

The excised mass was a renal cell carcinoma measuring 15 cm × 4 cm × 3 cm. The patient tolerated the surgical procedure well and was discharged from the hospital on the twelfth postoperative day.

Questions

I.   Fill in the Blank

Fill in the blank with the appropriate term.

  1. The transthoracic echocardiography revealed a right atrial mass. To what part of the circulatory system did the mass extend?

2. What were the findings obtained with the computerized tomography?

_____

_____

3. In what part of the body did the mass in question #1 originate?

_____

4. Were the aorta and pulmonary artery found to be normal?

_____

II.   Matching

Match the term to its meaning. (The same meaning may be used more than once.)
Insert the appropriate letter in the space next to the question number.

Choices:

_____ **1.** angiography
_____ **2.** dyspnea
_____ **3.** nephrectomy
_____ **4.** prolapse
_____ **5.** regurgitation
_____ **6.** ventricle
_____ **7.** echocardiography

a. labored breathing
b. x-ray procedure to view the body's blood vessels
c. a falling or dropping down of a body organ or part
d. removal of a kidney
e. backward flowing
f. chamber of the heart
g. using ultrasound to see heart structure

III.   Spell Check

Circle each incorrectly spelled term and write it correctly in the space provided.

1. angeogaphy   _____
2. ekocardiography _____
3. transthoracik   _____
4. regurgitatoin   _____
5. diastole   _____
6. nephrectomy   _____
7. prolapse   _____
8. transesophageal _____

I. Increasing Your Medical Terminology Word Power 3

1. Read the following report.
2. Prepare to answer the questions at the end of the section.
3. **Circle** all unfamiliar terms with a red pencil.
4. **Underline** familiar terms with a blue pencil.
5. Use your knowledge of word elements, a medical dictionary, and the key terms to find the meaning of unfamiliar terms.

Pulmonary Artery Sarcoma

Key Terms

angiography (an'-jē-OG-ra-fē)   refers to an x-ray of blood vessels and lymphatics

dyspnea (disp-NĒ-a)   labored breathing

effusion (e-FŪ-shyn)   escape of fluid into a body part, such as the pleural cavity

heparin (HEP-a-rin)   a clot-preventing (anti-coagulant) chemical

infarct (in-FARKT)   tissue or organ that undergoes destruction following a stoppage of its blood supply

intraluminal (in'-tra-LŪ-mi-nal)   within any tubular structure

pleuritic (ploo-RIT-ik)   related to inflammation of pleura (membranes that enfold both lungs)

pneumonectomy (nū'-mon-EK-tō-mē)   removal of a lung

polypoid (POL-i-poyd)   like a polyp (a tumor with a pedicle)

proximal (PROK-sim-al)   nearest to the point of attachment, center of the body, or point of reference

resection (rē-SEK-shun)   partial excision of a body structure

subscapular (sub-SKAP-ū-lar)   below the scapula (shoulder blade)

thoracic (thō-RAS-ik)   pertains to the chest

thoracotomy (thō'-rak-OT-ō-mē)   surgical excision of the chest wall

warfarin (WAR-fer-in)   a drug used to prevent blood clotting (coagulation)

C ASE HISTORY

A 71-year-old female was admitted to the medical center with a preliminary diagnosis of pulmonary arterial obstruction. The patient had been in relatively good health until approximately two months before admission, when an intermittent, nonproductive cough developed. Ten days prior to admission, she experienced left-sided subscapular pain after vacuuming her apartment. That evening the pain spread to the area just below her left breast. The next morning, the patient experienced an episode of sudden, severe pleuritic pain in the same area, accompanied by dizziness and sweating. Dyspnea or a loss of consciousness did not occur. The patient went to another medical facility, where she was told that her electrocardiogram was normal, but a chest radiograph showed a small, left-sided pleural effusion. She was given appropriate medications and discharged.

   The next day, the patient again felt left-sided pleuritic pain, this time with dyspnea and extreme weakness. She returned to the same medical facility, where she was admitted to the intensive care unit and given oxygen, heparin, and warfarin. Her symptoms improved markedly. A pulmonary angiographic examination revealed an intraluminal mass blocking the left pulmonary artery and involving the main and proximal right pulmonary arteries.

   During the next four days, the patient had a recurrence of her intermittent, nonproductive cough. On the eighth day, she was transferred to this center, where a thoracotomy was performed. In the resection, the proximal portion of the main pulmonary artery was opened and the incision was extended into the right pulmonary artery. A left pneumonectomy was performed during the procedure.

P ATHOLOGY

Pathological examination of the resected specimen taken during the thoracotomy showed a firm, jelly-like, polypoid mass measuring 9 cm in length and 3 cm in diameter. This mass was found within the pulmonary artery and apparently caused a significant narrowing of the vessel. A firm, hemorrhagic pulmonary infarct measuring 7.0 cm in length and 1.5 cm in diameter was also uncovered in the lower left lobe.

The patient was discharged five days later in good condition. Unfortunately, follow-up radiologic studies during the next seven months showed the development of several new pulmonary nodules. Chemotherapy was initiated, but proved to be unsuccessful. The patient's health took a turn for the worse, and she died three weeks later.

Questions

I.   Fill in the Blank

Fill in the blank with the appropriate term.

1. Where was the patient's pain? _____
2. At the second health care facility, what was given to the patient to relieve her discomfort? _____
3. What parts of the body did the intraluminal mass block? _____
4. What were the pathological findings obtained with the patient's resected specimen? _____

II.   Matching

Match the term to its meaning. (The same meaning may be used more than once.) Insert the appropriate letter in the space next to the question number.

Choices:

_____ 1. effusion	**a.** a clot-preventing chemical
_____ 2. heparin	**b.** escape of fluid into a body part
_____ 3. infarct	**c.** within any tubular structure
_____ 4. intraluminal	**d.** a tissue area that undergoes destruction following the stoppage of its blood supply
_____ 5. pneumonectomy	
_____ 6. polypoid	
_____ 7. resection	**e.** removal of a lung
_____ 8. subscapular	**f.** partial excision of a body structure
_____ 9. thoracic	**g.** below the shoulder blade
_____ 10. thoracotomy	**h.** pertains to the chest
	i. surgical excision of the chest wall
	j. tumor with no stem

III.   Spell Check

Circle each incorrectly spelled term and write it correctly in the space provided.

1. effusion   _____
2. dyspnea   _____
3. pluritic   _____
4. thorakotomy   _____
5. subsapular   _____
6. proximal   _____
7. pneumonectomy _____
8. infarkt   _____

Term Search Challenge

Locate 16 terms in the puzzle.

1. Write the specific term next to its definition. Then find that term in the puzzle diagram and circle it.
2. Terms may be read from left to right, backward, up, down, or diagonally.
3. If a term appears more than once, circle it only once. (A term may be found inside others.)
4. Check your answers.

Clues:

1. abbreviation for biopsy _____
2. term for new growth _____
3. abbreviation for cancer _____
4. combining form for cancerous _____
5. the study of drugs and their actions _____
6. terms for written plan _____
7. method _____
8. life-threatening tumor _____
9. suffix for growth or tumor _____
10. term for localized tumor cells that have not invaded neighboring structures _____
11. short version of Papanicolaou _____
12. abbreviation for deoxyribonucleic acid _____
13. use of extreme cold for surgery _____
14. tumor of leukocytes _____
15. spreading process of cancer _____
16. malignant tumor of muscle _____

Term Search Puzzle

B	X	O	S	A	R	D	O	M	A	O	D	A	L	M	P
E	C	A	T	L	M	N	N	N	E	G	P	L	L	L	R
M	I	C	L	D	A	A	I	I	N	S	I	T	U	D	O
O	L	E	U	K	E	M	I	A	L	D	E	X	M	A	T
O	M	Y	C	O	S	A	R	C	O	M	A	D	N	R	O
M	M	E	T	A	S	T	A	S	I	S	T	I	O	I	C
P	H	A	R	M	A	C	O	L	O	G	Y	A	T	T	O
O	N	E	O	P	L	A	S	M	M	L	T	G	Y	O	L
M	A	L	I	G	N	A	N	T	Y	U	T	S	D	T	P
A	C	R	Y	O	S	U	R	G	E	R	Y	T	M	N	A
R	G	P	S	R	D	R	S	T	A	N	I	T	Y	T	P
Y	A	L	C	O	N	O	C	O	G	E	N	E	N	I	P
O	L	E	O	G	N	N	A	D	A	R	G	O	G	L	C
C	A	R	C	I	N	O	M	O	D	A	L	I	T	Y	A

The Integumentary System

By a jungle river an alligator sleeps and sleeps, can risk it because besides the built-in defenses that all of us have it has that other barricade . . . . Humans have this outer barricade too, the skin, gentle, soft, yet doing rough work . . . . Skin is a defense against assault of many kinds . . . .

—Gustav Eckstein, *The Body Has a Head*

INFORMATIONAL CHALLENGE

A. Structure and Functions of the Skin

I.   Fill in the Blank

Fill in the blank with the appropriate term.

1. What is the tough, protective protein associated with the skin? _____.

2. List in order, beginning at the surface, the layers of the epidermis: _____, _____, _____, _____, and _____.

3. Sebaceous glands secrete _____.

4. The three types of glands found in the skin are _____, _____, and _____.

5. The pigment found in melanocytes is _____.

II.   Matching 1: Epidermis Layers (Strata)

Match the term to its meaning. (The same meaning may be used more than once.) Insert the appropriate letter in the space next to the question number.

_____ **1.** outermost layer
_____ **2.** new cell growth
_____ **3.** contains large amounts of keratin
_____ **4.** layer containing corneocytes
_____ **5.** a thin layer found only in the palms and soles
_____ **6.** cells tightly attached to one another by spinelike processes
_____ **7.** contains melanocytes

Choices:

a. stratum corneum
b. stratum lucidum

    c. stratum granulosum

    d. stratum spinosum

    e. stratum germinativum

III.   Matching 2: Skin Functions

Match the term to its meaning. (The same meaning may be used more than once.) Insert the appropriate letter in the space next to the question number.

Choices:

_____ **1.** protects against sun damage

_____ **2.** sensitive to pressure

_____ **3.** sensitive to touch

_____ **4.** binds epidermis to underlying tissue

_____ **5.** protects against certain chemicals, physical factors, and microbes

a. subcutaneous layer

b. melanin

c. Pacinian corpuscle

d. Meissner's corpuscle

e. keratin

IV.   Spell Check

Circle each incorrectly spelled term and write it correctly in the space provided.

1. strata   _____

2. stratim   _____

3. keretin   _____

4. germinativum   _____

5. basel   _____

6. melanin   _____

7. albinism   _____

8. sudoriferous   _____

9. spinosum   _____

10. granuleosum   _____

11. keratinohylalin   _____

12. cornocytes   _____

13. elieden   _____

14. cerumenous   _____

V.   Vision Quiz: Human Skin

Figure 11-11 shows a longitudinal section of human skin. Identify and write the name of the numbered components in the spaces provided.

1. _____

2. _____

3. _____

4. _____

5. _____

6. _____

7. _____

8. _____

9. _____

10. _____

11. _____

12. _____

13. _____

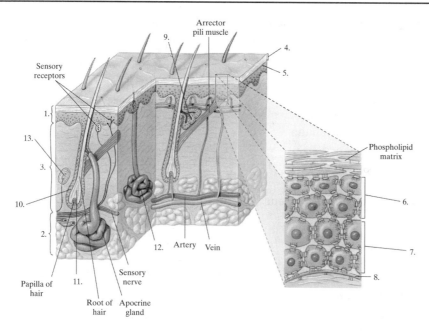

FIGURE 11-11   Vision Quiz. The microscopic features of human skin.

B. *Structure and Organization of the Hair and Nails*

I.   Matching 1: Structure and Organization of Human Hair

Match the term to its meaning. (The same meaning may be used more than once.)
Insert the appropriate letter in the space next to the question number.

Choices:

_____ **1.** pulls on hair follicles to
        make them erect
_____ **2.** component of hair shaft
_____ **3.** part of the hair found in
        the dermis
_____ **4.** consists of keratinized
        scalelike cells
_____ **5.** part of hair follicle
_____ **6.** located at the base of
        each follicle
_____ **7.** expressed hollow region
        in a bulb

a. root
b. internal root sheath
c. cuticle
d. arrector pili
e. medulla
f. bulb
g. cortex
h. dermal papilla

II.   Matching 2: Structure and Organization of the Nail

Match the term to its meaning. (The same meaning may be used more than once.)
Insert the appropriate letter in the space next to the question number.

_____ **1.** nail production occurs here
_____ **2.** cuticle
_____ **3.** whitish half-moon-shaped area of the proximal end of the nail
_____ **4.** part of the stratum corneum found below free edge of the nail

_____ **5.** part of the epidermis beneath the nail
_____ **6.** component of the nail

Choices:

    a. lunula
    b. eponychium
    c. hyponychium
    d. nail bed
    e. nail root
    f. nail body
    g. free projecting end

III.   Spell Check

Circle each incorrectly spelled term and write it correctly in the space provided.

    1. roote   _____
    2. medulla   _____
    3. kuticel   _____
    4. pilla   _____
    5. folicle   _____
    6. lunula   _____
    7. highonychium   _____
    8. eponychium   _____

C. Word Elements Used with the Skin, Nails, and Hair

I.   Matching: Word Elements and the Integumentary System

Match the term to its meaning. (The same meaning may be used more than once.) Insert the appropriate letter in the space next to the question number.

Choices:

_____ **1.** scaly	**a.** cutane/o	
_____ **2.** dry	**b.** seb/o	
_____ **3.** thorny	**c.** erythr/o	
_____ **4.** sebum	**d.** onych/o	
_____ **5.** sweat	**e.** steat/o	
_____ **6.** skin	**f.** ichthy/o	
_____ **7.** black	**g.** ungu/o	
_____ **8.** fat	**h.** acanth/o	
_____ **9.** white	**i.** xer/o	
_____ **10.** redness	**j.** melan/o	
_____ **11.** nail	**k.** hidr/o	
_____ **12.** horny	**l.** kerat/o	
	m. albin/o	

II.   Spell Check

Circle each incorrectly spelled term and write it correctly in the space provided.

    1. cutaineous   _____
    2. hidropoieis   _____

    3. icthoyd   _____

    4. melanoma   _____

    5. seborhagia   _____

    6. steetopathy   _____

    7. squamous   _____

    8. unguel   _____

III.   Word Analysis: Word Elements Used with the Skin, Nails, and Hair

Table 11-12 lists a number of terms with their pronunciations and definitions.

    1. Analyze each term.

    2. Circle all combining forms and word roots and label them **cf** and **wr**, respectively.

    3. Check your answers (shown in Table 11-17).

TABLE 11-12 WORD ANALYSIS: WORD ELEMENTS USED WITH THE SKIN, NAILS, AND HAIR

Term and Pronunciation	Definition
acanthoma (ak'-an-THŌ-ma)	noncancerous spiny tumor of the skin
albinism (AL-bin-iz-em)	absence of pigment
cutaneous (kū-TĀ-nē-os)	pertaining to the skin
dermal (DER-mal)	pertaining to the skin
erythematous (er'-i-THĒ-ma-tus)	pertaining to redness (rash)
hidropoiesis (hī'-drō-poy-Ē-sis)	formation of sweat
ichthyoid (IK-thē-oyd)	fishlike (scaly)
keratosis (ker'-a-TŌ-sis)	formation of horny growths (warts)
melanoma (mel'-a-NŌ-ma)	malignant, pigmented tumor (mole)
onychitis (on'-i-KĪ-tis)	inflammation of the nail bed
pilonidal (pī'-lō-NĪ-dal)	hair beneath the skin, forming a mass of cells or *nest*
seborrhea (seb'-or-Ē-a)	excessive discharge of sebum
squamous (SKWĀ-mus)	scalelike
steatopathy (stē-a-TŌP-a-thē)	disease of the sebaceous gland
trichoesthesia (trik'-ō-es-THĒ-zē-a)	sensation felt when a hair is touched
ungual (UNG-gual)	pertaining to the nails
xerasia (zē-RĀ-zē-a)	abnormal dry condition (of the hair)

D. Singular and Plural Forms

I.   Fill in the Blank 1

Fill in the blank with the appropriate term.

	Singular Form	**Plural Form**
1.	bulla	_____
2.	carbuncle	_____
3.	_____	maculae
4.	papule	_____
5.	_____	petechiae
6.	_____	pustulae
7.	vesicle	_____
8.	wheal	_____

II.   Fill in the Blank 2

Fill in the blank with the appropriate term.

1. An abnormally raised, thickened scar formed after surgery or injury is called a(n) _____.
2. A slit or crack-like sore is known as a(n) _____.
3. The plural form of bulla is _____.
4. A closed sac or pouch containing fluid is called a(n) _____.
5. A skin lesion enclosed within a limited area is referred to as being _____.
6. A tumorous growth with a thin surface layer is an example of a(n) _____.
7. A purplish-red, irregular spot on the skin is called a(n) _____.

III.   Matching: Signs and General Features of Diseases and Abnormalities Involving the Skin

Match the term to its meaning. (The same meaning may be used more than once.) Insert the appropriate letter in the space next to the question number.

Choices:

_____ **1.** fissure	**a.**	small, purplish hemorrhagic spot
_____ **2.** macule	**b.**	fluid-containing enclosed sac
_____ **3.** petechia	**c.**	slit or crack-like lesion
_____ **4.** pustule	**d.**	localized, inflamed region with a soft center and pus discharge
_____ **5.** cyst	**e.**	round, circumscribed, generally flat spot on the skin
_____ **6.** cicatrix	**f.**	small, elevated, pus-containing skin lesion
_____ **7.** furuncle	**g.**	deep skin sore or ulcer, usually with a hardened border and pus drainage
_____ **8.** ulcer	**h.**	scar left by a healed wound
_____ **9.** carbuncle	**i.**	rounded or irregularly shaped depression in the skin

IV.   Spell Check

Circle each incorrectly spelled term and write it correctly in the space provided.

1. bleb   _____
2. ulser   _____
3. pupual   _____
4. weal   _____
5. petechia   _____
6. maculae   _____
7. polpy   _____
8. viteligo   _____
9. pustule   _____

E. Skin Injuries

I.   Fill in the Blank

Fill in the blank with the appropriate term.

1. The accumulation of the blood under the skin caused by a severe blood vessel injury is called a(n) _____.
2. A term for a bruise is _____.
3. When tissue damage occurs without an actual break in the skin, the wound is referred to as being _____.
4. List five general open wound types: _____, _____, _____, _____, and _____.
5. Which type of burn is the mildest? _____.
6. The system used to determine the extent of burns on the body surface is called _____.

II.   Matching

Match the term to its meaning. (The same meaning may be used more than once.)
Insert the appropriate letter in the space next to the question number.

Choices:

_____ 1. hematoma
_____ 2. incision
_____ 3. avulsion
_____ 4. contusion
_____ 5. abrasion
_____ 6. ecchymosis
_____ 7. laceration
_____ 8. third-degree burn
_____ 9. first-degree burn
_____ 10. puncture
_____ 11. second-degree burn

a. bruise
b. irregularly formed hemorrhage in the skin
c. accumulation of blood beneath the skin due to severe injury
d. superficial wound from a scrape or scratch
e. wound caused by a smooth cut
f. wound with a skin flap
g. deeply penetrating wound
h. jagged cut
i. burn characterized by redness and pain only
j. burn characterized by redness, pain, edema, and blisters
k. burn extending from epidermis into the subcutaneous fat and with charring of the skin
l. full-thickness burn

III.   Spell Check

Circle each incorrectly spelled term and write it correctly in the space provided.

1. contuson   _____
2. abrasion   _____
3. insision   _____
4. laseration   _____
5. avulsion   _____
6. echymoses   _____
7. hemtoma   _____
8. bruise   _____

F. Common Skin Diseases

I.   Fill in the Blank

Fill in the blank with the appropriate term.

1. The two categories into which skin diseases may be divided are _____ and _____.
2. The malignant tumor that may be associated with AIDS is _____.
3. A tumor of melanocytes is called _____.
4. A benign neoplastic growth of melanocytes is called _____.

II.   Matching

Match the term to its meaning. (The same meaning may be used more than once.) Insert the appropriate letter in the space next to the question number.

Choices:

_____ 1. connective tissue tumors
_____ 2. squamous-cell carcinoma
_____ 3. Kaposi's sarcoma
_____ 4. basal cell carcinoma
_____ 5. malignant melanoma
_____ 6. sweat-gland adenocarci-noma
_____ 7. epidermoid carcinoma
_____ 8. nevus

a. malignant tumor consisting of cells similar to epidermis cells
b. benign tumors in the dermis
c. a multifocal malignant tumor characterized by bluish-red or brown nodules; may be found with AIDS
d. malignant tumor of squamous cells
e. tumor of the melanin-producing cells
f. sudoriferous malignant tumor
g. birthmark
h. squamous cell malignant tumor

III.   Spell Check

Circle each incorrectly spelled term and write it correctly in the space provided.

1. basel   _____
2. carcinoma   _____
3. Kaposhe's   _____
4. melanoma   _____
5. malignent   _____
6. epidermoyd   _____
7. adenocarcinoma _____
8. sguamous   _____

G. Skin Infections

I.   Fill in the Blank

Fill in the blank with the appropriate term.

    1. Pus-producing disease agents are also referred to as being

    _____.

    2. The general term used to indicate the several types of fungus infections of the skin, nails, and hair is _____.

    3. Ringworm of the foot also is known as _____.

II.   Matching

Match the term to its meaning. (The same meaning may be used more than once.)
Insert the appropriate letter in the space next to the question number.

Choices:

_____ **1.** carbuncle	**a.** inflamed skin area resulting in necrosis and pus formation
_____ **2.** dermatophytosis	**b.** fungal skin infection
_____ **3.** acne vulgaris	**c.** acute inflammatory destructive disease of the skin
_____ **4.** tinea pedis	**d.** common form of acne
_____ **5.** pyoderma	**e.** ringworm of the feet

III.   Spell Check

Circle each incorrectly spelled term and write it correctly in the space provided.

    1. teenea _____

    2. karbuncle _____

    3. dermatites _____

    4. impetigo _____

    5. pyoderma _____

    6. acknee _____

    7. cellulitis _____

    8. ekzema _____

    9. pustule _____

    10. dermatophytosis _____

H. Signs of Nail Disease and Abnormalities

I.   Fill in the Blank

Fill in the blank with the appropriate term.

    1. How are nail dyschromias classified? _____

    2. Six causes of nail dyschromia are _____, _____,

    _____, _____, _____,

    and _____.

II.   Matching

Match the term to its meaning. (The same meaning may be used more than once.)
Insert the appropriate letter in the space next to the question number.

Choices:

_____ **1.** excessive horny layer
     growth

a. onychia

b. dyschromia

_____ **2.** nail bed inflammation

c. hyperkeratosis

_____ **3.** nail discoloration

d. paronychia

_____ **4.** white streaks on nails

e. leukonychia

_____ **5.** disease state around nail

III.   Spell Check

Circle each incorrectly spelled term and write it correctly in the space provided.

1. dyskromia   _____

2. discoloration   _____

3. hyperkeratosis   _____

4. leukonickea   _____

5. onychia   _____

6. paranychia   _____

7. inflamed   _____

8. striata   _____

IV.   Word Analysis: Signs of Nail Disease and Abnormalities

Table 11-13 lists a number of terms with their pronunciations and definitions.

TABLE 11-13   WORD ANALYSIS: SIGNS OF NAIL DISEASE AND ABNORMALITIES

Term and Pronunciation	Definition
dyschromia (dis-KRŌ-mē-a)	discoloration of nails
hyperkeratosis (hī'-per-ker'-a-TŌ-sis)	excessive growth of horny layer of epidermis
leukonychia (lū-kō-NIK-ē-a)	white streaks on the nails
onychia (ō-NIK-ē-a)	inflamed condition of the nail bed
paronychia (par-ō-NIK-ē-a)	diseased state around the nail

1. Analyze each term.

2. Circle all combining forms and word roots and label them **cf** and **wr**, respectively.

3. Check your answers (shown in Table 11-18).

I. Surgical Procedures Involving the Skin

I.   Matching 1: Operative Procedures

Match the term to its meaning. (The same meaning may be used more than once.) Insert the appropriate letter in the space next to the question number.

Choices:

_____ **1.** drainage

a. skin grafting

_____ **2.** cryosurgery

b. use of extreme cold to destroy a lesion

_____ **3.** dermabrasion

_____ **4.** curettage

_____ **5.** replacement of injured tissue with normal tissue

c. scraping a superficial lesion with a curet

d. removal of moles or scars with abrasives

e. withdrawal of fluid from a wound

II.   Matching 2: Operative Procedures

Match the term to its meaning. (The same meaning may be used more than once.) Insert the appropriate letter in the space next to the question number.

Choices:

_____ **1.** débridement

_____ **2.** liposuction

_____ **3.** excision

_____ **4.** escharotomy

_____ **5.** rhytidectomy

a. surgical removal of burned tissue

b. surgical removal

c. removal of subcutaneous fat with high-powered suction

d. removal of skin wrinkles by plastic surgery

e. removal of damaged tissue by excision

III.   Spell Check

Circle each incorrectly spelled term and write it correctly in the space provided.

1. boipsy   _____

2. ciryosurgery   _____

3. curretage   _____

4. débridement   _____

5. dermabrasion   _____

6. echarotomy   _____

7. lipposuction   _____

8. rytidektomy   _____

J. Medical Vocabulary Building

I.   Matching

Match the term to its meaning. (The same meaning may be used more than once.) Insert the appropriate letter in the space next to the question number.

Choices:

_____ **1.** anhidrosis

_____ **2.** hidradenitis

_____ **3.** hyperhidrosis

_____ **4.** hypodermoclysis

_____ **5.** senile keratosis

_____ **6.** thermanesthesia

_____ **7.** acrochordon

_____ **8.** wen

a. inflammation of sweat glands

b. complete absence of sweating

c. excessive sweating

d. dry skin and localized scaling in the elderly, caused by excessive sun exposure

e. injection of fluids for rapid fluid replacement

f. inability to distinguish between heat and cold sensations

g. small outgrowth of epidermal and dermal tissue

h. sebaceous cyst

II.   Spell Check

Circle each incorrectly spelled term and write it correctly in the space provided.

1. wenn   _____
2. keratosis   _____
3. hidratenitis   _____
4. hyperhidrosis   _____
5. akrocordon   _____
6. thermanesthesia   _____
7. hyopdermoclysis   _____
8. anhidrosis   _____

K. Abbreviations

I.   Matching: Abbreviations Used with the Integumentary System

Match the term to its meaning. (The same meaning may be used more than once.) Insert the appropriate letter in the space next to the question number.

Choices:

_____ 1. UV   a. ointment
_____ 2. ung   b. ultraviolet
_____ 3. T   c. temperature
_____ 4. TTS   d. skin draft
_____ 5. subq   e. incision and drainage
_____ 6. I&D   f. intradermal
_____ 7. H   g. dermatology
_____ 8. Hx   h. history
_____ 9. ID   i. transdermal therapeutic system
_____ 10. SG   j. subcutaneous
_____ 11. derm   k. hypodermic
                      l. skin graft

L. Increasing Your Medical Terminology Word Power 1

1. Read the following report.
2. Prepare to answer the questions at the end of the section.
3. Circle all unfamiliar terms with a red pencil.
4. Underline familiar terms with a blue pencil.
5. Use your knowledge of basic word elements, a medical dictionary, and the key terms to find the meaning of unfamiliar terms.

Melanomas

Key Terms

actinic keratoses (ak-TIN-ik ker-a-TŌ-sēz)   pertains to the formation of horny growths caused by sunlight or other form of radiant energy

excision (ek-SI-zhun)   surgical removal

histopathology (his'-tō-pa-THOL-ō-jē)   the study of diseased tissue

lymph (limf) node   accumulation of lymphatic tissue found at certain points in the lymphatic system

malignancy (ma-LIG-nan-sē)   cancerous growth or condition

melanoma (mel'-a-NŌ-ma)   pigmented growth (tumor) that may be benign or malignant

metastasis (me-TAS-ta-sis)   movement of cancers from one part of the body to another abbreviation for millimeter *mm.*

nevus (NĒ-vus)   benign, pigmented skin tumor

palliative (PAL-ē-a-tiv)   relieving or easing without curing

plantar (PLAN-tar)   pertaining to the sole of the foot

retinoid (RET-i-noyd)   form of vitamin A

subungual (sub-UNG-gual)   beneath the nail

symmetric (sim-ET-rik)   corresponding parts on opposite sides of a body

variegation (ver-ē-a-GĀ'-shun)   a streaking or spotting with color

Introduction

Melanoma is perhaps the clearest example of a cancer in which early treatment is the key to survival. Diagnosed when the malignant cells are restricted to the epidermis, cutaneous melanoma is nearly 100 percent curable by excision. But by the time the malignancy has spread to regional lymph nodes, patients have a 50 percent five-year survival. Once the disease has metastasized to distant body sites, treatment is palliative. Unfortunately, most such situations end in death, usually within a matter of months.

Prevention of melanoma is complicated by resistance on the part of individuals to making important lifestyle changes. Enough is known about risk factors, particularly among populations with the highest risk, that prevention is possible with early detection.

Most melanoma patients are young to middle-aged adults; the median age at diagnosis is approximately 45 years. Historically, the disease has been rare in children, but increases are being reported. Men and women are at roughly equal risk, although women tend to have a better overall survival.

Both lifestyle and genetics appear to play roles in melanoma development. Table 11-14 lists most of the risk factors associated with susceptibility for cutaneous melanoma.

TABLE 11-14   RISK FACTORS FOR CUTANEOUS MELANOMA

Personal or family history of melanoma	Light skin type
History of intermittent acute exposure to sunlight	Blue or green eyes
History of severe sunburns (three or more) during childhood and adolescence	Blond or red hair
Large number of moles	Northern European ancestry of person living in areas of intense sunlight
Clinically atypical moles	

B EHAVIORAL FACTORS

Behavioral risk factors also include a history of severe sun exposure during childhood and adolescence. Indeed, three severe sunburns early in life are enough to increase a person's subsequent risk of cutaneous melanoma. Melanoma rates also correlate positively with various socioeconomic factors, including education level, income, and profession. Interestingly, people who work outdoors are at somewhat lower risk, perhaps because tanning associated with chronic sun exposure provides some protection. People who work indoors and get short, intense sun exposure during activities such as skiing, golf, and sailing seem to have a higher incidence of melanomas. Thus, it appears that acute intermittent exposure is responsible for the damage, perhaps in combination with damaging sunburns early in life.

Primary melanomas also can occur on parts of the body that do not receive substantial amounts of sun exposure, such as the palms and plantar surfaces, mucosa, perianal skin, and internal sites. Causes here can include various other carcinogens or changes in the atmosphere, especially a decrease in atmospheric ozone.

Factors shown not to be associated with increased risk include diet, intake of vitamin D and retinoids, increased alcohol consumption, hormone use in women, tobacco smoking, skin hygiene, and use of hair dyes.

*G*ENETIC FACTORS

Genetically determined risk factors for melanoma include fair skin, an inability to tan, blond or red hair, blue or green eyes, and freckles. Lighter skin doubles a person's risk. Blond hair increases the risk by 60 percent. Women with red hair have three times the risk of age-matched controls.

*C*LINICAL FEATURES

A general approach to identifying pigmented lesions that may be malignant is the well-known **ABCD** guideline (Table 11-15). Benign nevi tend to be flat, hairless,

TABLE 11-15   CLINICAL WARNING SIGNS OF MELANOMA: THE ABCD GUIDELINE

A	Asymmetrical shape of a mole
	Appearance of a new pigmented lesion
B	Borders are notched and/or irregular
	Bleeding of a mole
C	Color of mole varies or contains blue, gray, pink, red, or white areas
D	Diameter of a mole exceeding 2 mm in any direction and in combination with other warning signs

round or oval, less than 6 mm in diameter, and symmetrical, with borders that are usually smooth. Pigmentation is generally even, although there are sometimes color variations, especially in shades of brown. Physicians should be suspicious of moles that are asymmetrical or exhibit notched borders or color variations, regardless of size. Suspicious colors include gray, blue, white, pink, or red in a brown, tan, or black lesion (Figure 11-12).

Variation is thought to be caused by varying depths of melanin in the skin (the deeper the pigment, the more bluish it appears) and by differing degrees of inflammation and vascular dilation.

Moles that bleed should also be viewed with suspicion. A diameter exceeding 6 mm can be a warning sign, but diameter by itself is not a reliable indicator.

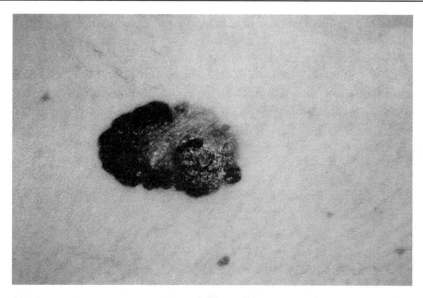

FIGURE 11-12   The appearance of a lesion in the case of a melanoma.

Children, especially adolescents, frequently have nevi with irregular borders, multiple shades of pigment, or both. Most are normal variants of benign nevi, but any nevus that arouses clinical suspicion or is of concern to the patient should be removed. All nevi should be sent for pathologic examination.

C LASSIC TYPES OF MELANOMAS

Melanomas are categorized based on histopathology but are often distinguishable clinically. Establishing the category is important, since prognosis differs somewhat for each pattern. Table 11-16 lists and briefly describes the major types.

TABLE 11-16   CLASSIC TYPES OF MELANOMAS

Type	General Features
superficial spreading melanoma	most common form; generally flat and less than 2 cm in diameter; as it evolves it changes in pigmentation, either darkening or changing to unusual colors; eventually cells penetrate deeper skin layers; often are curable
nodular melanoma	second most common form; has sharp borders; often blue to black in color; penetrates the dermis, extends above the skin surface, and tends to be round; reported to be somewhat more frequent in men than women
acral (AK-ral) lentiginous (len-TIG-i-nos) melanoma	an uncommon melanoma in white populations, but most common among blacks, Asians, and Hispanics; occurs on palms or soles, or sublingually, and may also develop on the rectum and vagina; irregular borders and pigment variegations are common; usually occurs in the elderly and on chronically sun-exposed skin areas. This type of melanoma is more aggressive than the superficial or nodular forms.

T HE MELANOCYTE AND THE MELANOMA CONNECTION

Cutaneous melanoma involves the transformation of pigment cells (*melanocytes*) by a mechanism that incorporates genetic abnormalities of regulatory proteins and the responses of cells to such proteins. One of the pathological processes in melanoma development may involve toxic substances formed by the pigments themselves. This mechanism may be especially important in light-skinned individuals.

Whatever triggers the transformation from pigment cell to melanoma, the cancer is not life threatening until it enters a vertical growth phase and invades the deeper skin layers and spreads lymphatically or hematogenously. The molecular and cellular biology of this phase is not well understood. Melanocytes are known to be capable of migration within the *stratum basale* of the epidermis, which may explain why melanoma cells metastasize so readily.

𝒫 REVENTION

For the foreseeable future, prevention and early diagnosis remain key in reducing the morbidity and mortality of melanoma.

Questions

I.   Matching 1: Terms Associated with Melanomas

Match the term to its meaning. (The same meaning may be used more than once.) Insert the appropriate letter in the space next to the question number.

Choices:

_____ **1.** cancerous growth or condition
_____ **2.** study of diseased tissue
_____ **3.** a horny growth
_____ **4.** a pigmented tumor
_____ **5.** surgical removal
_____ **6.** movement of cells, especially cancerous ones
_____ **7.** beneath the nail
_____ **8.** streaked or spotted coloration
_____ **9.** form of vitamin A
_____ **10.** concerning the sole of the foot

a. melanoma
b. keratosis
c. malignancy
d. histopathology
e. excision
f. metastasis
g. retinoid
h. subungual
i. plantar
j. variegation

II.   Matching 2: Classic Melanoma Types

Match the term to its meaning. (The same meaning may be used more than once.) Insert the appropriate letter in the space next to the question number.

_____ **1.** superficial spreading melanoma
_____ **2.** nodular melanoma
_____ **3.** acral lentiginous melanoma

Choices:

a. uncommon in white populations, but common among blacks, Asians, and Hispanics
b. sharp borders, often blue to black
c. more frequent in men
d. generally flat
e. changes in pigmentation during development
f. occurs sublingually

III.   Multiple Choice

Circle the best possible answer for each question.

1. Which of the following factors have not been found as risk factors for melanoma development?
    a. tobacco smoking
    b. light skin type
    c. family history of melanoma
    d. green eyes
    e. all of these

2. Which of the following are considered to be genetic factors in the development of melanomas?
    a. fair skin
    b. freckles
    c. inability to tan
    d. red hair
    e. all of these

IV.   Spell Check

Circle each incorrectly spelled term and write it correctly in the space provided.

1. keratoses   _____
2. ekscision   _____
3. maligancy   _____
4. melanoma   _____
5. metestasis   _____
6. nevus   _____
7. paliative   _____
8. retenoid   _____
9. subungual   _____
10. symetric   _____
11. varegation   _____
12. patient   _____

M. Increasing Your Medical Terminology Word Power 2

1. Read the following report.
2. Prepare to answer the questions at the end of the section.
3. Circle all unfamiliar terms with a red pencil.
4. Underline familiar terms with a blue pencil.
5. Use your knowledge of basic word elements, a medical dictionary, and the key terms to find the meaning of unfamiliar terms.

Eczema Vaccinatum

Key Terms

b.i.d. twice daily

confluent (KON-floo-ent) running together, as in situations when pustules combine

eczema vaccinatum (EK-zē-ma VAK-sin-āt-um) cutaneous inflammatory condition with the formation of a variety of skin lesions alone or in combination; occurs as a complication of vaccination or through contact with a recently vaccinated individual

immunoglobulin (im-ū-nō-GLOB-ū-lin)   protective proteins produced by the body's immune system

intermittent (in-ter-MIT-ent)   periodic

prophylactic (prō-feh-LAK-tik)   as a protective measure

pruritus (proo-Rī-tus)   severe itching

pustular (PUS-tū-lar)   lesions filled with pus

t.i.d.   three times a day

umbilicated (um-BIL-i-kā-ted)   central depressed point

Introduction and Overview

Eczema vaccinatum is a potentially fatal complication that occurs in persons with eczema and other forms of dermatitis. The condition usually occurs in young children under the age of five years. Typical signs and symptoms include high fever, toxicity, and widespread eruptions consisting of vesicular and pustular lesions. At first these lesions are superficial but they progress to vesicular and finally to pustular forms. Crusting develops by the seventh day of the illness, with crust shedding occurring within two weeks. In the majority of cases, full recovery occurs and skin lesions heal without scarring. However, death may result when extensive involvement of the internal organs occurs or if inflammation of the brain or encephalitis complicates the condition.

C ASE HISTORY

On August 14, 1999, an 18-month-old male was taken to the emergency room of a local medical center. The patient had a fever of 101–103 °F and exhibited a "chickenpox-like rash." The child was referred to the dermatology clinic for a physical examination and laboratory tests.

The physical examination showed multiple early vesicular lesions, and in some body areas the lesions progressed to an umbilicated pox stage. Confluent lesions were found in the ears, nape of the neck, midabdomen, elbows, and knees. Crusting of the isolated lesions was present, suggesting secondary bacterial infection. All other aspects of the physical examination were normal.

The patient's treatment included Alpha-Keri baths t.i.d. for pruritus and antibiotics for the secondary bacterial infection. Because of the severe nature of the itching, an anti-inflammatory cream was applied b.i.d., and the patient was placed in isolation and sedated. On the fourteenth hospital day, the patient was discharged.

Questions

I.   Fill in the Blank

Fill in the blank with the appropriate phrase.

1. On which body areas were confluent lesions found?   _____

    _____

2. What physical finding suggested the presence of a bacterial infection?

    _____

3. How often was the anti-inflammatory cream applied?

    _____

4. How many days did the patient spend in the hospital?

    _____

II.   Matching: Eczema Vaccinatum

Match the term to its meaning. (The same meaning may be used more than once.)
Insert the appropriate letter in the space next to the question number.

Choices:

_____ **1.** being poisonous
_____ **2.** severe itching
_____ **3.** having a central
           depression
_____ **4.** skin inflammation
_____ **5.** brain inflammation
_____ **6.** confined to the surface
_____ **7.** calmed, often by admin-
           istration of drugs
_____ **8.** small skin lesion filled
           with pus

a. encephalitis
b. superficial
c. pruritus
d. pustule
e. sedated
f. toxicity
g. dermatitis
h. umbilicated

III.   Spell Check

Circle each incorrectly spelled term and write it correctly in the space provided.

1. conflooent   _____
2. umbilicated   _____
3. profilactic   _____
4. puritis   _____
5. imunoglobulin _____
6. vaccinated   _____

N. *Increasing Your Medical Terminology Word Power 3*

1. Read the following report.
2. Prepare to answer the questions at the end of the section.
3. Circle all unfamiliar terms with a red pencil.
4. Underline familiar terms with a blue pencil.
5. Use your knowledge of basic word elements, a medical dictionary, and
      the key terms to find the meaning of unfamiliar terms.

Congenital Cutaneous Candidiasis

Key Terms

candidiasis (kan'-di-DĪ-a-sis)   infectious syndrome linked to the yeast *Candida al-bicans* (KAN-di-da, AL-bi-kans)

erythematous (er'-i-THEM-a-tus)   spreading area of redness

g   abbreviation for gram

gestation (jes-TĀ-shun)   time from conception to birth

lymphadenopathy (lim-fad'e-NOP-a-thē)   disease of the lymph nodes

macula (MAK-ū-la)   small spot or colored area

oral thrush (thrush)   a yeast infection of the mouth; characterized by the presence
of white patches in the mouth, fever, and gastrointestinal problems

papular (PAP-ū-ler)   elevated red areas on the skin

prognosis (prog-NŌ-sis)   prediction of the course and end of a disease, including
chances for recovery

pustular (PUS-tū-lar) lesions containing pus

sepsis (SEP-sis) disease caused by microorganisms and/or their products in the blood

syndrome (SIN-drōm) a group of signs and symptoms

systemic (sis-TEM-ik) pertaining to the entire body rather than to one of its parts

third trimester the final three months of pregnancy

topical local, confined to definite body area

𝒢 ENERAL BACKGROUND

Congenital cutaneous candidiasis is a rare but well-described infectious syndrome that occurs in newborn infants. The infection caused by the yeast *Candida albicans* typically presents in one of two ways. Infants who are delivered at term may present with typical erythematous papular and pustular eruptions. Whether treated or not, this clinical condition has a good prognosis and usually is not associated with systemic infection. Premature infants (those born earlier than 27 weeks gestation and with a birth weight of less than 1000 g) may also present with denuded areas of skin or a diffuse erythematous macular eruption that resembles a burn. Without treatment, these infants are more likely to have invasive disease with sepsis and poor prognosis.

For full-term infants, therapy limited to topical antifungal agents is appropriate. Because of the potential for invasive disease, systemic antifungal therapy should be considered for premature infants and those who have burn-like dermatitis. The usual drug of choice is amphotericin.

𝒞 ASE REPORT

A male infant who was born at full term exhibited a disseminated papular rash on his trunk, thighs, and face at the time of delivery. The pregnancy and delivery were uncomplicated with the exception of a vaginal yeast infection that appeared during the mother's third trimester. The infant remained well, but by the time he was four days of age skin lesions had become prominent on the extremities, including the palms and soles.

The remainder of the physical examination was remarkable only for the presence of oral thrush and diffuse lymphadenopathy. Attempts to culture bacteria and yeast from blood and urine specimens were unsuccessful.

𝒯 REATMENT AND OUTCOME

The infant was treated with topical ketoconazole, an antifungal agent. Ten days after treatment initiation, skin shedding occurred over most of the body, leaving a few residual pustules on the face.

Questions

I.   Fill in the Blank

Fill in the blank with the appropriate phrase.

1. The cause of congenital cutaneous candidiasis is _____ _____.

2. What type of eruption can be expected from infected infants who are delivered at term? _____

3. Does an infant delivered at term with congenital cutaneous candidiasis have a good or poor prognosis? _____.

4. The drug of choice in cases of congenital cutaneous candidiasis is

_____.

II.   Matching

Match the term to its meaning. (The same meaning may be used more than once.) Insert the appropriate letter in the space next.

Choices:

_____ **1.** sepsis
_____ **2.** syndrome
_____ **3.** gestation
_____ **4.** lymphadenopathy
_____ **5.** prognosis
_____ **6.** third trimester
_____ **7.** topical

a. definite body area
b. prediction of the outcome of a disease
c. disease of the lymph nodes
d. group of signs and symptoms
e. the last three months of pregnancy
f. time from conception to birth
g. microorganisms and/or their products in the blood

III.   Spell Check

Circle each incorrectly spelled term and write it correctly in the space provided.

1. sepsis   _____
2. lymphadenopathy _____
3. erythematos   _____
4. topikal   _____
5. postular   _____
6. progknowsis   _____

Term Search Challenge

Locate 14 terms in the puzzle.

1. Write the specific term next to its definition. Then find that term in the puzzle and circle it.
2. Terms may be read from left to right, backward, up, down, or diagonally.
3. If a term appears more than once, circle it only once. (A term or abbreviation may be found inside others.)
4. Check your answers.

Clues:

1. Secretion of sebaceous glands _____
2. Glands that secrete sweat _____
3. Another term for earwax _____
4. Term pertaining to redness _____
5. A malignant, pigmented tumor _____
6. Inflammation of the nail bed _____
7. Pertaining to the nails _____
8. A scar left by a healed wound _____
9. Enclosed within a limited area _____
10. A small, purplish hemorrhagic spot _____
11. A benign skin tumor _____
12. The general term to designate ringworm _____
13. Removal of a small amount of tissue for diagnosis _____
14. Excessive discharge or flow of sebum _____

Term Search Puzzle

```
S   E   B   U   M   U   N   G   U   L   A   C   C
U   E   G   Y   U   U   B   I   O   P   S   Y   I
D   P   A   T   R   P   A   T   T   H   O   G   R
O   T   H   A   E   N   E   V   U   S   T   O   C
R   T   H   A   C   I   C   A   T   R   I   X   U
I   M   E   L   A   D   R   A   M   A   S   I   M
F   M   E   L   A   N   O   M   A   N   S   I   S
E   P   E   T   E   C   H   I   A   X   E   R   C
R   T   I   N   E   A   H   I   A   I   I   A   R
O   N   Y   C   H   I   T   I   S   C   A   I   I
U   C   E   R   U   M   S   K   I   N   S   B
S   E   B   O   R   R   H   E   A   S   K   I   E
E   R   Y   T   H   E   M   A   T   O   U   S   D
```

CHAPTER 12

The Muscular System

"The human heart… No other type of muscle has the stamina of that fist-sized, four-chambered pump."

—Rick Weiss

INFORMATIONAL CHALLENGE

A. Muscle Structure and Function

I.   Fill in the Blank

Fill in the blank with the appropriate term.

   1. The three types of muscle tissue are _____, _____, and _____.
   2. _____ muscle is voluntary, while _____ muscle is involuntary.
   3. The point of attachment of a muscle is called an _____, and the location where the muscle ends is called an _____.
   4. One type of tendon that attaches muscle to bone is called a(n) _____.

II.   Matching: Muscle Action

Match the term to its meaning. (The same meaning may be used more than once.) Insert the appropriate letter in the space next to the question number.

Choices:

_____ **1.** synergistic
_____ **2.** antagonistic
_____ **3.** adductor
_____ **4.** abductor

a. muscle that performs an opposite movement
b. muscles that work together to perform a function
c. muscles that pull away from the body's medial plane
d. muscles that pull toward the body's medial plane.

III.   Spell Check

Circle each incorrectly spelled term and write it correctly in the space provided.

   1. fasci   _____
   2. fusyform   _____

3. tenden   _____
4. actin   _____
5. myosen   _____
6. sinergistic _____
7. antagonistic _____
8. insertion   _____
9. asetolcholine _____
10. aponeurosis _____

IV.   Vision Quiz: Muscle Origins and Insertion Points

Figure 12-5 shows the biceps and the triceps. Identify and write the origin and insertion points for each muscle in the spaces provided.

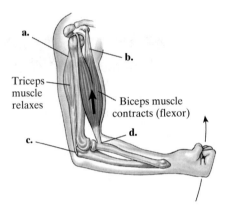

FIGURE 12-5   Vision Quiz. Examples of synergistic and antagonistic muscles. The biceps are antagonistic to the triceps.

1. biceps origin _____
2. origin triceps _____
3. biceps insertion _____
4. triceps insertion _____

B. Muscle Naming

I.   Spell Check

Circle each incorrectly spelled term and write it correctly in the space provided.

1. gastronemius _____
2. sartorus   _____
3. oblique   _____
4. frontalis   _____
5. pectorelis _____
6. deltoid   _____
7. biseps   _____
8. trapezius   _____
9. glooteus   _____
10. latisimus _____

11. Achilez   _____

12. brachii   _____

II.   Vision Quiz: Muscle Identification

Figure 12-6 shows a posterior view of superficial muscles. Identify the numbered muscles and indicate their function in the spaces provided.

Muscle	**Function**
1. _____	
2. _____	
3. _____	
4. _____	
5. _____	
6. _____	
7. _____	
8. _____	
9. _____	

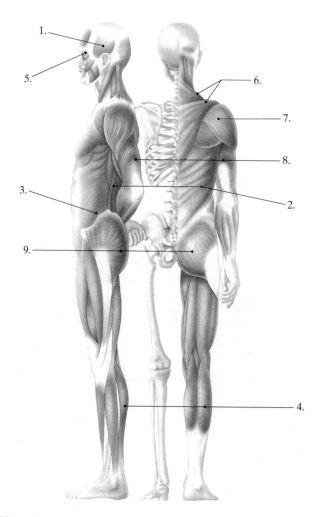

FIGURE 12-6   Vision Quiz. Posterior view of selected superficial skeletal muscles.

C. Word Roots and/or Combining Forms Used with Muscles and Related Structures

I.   Matching: Word Roots and/or Combining Forms Used with Muscles and Related Structures

Match the term to its meaning. (The same meaning may be used more than once.) Insert the appropriate letter in the space next to the question number.

Choices:

_____ **1.** leiomy/o	**a.** tendon
_____ **2.** myocardi/o	**b.** fascia
_____ **3.** fasci/o	**c.** smooth muscle
_____ **4.** rhabd/o	**d.** striated
_____ **5.** sarc/o	**e.** muscle
_____ **6.** myos/o	**f.** heart muscle
_____ **7.** tend/o	**g.** flesh/muscle

II.   Spell Check

Circle each incorrectly spelled term and write it correctly in the space provided.

1. fascial   _____
2. lieomyoma   _____
3. myelgia   _____
4. rabdomyoma   _____
5. sarcogenic   _____
6. tendeplasty   _____
7. tendinitis   _____
8. myocitis   _____

III.   Word Analysis: Prefixes, Word Roots, Combining Forms, and Suffixes Used with Muscles and Related Structures

Table 12-7 lists a number of terms with their pronunciations and definitions.

1. Analyze each term.
2. Circle all combining forms and word roots and label them **cf** and **wr**, respectively.
3. Check your answers (shown in Table 12-9).

TABLE 12-7 WORD ANALYSIS: PREFIXES, WORD ROOTS, COMBINING FORMS, AND SUFFIXES USED WITH MUSCLES AND RELATED STRUCTURES

Term and Pronunciation	Definition
fascial (FASH-ē-al)	pertaining to fascia
leiomyoma (lī'-ō-mī-Ō-ma)	smooth-muscle tumor
myalgia (mī-AL-jē-a)	muscle pain
myositis (mī'-ō-SĪ-tis)	muscle inflammation
rhabdomyoma (rab'-dō-mī-Ō-ma)	striated-muscle tumor

(Continued)

TABLE 12-7   (CONTINUED)

Term and Pronunciation	Definition
sarcogenic (sar'-kō-JEN-ik)	producing flesh or muscle
tendoplasty (TEN-dō-plas-tē)	surgical repair of a tendon
tendinitis (ten'-din-Ī-tis)	tendon inflammation

D. Abnormal and Pathological Conditions and Operative and Diagnostic Procedures

I.   Matching 1: Abnormal and Pathological Conditions

Match the term to its meaning. (The same meaning may be used more than once.) Insert the appropriate letter in the space next to the question number.

Choices:

_____ **1.** contracture
_____ **2.** paralysis
_____ **3.** fibromyositis
_____ **4.** fasciitis (or fascitis)
_____ **5.** myositis
_____ **6.** poliomyelitis
_____ **7.** graphospasm
_____ **8.** myopathy
_____ **9.** myokymia
_____ **10.** tenosynovitis

a. fascia inflammation
b. inflammation of both skeletal muscle and associated connective tissue
c. any muscle disease
d. muscle inflammation
e. writer's cramp
f. temporary or permanent loss of muscle function
g. polio virus infection resulting in muscle paralysis
h. tendon and synovia sheath inflammation
i. quivering movement of muscle
j. permanent shortening of muscle caused by paralysis

II.   Matching 2: Operative and Diagnostic Procedures

Match the term to its meaning. (The same meaning may be used more than once.) Insert the appropriate letter in the space next to the question number.

Choices:

_____ **1.** muscle biopsy
_____ **2.** myoplasty
_____ **3.** myorrhaphy
_____ **4.** myotasis
_____ **5.** electromyography
_____ **6.** tenosynovectomy
_____ **7.** tenodesis
_____ **8.** tenoplasty

a. test to measure muscle function
b. stretching of a muscle
c. surgical removal of muscle tissue
d. surgical tendon repair
e. surgical binding or fixation of a tendon
f. surgical muscle repair
g. suturing muscle
h. surgical excision of a tendon sheath

III.   Spell Check

Circle each incorrectly spelled term and write it correctly in the space provided.

1. contrachur   _____
2. grafospasm   _____
3. distrofy   _____
4. atrophy   _____
5. dejeneration   _____
6. miokymia   _____
7. poliomylitis   _____
8. myoplasty   _____
9. myorhaphy   _____
10. myotasis   _____
11. tendoesis   _____
12. tenosinovectomy   _____

IV.   Word Analysis: Abnormal and Pathological Conditions and Operative and Diagnostic Procedures

Table 12-8 lists a number of terms with their pronunciations and definitions.

TABLE 12-8   WORD ANALYSIS: ABNORMAL AND PATHOLOGICAL CONDITIONS AND OPERATIVE AND DIAGNOSTIC PROCEDURES

Term and Pronunciation	Definition
electromyography (ē-lek'-trō-mī-OG-ra-fē)	test used to measure muscle function
fibromyositis (fī'-brō-mī-ō-SĪ-tis)	inflammation of both skeletal muscle and associated connective tissue; frequently occurs in the lumbar region
graphospasm (GRAF-ō-spaz-em)	writer's cramp
myopathy (mī-OP-a-thē)	any muscle disease
myoplasty (mī-ō-PLAS-tē)	surgical muscle repair
myorrhaphy (mī-OR-a-fē)	stitching or suturing of a muscle
myositis (mī-ō-SĪ-tis)	inflammation of muscle
tenodesis (ten-OD-ē-sis)	surgical binding or fixation of a tendon; usually a tendon is transferred to a new origin in the procedure
tenoplasty (TEN-ō-plas-tē)	surgical tendon repair
tenosynovectomy (ten'-ō-sin-ō-VEK-tō-mē)	surgical removal or excision of a tendon sheath

1. Analyze each term.
2. Circle all combining forms and all word roots and label them **cf** and **wr**, respectively.
3. Check your answers (shown in Table 12-10).

E. Medical Vocabulary Building

I.   Matching: Medical Vocabulary Building

Match the term to its meaning. (The same meaning may be used more than once.)
Insert the appropriate letter in the space next to the question number.

Choices:

_____ **1.** brachialgia   **a.** arm pain
_____ **2.** fasciectomy   **b.** suture of an aponeurosis
_____ **3.** myoid   **c.** resembling muscle
_____ **4.** myoma   **d.** surgical excision of fascia
_____ **5.** myotome   **e.** muscle tissue destruction
_____ **6.** sarcitis   **f.** an instrument used to cut muscle
_____ **7.** voluntary   **g.** muscle tissue inflammation
_____ **8.** flaccid   **h.** an action within an individual's
_____ **9.** involuntary   control
_____ **10.** aponeurorrhaphy   **i.** lacking muscle tone
                              j. an action independent of one's
                                  control

II.   Spell Check

Circle each incorrectly spelled term and write it correctly in the space provided.

1. flascid   _____
2. myotome   _____
3. brachialgea   _____
4. sarsitis   _____
5. myoyd   _____
6. aponeurorrhaphy   _____

F. Abbreviations

I.   Matching: Abbreviations

Match the term to its meaning. (The same meaning may be used more than once.)
Insert the appropriate letter in the space next to the question number.

Choices:

_____ **1.** above knee   **a.** BK
_____ **2.** below knee   **b.** AK
_____ **3.** Ca   **c.** TJ
_____ **4.** full range of motion **d.** calcium
_____ **5.** musculoskeletal   **e.** sh
_____ **6.** physical medicine   **f.** PM
_____ **7.** shoulder   **g.** MS
_____ **8.** triceps jerk   **h.** FROM

II. Definitions

Define the following abbreviations.

1. AE   _____
2. PMR   _____
3. IM   _____
4. ADP   _____
5. LOM   _____
6. TBW   _____
7. Ht   _____
8. ROM   _____

G. Increasing Your Medical Terminology Word Power 1

1. Read the following report.
2. Prepare to answer the questions at the end of the section.
3. Circle all unfamiliar terms with a red pencil.
4. Underline familiar terms with a blue pencil.
5. Use your knowledge of word elements, a medical dictionary, and the key terms to find the meaning of unfamiliar terms.

Hypertrophic Osteoarthropathy Syndrome

Key Terms

adenosarcoma (ad-e-nō-sar-KŌ-ma)   a tumor having features of glandular and muscular tissues

bronchoscopy (bron-KOS-kō-pē)   examination of the bronchi with the use of a bronchoscope, an instrument that passes through the windpipe to allow viewing of the respiratory passages

clubbing   common sign in diseases of the lungs and appears as a curving of the nails accompanied by the enlargement of the soft tissues of the fingers and toes

diarrhea (dī-a-RĒ-a)   frequent passage of watery bowel movements

edema (e-DĒ-ma)   accumulation of fluid in the tissues

hypertrophic (hī-per-TROF-ik)   pertaining to an increase in the size of an organ or structure; does not involve tumor formation

lobectomy (lō-BEK-tō-mē)   surgical removal of a lobe from any organ or gland

osteoarthropathy (os'-tē-ō-ar-THROP-a-thē)   any disease involving the joints and bones

periostitis (per-ē-os-TĪ-tis)   pertaining to an inflammation of the membrane covering a bone except at its articulations

roentgenogram (rō-ent-JEN-ō-gram)   a film produced by a type of x-ray

G ENERAL BACKGROUND

The hypertrophic osteoarthropathy syndrome is characterized by the presence of periostitis, new bone formation, arthritis, and clubbing of the digits. The syndrome can also accompany cardiac disease, liver disease, gastrointestinal diseases producing acute diarrhea, and various other conditions. In its primary form clubbing, bone changes, increased sweating of the palms and soles, and a pronounced thickening of the skin of the face, forehead, and scalp occur. While clubbing is associated with periostitis of the distal ends of the long bones, the roentgenogram is the key to the correct diagnosis. The ulna and radius are involved in 80 percent of cases, and the tibia and fibula in 74 percent.

A unique feature of this syndrome is the presence of lower-extremity edema and bone pain. These rheumatic signs and symptoms are controlled with aspirin.

$\mathcal{T}$HE CASE HISTORY

A 38-year-old male was admitted to the medical center showing a mild edema and *arthralgia* (ar-THRAL-jē-a). The patient indicated that he never had arthritis and that both conditions improved with the elevation of his feet and the use of anti-inflammatory agents such as ordinary aspirin. Being a heavy smoker, the patient had smoked two packs of cigarettes per day since the age of eighteen.

The patient was principally admitted to the hospital for an evaluation of a 2 cm lesion about the size of a small coin, which was discovered in chest films of the left lung. A bronchoscopic biopsy of the lesion showed an adenocarcinoma. After the ruling out of metastases, a left upper lobectomy was done. Clubbing of the fingers and toes resolved within three months after the operation.

Questions

I.   Fill in the Blank

Fill in the blank with the appropriate term.

1. The meanings of the word elements in the term osteoarthropathy (osteo, arthro, and pathy) are _____.
2. Osteoarthropathy means _____.
3. The meanings of the word elements in the term arthralgia (arth and algia) are _____.
4. Arthralgia means _____.

II.   Matching

Match the term to its meaning. (The same meaning may be used more than once.) Insert the appropriate letter in the space next to the question number.

Choices:

_____ 1. clubbing
_____ 2. hypertrophic
_____ 3. rheumatoid arthritis
_____ 4. adenosarcoma
_____ 5. periostitis
_____ 6. lobectomy
_____ 7. bronchoscopy

a. glandular and muscular tissue tumor
b. inflammation of bone covering
c. curving of nails with fingertip enlargement
d. chronic form of crippling arthritis
e. increase in size of an organ
f. surgical removal of a lobe of an organ
g. procedure used to examine the respiratory passages

III.   Spell Check

Circle each incorrectly spelled term and write it correctly in the space provided.

1. adenosarcoma   _____
2. bronkescopy   _____
3. clubing   _____
4. diarhea   _____
5. edema   _____
6. hypertrofic   _____
7. lobektomy   _____
8. ostioarthropathy   _____
9. periostitis   _____
10. roentenogram   _____

H. Increasing Your Medical Terminology Word Power 2

1. Read the following report.
2. Prepare to answer the questions at the end of the section.
3. Circle all unfamiliar terms with a red pencil.
4. Underline familiar terms with a blue pencil.
5. Use your knowledge of word elements, a medical dictionary, and the key terms to find the meaning of unfamiliar terms.

Necrotizing Fasciitis

Key Terms

anesthesia (an'-es-THĒ-zē-a)   partial or complete loss of feeling with or without a loss of consciousness

crepitation (krep-i-TĀ-shun)   crackling sound

histology (his-TOL-ō-jē)   microscopic study of tissue

necrosis (nē-KRŌ-sis)   dead tissue surrounded by healthy parts

perirectal (per'-i-REK-tal)   around the rectum

postoperative   period following surgery

prognosis (prog-NŌ-sis)   prediction of the outcome of a disease and an estimate of the possibility for recovery

rectum (REK-tum)   lower part of the large intestine

superficial fascia (soo'-per-FISH-al FASH-ē-a)   fibrous covering that supports and separates muscles

debridement (dā-brēd-MON)   removal of dead or damaged tissue

tissue (TISH-ū)   group of similar cells that acts together

1 NTRODUCTION AND OVERVIEW

The disease state, *necrotizing fasciitis*, is a relatively rare, rapidly acting, soft-tissue infection. The superficial fascia are primarily involved. The infection often extends to the surrounding tissues and leads to their destruction. The necrotizing process is generally quite rapid and eventually involves the skin. The prognosis of necrotizing fasciitis depends to a large extent on the promptness of an accurate diagnosis and appropriate treatment. Effective treatment mainly consists of surgical debridement of all necrotic tissue and the administration of antibiotics and (if available) an enzyme to neutralize the tissue-destructive enzyme of the causative bacterium. Necrotizing fasciitis occurs postoperatively, after minor injury, or after inadequate care of perirectal abscesses or skin ulcers.

$\mathcal{T}$HE REVIEW

A review was conducted of 15 cases of necrotizing fasciitis that occurred over a 10-year period. The review involved all medical records, surgical summaries, biopsy (BĪ-op-sē) and autopsy (AW-top-sē) reports, and histologic slides used for diagnosis. The histologic findings included necrosis of superficial fascia, presence of microorganisms within the destroyed fascia, and an absence of muscle involvement.

The patients in the study were compared with respect to age, underlying disease, specific signs and symptoms, antibiotic administration, and supportive care. The particular signs of several patients were nonspecific and included edema or tissue swelling, erythema (redness), skin necrosis, skin ulcerations, blisters, local loss of feeling (anesthesia), occasional crepitation from involved areas, and a slight fever. The average age of the patients was 54.1 years with a range of 18 to 83. In the majority of cases, the initiating cause was a minor cut. Diagnosis was based on histologic examination and isolation of several microorganisms associated with skin and related tissue infections. The mortality rate was 45.5 percent.

This study clearly showed that the diagnosis of necrotizing fasciitis early in the development of the disease was difficult. It is also quite obvious from this study that rapid, life-saving surgical debridement of the necrotic tissue requires early recognition and diagnosis of necrotizing fasciitis and its differentiation from other diseases.

Questions

I.   Matching

Match the term to its meaning. (The same meaning may be used more than once.) Insert the appropriate letter in the space next to the question number.

Choices:

_____ **1.** debridement
_____ **2.** fascia
_____ **3.** crepitation
_____ **4.** superficial
_____ **5.** necrotic
_____ **6.** fasciitis
_____ **7.** edema
_____ **8.** anesthesia

a. excessive fluid in tissue
b. connective tissue layer covering muscles
c. inflammation of fascia
d. tissue that is dying or dead
e. crackling sound
f. surgical removal of dead tissue
g. limited to the surface
h. loss of feeling

II.   Spell Check

Circle each incorrectly spelled term and write it correctly in the space provided.

1. edeema _____
2. fashitis _____
3. necrotic _____
4. debridement _____
5. fashea _____
6. superficial _____

I. Increasing Your Medical Terminology Word Power 3

1. Read the following report.
2. Prepare to answer the questions at the end of the section.
3. Circle all unfamiliar terms with a red pencil.
4. Underline familiar terms with a blue pencil.
5. Use your knowledge of word elements, a medical dictionary, and the key terms to find the meaning of unfamiliar terms.

An Avulsed Phalanx Replacement with Tissue-Engineered Bone

Key Terms

allograft (AL-ō-graft)   transplant tissue from the same species, i.e., human to human

autograft (AW-tō-graft)   graft transferred from one part of a patient's body to another

autologous (aw-TOL-ō-gus)   something having its origin within an individual

avulsion (a-VUL-zhun)   bone or tissue that is torn but still attached

demineralized   loss of mineral salts, such as calcium, from bones

graft   tissue that is transplanted in a part of the body

inert   inactive; having little or no ability to react

matrix (MĀ-triks)   basic substance from which a structure or object is made

pedicle (PED-i-kl)   stemlike structure that attaches a new growth

polypeptide   protein-like compound; formed by the union of several amino acids

vascularized (VAS-kū-lar-īzd)   pertaining to development of new blood vessels in a structure

G ENERAL BACKGROUND

For several years, various approaches have been used to replace bone lost to trauma or disease. Attempts have included joint reconstruction with newly amputated or cadaveric allografts. In more recent years, *autografts* and *allografts* have been used extensively to replace bone. Several natural or synthetic bone substitutes have also been used, alone or in conjunction with demineralized bone, as vascularized or nonvascularized grafts. In addition, there have been numerous reports about the use of polypeptides or demineralized bone powder to stimulate bone development.

More recently, living cells have been implanted in conjunction with inert materials. In this type of tissue engineering, living cells are implanted in a recipient after the cells are seeded in some type of *supportive structure* (**template**) that guides its regeneration. The template is designed and constructed so that cells can be nourished as they generate a new matrix, blood vessel development occurs, and function is restored.

C ASE REPORT

A 40-year-old male in whom the dorsal skin, nail, nail bed, extensor tendon, and distal phalanx of the right thumb had been torn off in a machine accident presented for treatment. The patient was right-handed. The medical history of the patient was unremarkable.

Within one hour after the injury, the patient's wound was debrided and covered with a pedicle of abdominal skin. The pedicle was partially dissected from the abdomen on postoperative days 8 and 14, and the flap of skin on the thumb was completely separated from the abdomen on postoperative day 18. The donor site of the patient healed well, as did the abdominal skin attached to the thumb.

The possibility of generating a tissue-engineered phalanx was discussed with the patient. The patient agreed to the procedure, and signed an informed consent form. A plan was subsequently developed for the procedure to replace the avulsed phalanx.

Questions

I.   Fill in the Blank

Fill in the blank with the appropriate term.

1. Tissue transplanted from one part of an individual's body to another part is called a(n) _____.

2. A substance with little or no ability to react is referred to as being _____.

3. A protein-like compound formed by the union of several amino acids is called a(n) _____.

4. Tissue that is transplanted or implanted in a part of the body for purposes of repairing a defect or part replacement is called a(n) _____.

II.   Spell Check

Circle each incorrectly spelled term and write it correctly in the space provided.

1. avulsun   _____
2. autologus   _____
3. matrix   _____
4. demineralized _____
5. vascularized   _____
6. alograft   _____

Term Search Challenge

Locate 13 terms in the puzzle.

1. Write the specific term next to its definition. Then find that term in the puzzle diagram and circle it.

2. Term may be read from left to right, backward, up, down, or diagonally.

3. If a term appears more than once, circle it only once. (A term or abbreviation may be found inside others.)

4. Check your answers.

Clues:

1. Muscles that work together to perform a particular action

_____

2. A muscle's point of attachment _____

3. The word root for smooth muscle _____

4. The word root for fascia _____

5. Two word roots for muscle _____

6. Suffix for inflammation _____

7. The term used for any muscle disease _____

8. A permanent shortening of one or more muscles

_____

9. The term for writer's cramp _____

10. The three types of muscles _____

Term Search Puzzle

```
S   Y   N   E   R   G   I   S   T   I   C   E   G
K   O   C   O   M   P   A   C   T   N   A   P   R
E   S   M   O   O   T   H   S   L   E   R   I   A
L   T   U   T   R   N   D   O   N   M   D   P   P
E   E   N   E   I   T   I   S   A   Y   I   Y   H
T   O   L   O   G   G   A   T   A   O   A   S   O
A   C   L   E   I   O   M   Y   I   P   C   I   S
L   Y   Y   O   N   T   E   O   C   A   A   S   P
F   T   G   G   C   Y   T   N   E   T   T   S   A
A   E   M   Y   O   S   I   I   G   H   L   A   S
S   A   Y   P   E   N   D   I   C   Y   L   A   M
C   E   O   N   O   S   S   E   O   L   S   S   D
I   N   O   I   T   I   S   U   C   E   T   R   I
S   I   C   O   N   T   R   A   C   T   U   R   E
```

The Skeletal System

"The invisible in us has suddenly become visible."

—Jan Lindberg, Karolinska Institute

INFORMATIONAL CHALLENGE

A. Skeletal System Functions and Bone Organization

I.   Fill in the Blank

Fill in the blank with the appropriate term.

1. The five major functions of the skeletal system are _____, _____, _____, _____, and _____.
2. The specialty that deals with the study of bones is called _____.
3. Another term for a joint is _____.
4. Two portions into which the human skeleton is conveniently divided are _____.
5. The two bone categories that are based on the distribution and size of the spaces between hard regions are _____, and _____.
6. The unspecialized cells that give rise to osteoblasts are known as _____ cells.

II.   Matching: Bone's Internal Organization

Match the term to its meaning. (The same meaning may be used more than once.) Insert the appropriate letter in the space next to the question number.

Choices:

_____ 1. osteocytes
_____ 2. lacunae
_____ 3. ossification
_____ 4. osteoblasts
_____ 5. hydroxyapatites
_____ 6. osteoclast
_____ 7. cancellous

a. small cavities in bone tissue
b. mineral salts in bone
c. removes dead or unwanted bone tissue
d. mature bone cells that help main bone
e. immature bone cells
f. bone formation
g. spongy bone

III.   Spell Check

Circle each incorrectly spelled term and write it correctly in the space provided.

1. artikulation   _____
2. osteology   _____

3. hemetopoisis _____

4. skeletel _____

5. oseous _____

6. osteocyte _____

7. lacunae _____

8. lammella _____

9. canaleculi _____

10. osteoblast _____

11. spongy _____

12. axiel _____

13. torso _____

14. appendicular _____

B. Skeletal Organization

I.   Vision Quiz 1: The Human Skeleton

Figure 13-14 shows the human skeleton. Identify and write the name of the numbered structures in the spaces provided.

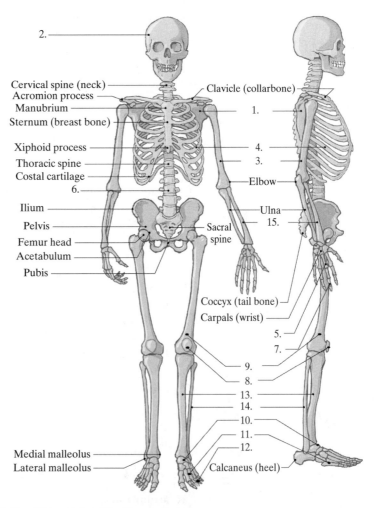

FIGURE 13-14   Vision Quiz 1. The Human Skeleton.

Choices:

1. _____	**a.** skull: provides protection for the brain and forms the face's framework
2. _____	**b.** scapula: large triangular bone that is joined to the longest bone of the arm
3. _____	**c.** humerus: the longest bone of the arm
4. _____	**d.** ribs: support the chest wall and protect the heart and lungs
5. _____	**e.** part of the spine or vertebral column: protects the spinal cord
6. _____	**f.** metacarpals: bones of the hand
7. _____	**g.** phalanges: bones of the fingers
8. _____	**h.** patella: kneecap
9. _____	**i.** femur: thigh bone
10. _____	**j.** metatarsals: bones of the feet
11. _____	**k.** tarsals: bones of the ankles
12. _____	**l.** phalanges: toe bones
13. _____	**m.** fibula: the outer and smaller bone of the leg from the ankle to the knee
14. _____	**o.** radius: the outer and shorter bone of the arm
15. _____	

II.   Vision Quiz 2: The Axial Skeleton

List by number all of the axial skeleton components shown in Figure 13-14 in the space provided. _____

III.   Spell Check

Circle each incorrectly spelled term and write it correctly in the space provided.

1. vertebrel   _____
2. metakarpel   _____
3. kranium   _____
4. hyoid   _____
5. clavicle   _____
6. shapula   _____
7. thorax   _____
8. humorus   _____
9. patella   _____
10. tarsal   _____
11. falanges   _____
12. fibulla   _____

C. *The Properties of Bone*

I.   Fill in the Blank

Fill in the blank with the appropriate term.

1. Five general types of bones found in the human skeleton are

_____, _____, _____, _____,

_____.

II.   Matching: Long Bone Organization

Match the term to its meaning. (The same meaning may be used more than once.)
Insert the appropriate letter in the space next to the question number.

Choices:

_____ **1.** consists of a layer of os-
            teoblasts lining the
            medullary cavity

_____ **2.** portion of the long bone
            that contains yellow mar-
            row

_____ **3.** the end of the long bone

_____ **4.** the hyaline cartilage cov-
            ering the epiphysis

_____ **5.** main portion of the long
            bone

_____ **6.** the covering around the
            bone

a. diaphysis
b. epiphysis
c. endosteum
d. medullary cavity
e. periosteum
f. articular cartilage

III.   Spell Check

Circle each incorrectly spelled term and write it correctly in the space provided.

1. sesamoid   _____
2. patella   _____
3. vertibrae   _____
4. diafysis   _____
5. marow   _____
6. endostium   _____
7. articular   _____
8. perriosteum   _____
9. cancellous   _____
10. Voklman's   _____

D. Bone Markings

I.   Fill in the Blank

Fill in the blank with the appropriate term.

1. Sites where blood vessels and nerves either penetrate or lie along the
     side of a bone are _____ and _____.

2. Locations where tendons and ligaments attach and where neighboring
     bones articulate are referred to as _____.

II.   Spell Check

Circle each incorrectly spelled term and write it correctly in the space provided.

1. alveolis   _____
2. fossa   _____
3. sulkus   _____
4. fissur   _____
5. foramen   _____
6. meatis   _____

7. trochanter _____
8. tuberosite _____
9. condyle _____
10. faset _____
11. tubercle _____
12. trochleea _____

E. Bones of the Body (The Skull, Sinuses, and Hyoid)

I. Fill in the Blank

Fill in the blank with the appropriate term.

1. Four major components of the axial skeleton are _____,

_____, _____, _____

2. The skull is composed of the _____ and _____
bones.

3. In a newborn infant, cranial bones not completely joined exhibit soft
spots or _____.

4. The eight bones that form the basic shape of an individual's face are

_____, _____, _____, _____,

_____, _____, _____, and

_____.

II. Matching: Cranial Bones

Match the term to its meaning. (The same meaning may be used more than once.)
Insert the appropriate letter in the space next to the question number.

Choices:

_____ 1. frontal bone
_____ 2. parietal bones
_____ 3. temporal bones
_____ 4. occipital bone
_____ 5. sphenoid bone
_____ 6. ethmoid bone

a. forms the roof of the nasal cavity
b. forms the anterior base of the
cranium
c. forms the back and most of the
skull's base
d. forms the lower sides of the cranium
e. form the upper sides and roof of the
cranium
f. forms the forehead, nasal cavity,
roof, and bony sockets that contain
the eyeballs.

III. Spell Check

Circle each incorrectly spelled term and write it correctly in the space provided.

1. vertibral _____
2. kranium _____
3. fasial _____
4. mastication _____
5. frontanelles _____
6. pareitals _____
7. occipital _____
8. etmoid _____

9. temporals   _____

10. sphenoid   _____

IV.   Vision Quiz 1: Cranial Bones

Figure 13-15 shows the cranial bones. Identify the numbered bone by matching it to one of the choices given. Insert the appropriate letter in the space provided next to each question number.

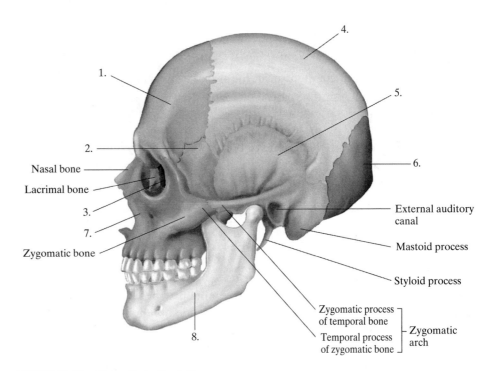

FIGURE 13-15   Vision Quiz. Cranial bones.

Choices:

1. _____   **a.** frontal bone
2. _____   **b.** sphenoid bone
3. _____   **c.** parietal bone
4. _____   **d.** ethmoid bone
5. _____   **e.** temporal bone
6. _____   **f.** maxillary bone
7. _____   **g.** occipital bone
8. _____   **h.** mandible

V.   Vision Quiz 2: Facial Bones

Figure 13-16 shows a frontal view of the skull. Identify the numbered facial bone by matching it to one of the choices given. Insert the appropriate letter in the space provided next to each question number.

Choices:

1. _____   **a.** frontal bone
2. _____   **b.** nasal bone

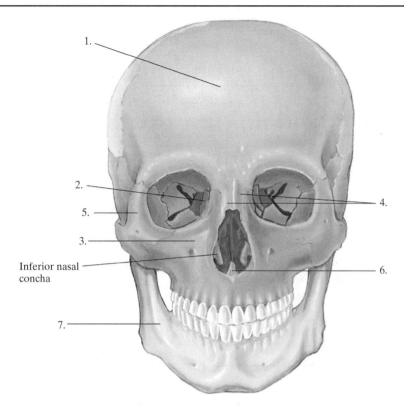

1.

2.

5.

3.

Inferior nasal
concha

7.

4.

6.

FIGURE 13-16   Vision Quiz. Facial bones.

3. _____   **c.** zygomatic bone
4. _____   **d.** lacrimal bone
5. _____   **e.** vomer
6. _____   **f.** maxilla
7. _____   **g.** mandible

F. Vertebral Column and Vertebra Structure

I.   Fill in the Blank

Fill in the blank with the appropriate term.

1. The fibrocartilage located between vertebral bodies is called an

_____ _____.

2. The bone that connects the breastbone to each shoulder bone is called
the _____.

3. The total number of ribs in the human body is _____.

4. Another name for the shoulder bone is the _____.

5. The lower portion of the breastbone or sternum is called the

_____.

II.   Spell Check

Circle each incorrectly spelled term and write it correctly in the space provided.

1. vertebrae   _____

2. thorasic   _____

3. lumber _____

4. sacral _____

5. cocygeal _____

6. spinus _____

7. pedicles _____

8. leminae _____

9. sternem _____

10. skapula _____

11. manubrium _____

12. xifoid _____

III.   Vision Quiz: Vertebral Column

Figure 13-17 shows a vertebral column. Identify the numbered region or related structure by matching it to one of the choices given. Insert the appropriate letter in the space provided next to each question number.

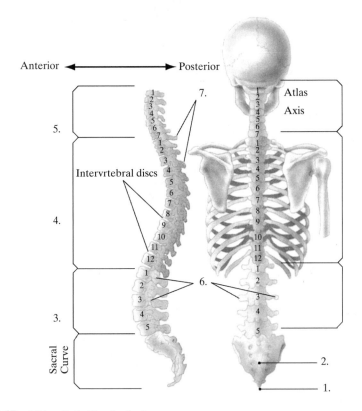

FIGURE 13-17   Vision Quiz. Vertebral column.

1. _____

2. _____

3. _____

4. _____

5. _____

6. _____

7. _____

8. _____

Choices:

a. cervical vertebrae

b. transverse processes

c. thoracic vertebrae

d. spinous processes

e. lumbar vertebrae

f. intervertebral foramina

g. sacrum

h. coccyx

G. *The Pelvic Girdle and Upper and Lower Extremities*

I.   Fill in the Blank

Fill in the blank with the appropriate term.

   1. The pectoral girdle consists of two _____ and two
         _____.

   2. Each coxa or hip bone consists of one _____, one
         _____, and one _____.

   3. The bones of one hip bone fuse in the region known as the
         _____.

II.   Matching: Pelvic and Pectoral Girdles and the Upper and Lower
        Extremities Parts

Match the term to its meaning. (The same meaning may be used more than once.)
Insert the appropriate letter in the space next to the question number.

                                        Choices:

_____ **1.** pubic symphysis   **a.** pectoral girdle
_____ **2.** humerus   **b.** pelvic girdle
_____ **3.** patella   **c.** lower extremities (legs)
_____ **4.** tibia   **d.** upper extremities (arms)
_____ **5.** carpals
_____ **6.** olecranon
_____ **7.** lateral malleolus
_____ **8.** tarsals

III.   Fill in the Blank: Singular and Plural Forms

Fill in the blank with the appropriate term.

	Singular	**Plural**
1.	_____	scapulae
2.	clavicle	_____
3.	_____	phalanges
4.	carpal	_____
5.	tarsal	_____

IV.   Spell Check

Circle each incorrectly spelled term and write it correctly in the space provided.

   1. scapular   _____
   2. clavecle   _____
   3. acromion   _____
   4. humeris   _____
   5. ulna   _____
   6. carpel   _____
   7. coxal   _____
   8. olecranon   _____
   9. flanges   _____
   10. ischeum   _____
   11. sacroilliac _____

12. tibia   _____

13. tarsis   _____

14. calcaneus   _____

15. fibula   _____

16. patela   _____

V.   Vision Quiz: The Human Hand

Figure 13-18 shows a view of the hand. Identify and write the name of the numbered part in the spaces provided.

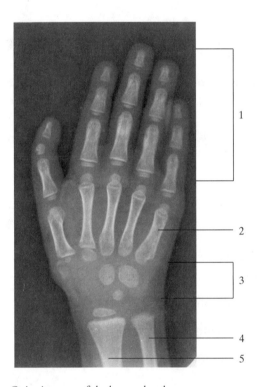

FIGURE 13-18   Vision Quiz. An x-ray of the human hand.

1. _____

2. _____

3. _____

4. _____

5. _____

H. Word Roots and/or Combining Form for Bones and the Skeleton

I.   Fill in the Blank

Fill in the blank with the appropriate term.

1. Two combining forms for vertebra are _____ and

_____

2. The combining form for bone is _____

3. The combining form for the spinal column is _____

II.   Matching: Combining Forms for Bones and/or the Skeleton

Match the term to its meaning. (The same meaning may be used more than once.)
Insert the appropriate letter in the space next to the question number.

                                          Choices:

_____ **1.** scoli/o   **a.** crooked
_____ **2.** lamin/o   **b.** flattened
_____ **3.** chondr/o   **c.** cartilage
_____ **4.** lumb/o   **d.** lower back
_____ **5.** myel/o   **e.** bone marrow

III.   Spell Check

Circle each incorrectly spelled term and write it correctly in the space provided.

1. condrogensis   _____
2. laminitis   _____
3. lumber   _____
4. myelopathy   _____
5. rakigraph   _____
6. scoliosis   _____
7. spondylodinea   _____
8. vertebrectomy   _____

IV.   Word Analysis: Word Roots, Combining Forms, and Suffixes for Bones and Skeleton

Table 13-10 lists a number of terms with their pronunciations and definitions.

TABLE 13-10   WORD ANALYSIS: WORD ROOTS, COMBINING FORMS, AND SUFFIXES FOR BONES AND SKELETON

Term and Pronunciation	Definition
chondrogenesis (kon'-drō-JEN-e-sis)	cartilage formation
laminitis (lam-in-Ī-tis)	inflammation of a lamina
lumbar (LUM-bar)	pertaining to lower back
myelopathy (mī-e-LOP-a-thē)	any pathological condition of the spinal cord
osteogenesis (os'-tē-ō-JEN-ē-sis)	bone formation
rachigraph (RĀ-ki-graf)	instrument for outlining the curves of the spine
scoliosis (sko'-lē-Ō-sis)	lateral curvature of the spine
spondylodynia (spon'-di-lō-DIN-ē-a)	pain in a vertebrae
vertebrectomy (ver-tē-BREK-tō-mē)	excision of a vertebra or a part of one

1. Analyze each term.
2. Circle all combining forms, word roots, and suffixes and label them **cf**, **wr**, and **s** respectively.
3. Check your answers (shown in Table 13-13).

I. *Word Roots and/or Combining Forms for Specific Bones*

I.   Matching: Word Roots and/or Combining Forms for Specific Bones

Match the term to its meaning. (The same meaning may be used more than once.) Insert the appropriate letter in the space next to the question number.

Choices:

_____ **1.** pelvic	**a.** clavicul/o
_____ **2.** wrist bones	**b.** mandibul/o
_____ **3.** ribs	**c.** carp/o
_____ **4.** clavicle	**d.** pelvi
_____ **5.** lower jaw bone	**e.** maxillo/o
_____ **6.** upper jaw bone	**f.** cost/o
_____ **7.** skull bones	**g.** crani/o

II.   Spell Check

Circle each incorrectly spelled term and write it correctly in the space provided.

    1. carpoptoesis   _____
    2. clavicular   _____
    3. costectemy   _____
    4. craniomelacia   _____
    5. fibular   _____
    6. humeral   _____
    7. mandibular   _____
    8. maxilitis   _____
    9. patellar   _____
  10. radiel   _____
  11. pubik   _____
  12. scapulectomy   _____

III.   Word Analysis: Word Roots, Combining Forms, and Suffixes for Specific Bones

Table 13-11 lists a number of terms with their pronunciations and definitions.

TABLE 13-11   WORD ANALYSIS: WORD ROOTS, COMBINING FORMS, AND SUFFIXES FOR SPECIFIC BONES

Term and Pronunciation	Definition
carpoptosis (kar'-pop-TŌ-sis)	sagging wrist; wrist drop
clavicular (kla-VIK-ū-lar)	pertaining to the clavicle
costectomy (kos-TEK-tō-mē)	surgical excision of a rib

(Continued)

TABLE 13-11   (CONTINUED)

Term and Pronunciation	Definition
craniomalacia (krā'-nē-ō-ma-LĀ-shē-a)	softening of the skull bones
fibular (FIB-ū-lar)	pertaining to the fibula
humeral (HŪ-mer-al)	pertaining to the humerus
mandibular (man-DIB-ū-lar)	pertaining to the mandible (lower jaw bone)
maxillitis (maks'-il-Ī-tis)	inflammation of the maxilla (upper jaw bone)
patellar (pa-TEL-ar)	pertaining to the kneecap
pelvioplasty (PEL-vi-ō-plas'-tē)	surgical repair of the pelvis
pubic (PŪ-bik)	pertaining to the pubis
radial (RĀ-dē-al)	pertaining to the radius
scapulectomy (skap'-ū-LEK-tō-mē)	surgical excision of the scapula
tibiofemoral (tib'-i-ō-FE-mor-al)	pertaining to the tibia and femur

1. Analyze each term.
2. Circle all combining forms, word roots, and suffixes, and label them **cf**, **wr**, and **s**, respectively.
3. Check your answers (shown in Table 13-14).

J. Skeletal Injuries and Disorders

I.   Fill in the Blank

Fill in the blank with the appropriate term.

1. The two major categories of fractures are _____, and _____.
2. The procedure used to set a fracture is called a _____ _____.
3. The procedure requiring exposure of the fracture before it is set is called _____ _____.
4. The condition resulting when one bone end forming a joint is displaced from its normal position is known as a _____.
5. _____ are injuries in which ligaments are stretched and partially torn.
6. _____ are injuries to soft tissue that occur around a joint.

II.   Matching 1: Fracture Types

Match the term to its meaning. (The same meaning may be used more than once.)
Insert the appropriate letter in the space next to the question number.

_____ **1.** break across the long axis of the bone
_____ **2.** a break occurs in the overlying skin

_____ **3.** transverse fracture only on one side of the bone
_____ **4.** the break line crosses the bone at an angle to the shaft
_____ **5.** fracture line has appearance of a coil
_____ **6.** broken ends of a fracture are jammed into one another
_____ **7.** bone is fragmented into more than two pieces
_____ **8.** a fracture of the distal end of the fibula
_____ **9.** a fracture of the distal end of the radius
_____ **10.** a completely internal breakage of bone

Choices:

a. compound fracture	**f.** comminuted fracture
b. greenstick fracture	**g.** impacted fracture
c. spiral fracture	**h.** Colle's fracture
d. transverse fracture	**i.** Pott's fracture
e. oblique fracture	**j.** closed fracture

III.   Matching 2: Spine Abnormalities and Injuries

Match the term to its meaning. (The same meaning may be used more than once.)
Insert the appropriate letter in the space next to the question number.

Choices:

_____ **1.** herniated disk   **a.** rupture of an intervertebral disk that
_____ **2.** sciatica   causes severe low back pain
_____ **3.** hyperlordosis   **b.** bulging of a disk's center through its
_____ **4.** quadriplegia   covering
_____ **5.** kyphosis   **c.** paralysis of all extremities
                                      d. increased incurving of the lumbar
                                            spine
                                      e. associated with hunch back condition

IV.   Spell Check

Circle each incorrectly spelled term and write it correctly in the space provided.

1. comminuted _____
2. kifosis _____
3. skoliosis _____
4. oblique _____
5. Pott's _____
6. frakture _____
7. tranferse _____
8. herniated _____
9. siatica _____
10. qadriplegia _____

K. Bone and Related Skeletal Abnormalities and/or Pathological States

I.   Fill in the Blank

Fill in the blank with the appropriate term.

1. The most common and abundant component found in connective
tissue is _____.

2. A major feature of rheumatic diseases is the destruction of tissue by
_____.

3. The study of bone diseases is called _____.

4. The diagnosis and treatment of the variety of diseases and abnormalities involving the musculoskeletal system is known as _____.

II.   Matching: Rheumatic Diseases and Bone Abnormalities

Match the term to its meaning. (The same meaning may be used more than once.) Insert the appropriate letter in the space next to the question number.

Choices:

_____ **1.** arthritis
_____ **2.** ankylosing spondylitis
_____ **3.** ankylosis
_____ **4.** arthropathy
_____ **5.** osteoporosis
_____ **6.** spina bifida
_____ **7.** polydactyly
_____ **8.** talipes
_____ **9.** rickets

a. inflammation and fusion of the lumbar region of the spine
b. stiff joint
c. any joint disease
d. inflammation of the joints
e. abnormal bone formation in children due to vitamin D deficiency
f. genetic vertebral column defect
g. extra digits
h. club foot
i. porous bone

III.   Spell Check

Circle each incorrectly spelled term and write it correctly in the space provided.

1. polydaktyly   _____
2. osteoma   _____
3. reumatiod   _____
4. talepis   _____
5. gowt   _____
6. ankylosing   _____
7. spondilitis   _____
8. orthopedics   _____
9. osteomalacia   _____
10. rickets   _____
11. spina bifida   _____
12. artheritis   _____
13. arthopothy   _____
14. osteoporosis   _____

L. Joints

I.   Fill in the Blank

Fill in the blank with the appropriate term.

1. The study of joints is called _____.
2. Another term for a joint is an _____.
3. A _____ joint has a joint cavity and ligaments to support articulating bones.

4. Flat, closed sacs filled with synovial fluid and found in spaces between tendons, ligaments, and bones are called _____.

5. Give an example of a location where each of the following joints can be found.
   a. synarthroses _____
   b. amphiarthroses _____
   c. diarthroses _____

II.   Matching: Functional Categories of Joints

Match the term to its meaning. (The same meaning may be used more than once.) Insert the appropriate letter in the space next to the question number.

Choices:

_____ **1.** immovable joints   **a.** amphiarthroses
_____ **2.** freely movable joints   **b.** synarthroses
_____ **3.** slightly movable joints   **c.** diarthroses

III.   Spell Check

Circle each incorrectly spelled term and write it correctly in the space provided.

1. imovable   _____
2. amfiarthoses   _____
3. articulation   _____
4. diartroses   _____
5. synarthrotic   _____
6. amphiarthrotic   _____
7. fibros   _____
8. cartilaginous   _____
9. sinoviel   _____
10. bursa   _____

M. *Operative and/or Diagnostic Procedures*

I.   Matching 1: Operative and/or Diagnostic Procedures

Match the term to its meaning. (The same meaning may be used more than once.) Insert the appropriate letter in the space next to the question number.

Choices:

_____ **1.** arthrotomy   **a.** partial or complete removal of a limb
_____ **2.** arthroscopy
_____ **3.** arthrolysis   **b.** surgical breaking of a stiff joint
_____ **4.** arthroclasia   **c.** visual examination of a joint's interior
_____ **5.** arthroplasty   **d.** reshaping of a diseased joint
_____ **6.** amputation   **e.** surgical opening of a joint
_____ **7.** arthrography   **f.** surgical restoring of a joint's mobility
                               g. roentgenography of a joint

II.   Matching 2: Operative and/or Diagnostic Procedures

Match the term to its meaning. (The same meaning may be used more than once.) Insert the appropriate letter in the space next to the question number.

Choices:

_____ **1.** bone transplantation
_____ **2.** osteotomy
_____ **3.** bone scan
_____ **4.** chondroplasty
_____ **5.** capsulotomy
_____ **6.** laminectomy
_____ **7.** tenotomy
_____ **8.** sequestrectomy

a. use of radioactive material to determine cancer spread in the body
b. surgical repair of cartilage
c. surgical cutting through bone
d. surgical cutting of a capsule
e. insertion of a bone to replace destroyed bone
f. surgical removal of a piece of dead bone
g. removal of the posterior part of a vertebral arch
h. surgical cutting of a tendon

III.   Spell Check

Circle each incorrectly spelled term and write it correctly in the space provided.

1. amputashun _____
2. arthroklasia _____
3. arthrography _____
4. arthrolysis _____
5. arthroplasty _____
6. arthrotomy _____
7. kapsulectomy _____
8. capsulotomy _____
9. condroplasty _____
10. laminectomy _____
11. ostiotomy _____
12. sequestrectomy _____
13. tennotomy _____
14. arthroscope _____

IV.   Word Analysis: Word Roots, Combining Forms, and Suffixes

Table 13-12 lists a number of terms with their pronunciations and definitions.

TABLE 13-12   WORD ANALYSIS: WORD ROOTS, COMBINING FORMS, AND SUFFIXES

Term and Pronunciation	Definition
arthredema (ar-thrē-DĒ-ma)	a swelling (edema) of a joint
arthroclasia (ar-thrō-KLĀ-zē-a)	surgical breaking of a stiff joint to provide for movement
arthrography (ar-THROG-ra-fē)	roentgenography (rent-gen-OG-ra-fē) or x-raying of a joint
arthrolysis (ar-THROL-i-sis)	surgically restoring joints' mobility
arthroplasty (AR-thrō-plas-tē)	surgical joint repair; may require the reshaping or reconstruction of a diseased joint

(Continued)

TABLE 13-12 (**CONTINUED**)

Term and Pronunciation	Definition
arthroscopy (ar-THROS-kō-pē)	visual examination of the inside of a joint; requires use of an arthroscope
arthrotomy (ar-THROT-ō-mē)	surgical opening of a joint
capsulotomy (kap'-sū-LOT-ō-mē)	surgical cutting of a capsule enclosing a joint
chondroplasty (KON-drō-plas-tē)	surgical repair of cartilage
laminectomy (lam-i-NEK-tō-mē)	excision or surgical removal of the posterior part of a vertebral arch
osteotomy (os-tē-OT-ō-mē)	surgical cutting through a bone
tenotomy (te-NOT-ō-mē)	surgical cutting of a tendon

1. Analyze each term.
2. Circle all combining forms, word roots, and suffixes, and label them **cf**, **wr**, and **s**, respectively.
3. Check your answers (shown in Table 13-15).

N. Medical Vocabulary Building

I.   Matching: Medical Vocabulary Building

Match the term to its meaning. (The same meaning may be used more than once.) Insert the appropriate letter in the space next to the question number.

Choices:

_____ 1. achillobursitis
_____ 2. acroarthritis
_____ 3. arthedema
_____ 4. cleidorrhexis
_____ 5. coxofemoral
_____ 6. metacarpectomy
_____ 7. olecranal
_____ 8. patellapexy
_____ 9. rachialgia
_____ 10. vertebrosternal

a. inflammation of hand or feet joints
b. inflammation of the bursa over the Achilles' heel
c. joint swelling
d. pertaining to the hip and femur
e. rupture of the fetus clavicle to make delivery easier
f. surgical excision of one or more hand bones
g. pertaining to the elbow
h. spine pain
i. surgical fixation of the patella
j. pertaining to the vertebra and the sternum

II.   Spell Check

Circle each incorrectly spelled term and write it correctly in the space provided.

1. akroarthritis _____
2. clidorrhexis _____

   3. olecranal   _____

   4. arthedema   _____

   5. coxofemorel   _____

   6. rackialgia   _____

O. Abbreviations

I.   Matching 1: Abbreviations Associated with the Skeletal System

Match the term to its meaning. (The same meaning may be used more than once.)
Insert the appropriate letter in the space next to the question number.

Choices:

_____ **1.** Ca	**a.**	fracture
_____ **2.** IS	**b.**	limitation of motion
_____ **3.** LOM	**c.**	calcium
_____ **4.** P	**d.**	metacarpal-phalangeal
_____ **5.** Fx	**e.**	intercostal space
_____ **6.** MP	**f.**	phosphorus
_____ **7.** RA	**g.**	rheumatoid arthritis

II.   Matching 2: Abbreviations Associated with the Skeletal System

Match the term to its meaning. (The same meaning may be used more than once.)
Insert the appropriate letter in the space next to the question number.

Choices:

_____ **1.** RF	**a.**	range of motion
_____ **2.** CD	**b.**	orthopedics
_____ **3.** THR	**c.**	rheumatoid factor
_____ **4.** ROM	**d.**	congenital dislocation of the hip
_____ **5.** Ortho	**e.**	total hip replacement
_____ **6.** KD	**f.**	knee disarticulation
_____ **7.** TKR	**g.**	total knee replacement

III.   Spell Check

Circle each incorrectly spelled term and write it correctly in the space provided.

   1. extremite   _____

   2. intercostal   _____

   3. phosforus   _____

   4. disarticulation   _____

   5. derangement   _____

   6. proximal   _____

P. Increasing Your Medical Terminology Word Power 1

   1. Read the following report.

   2. Prepare to answer the questions at the end of the section.

   3. Circle all unfamiliar terms with a red pencil.

   4. Underline familiar terms with a blue pencil.

   5. Use your knowledge of word elements, a medical dictionary, and the
key terms to find the meaning of unfamiliar terms.

Paget's (PAJ-ets) Disease

Key Terms

bone scan   a shortened form of *scintiscan* (SIN-ti-skan); refers to a technique to determine the outline and function of bones into which radioactive substances are introduced.

etiology (ē-tē-OL-ō-jē)   cause of a disease

hypercalcemia (hī-per-kal-SĒ-mē-a)   excessive calcium in the blood

hypercalciuria (hī-per-kal-sē-Ū-rē-a)   excessive calcium in the urine

neoplastic (nē-ō-PLAS-tik)   new, abnormal tissue formation

paget's disease   skeletal disease of the elderly resulting in bone thickening and softening and a curvature or bowing of the long bones

rheumatologic (roo'-ma-tō-LOJ-ik)   having rheumatism (ROO-ma-tiz-em), i.e., muscle inflammation, soreness, and stiffness and pain in the joints and associated structures

tibial bowing   curving of the tibia

I NTRODUCTION AND OVERVIEW

Paget's disease of the bone is a common, sometimes crippling, disorder. Unfortunately, the understanding of its etiology and pathogenesis is still incomplete. Paget's disease begins in middle age or later, is very slow to progress, and may give no problems other than those caused by the changes in size, shape, and direction of the diseased bones. Studies have shown that a localized, disorganized increase in osteoclastic bone resorption seems to be the primary event in the disease.

Paget's disease is usually symptomatic in middle-aged and elderly persons. Its prevalence in persons older than 40 years is about 3 percent, and men and women are affected equally. The disease can be detected readily by x-ray or, when active, by bone scan. Paget's disease can involve any bone, but it has a high incidence of involvement with those of the axial skeleton.

F EATURES OF THE DISEASE

About 10 percent to 20 percent of patients have signs and symptoms such as bone pain, deformity, and fractures. The commonest sites involved are the sacrum, spine, femurs, skull, sternum, and pelvis. Paget's disease often begins as breaking apart of the bone.

The bony deformities of Paget's disease are caused by abnormal remodeling of weight-bearing bones and include tibia bowing and skull defects. The complications of Paget's disease may be grouped into the following four categories: rheumatologic, neurologic, metabolic, and neoplastic. Rheumatologic complications are common. Osteoarthritis may be a finding or may result from abnormal stresses. With respect to the neurologic complications, the brain, spinal cord, and peripheral nerves are all at risk for involvement. Metabolic complications appear as a net increase in bone restoration. Locally this may reveal itself as rapid bone softening and destruction, and systematically it may present as hypercalciuria and hypercalcemia. The most severe complication of Paget's disease is the development of bone sarcoma. These tumors usually occur with swelling and increased pain. Radiologically, they often appear as destructive lesions.

Questions

I.   Fill in the Blank

Fill in the blank with the appropriate term.

1. Indicate the types of word elements in the term *hypercalcemia*.
 a. *hyper* is a _____
 b. *calc* is a _____
 c. *emia* is a _____
2. *Hypercalcemia* means _____.
3. Where is the tibia located? _____

II.   Matching: Paget's Disease

Match the term to its meaning. (The same meaning may be used more than once.) Insert the appropriate letter in the space next to the question number.

Choices:

_____ **1.** etiology
_____ **2.** hypercalciuria
_____ **3.** hypercalcemia
_____ **4.** tibial bowing
_____ **5.** neoplastic
_____ **6.** Paget's disease

a. excess calcium in blood
b. tibia curving
c. pertains to new abnormal tissue formation
d. excess calcium in urine
e. cause
f. disease among the elderly with bone thickening and softening as well as curving of the long bones

III.   Spell Check

Circle each incorrectly spelled term and write it correctly in the space provided.

1. etialogy   _____
2. hyperkalcemia _____
3. hypercalciuria _____
4. kneoplastic   _____
5. rhumatologic   _____
6. tibeal   _____
7. calcium   _____
8. Paget's   _____

Q. *Increasing Your Medical Terminology Word Power 2*

1. Read the following report.
2. Prepare to answer the questions at the end of the section.
3. Circle all unfamiliar terms with a red pencil.
4. Underline familiar terms with a blue pencil.
5. Use your knowledge of word elements, a medical dictionary, and the key terms to find the meaning of unfamiliar terms.

Hypertrophic Osteoarthropathy Syndrome

Key Terms

adenosarcoma (ad-e-nō-sar-KŌ-ma)   tumor having features of glandular and muscular tissues

bronchoscopy (brong-KOS-kō-pē) examination of the bronchi with the use of a bronchoscope, an instrument that passes through the windpipe to allow viewing of the respiratory passages.

clubbing a common sign in diseases of the lungs and appears as curving of the nails accompanied by the enlargement of the soft tissues of the fingers and toes.

diarrhea (dī-a-RĒ-a) frequent passage of watery bowel movements

edema (e-DĒ-ma) accumulation of fluid in the tissues

hypertrophic (hī-per-TROF-ik) increase in the size of an organ or structure; does not involve tumor formation

lobectomy (lō-BEK-tō-mē) surgical removal of the lobe from any organ or gland

osteoarthropathy (os'-tē-ō-ar-THROP-a-thē) any disease involving the joints and bones

periostitis (per-ē-os-TĪ-tis) inflammation of the membrane covering a bone except at its articulations

roentgenogram (rō-ent-JEN-ō-gram) picture produced by a type of x-ray

G ENERAL BACKGROUND

The hypertrophic osteoarthropathy syndrome is characterized by the presence of periostitis, new bone formation, arthritis, and clubbing of the digits.

The syndrome can also accompany cardiac disease, liver disease, gastrointestinal diseases producing acute diarrhea, and other conditions. In its primary form, clubbing, bone changes, increased sweating of the palms and soles, and a pronounced thickening of the skin of the face, forehead, and scalp occur. While clubbing of the digits is a prominent feature of the syndrome, it is not always present. When clubbing is associated with periostitis of the distal ends of the long bone, the roentgenogram is the key to a correct diagnosis. The ulna and radius are involved in 80 percent of cases, and the tibia and fibula in 74 percent. A unique feature of this syndrome is the presence of lower-extremity edema and bone pain.

C ASE HISTORY

A 38-year-old male was admitted to the medical center showing mild edema and *arthralgia* (ar-THRAL-jē-a). The patient indicated that he never had arthritis and that both conditions improved with the elevation of his feet and the use of anti-inflammatory agents such as ordinary aspirin. A heavy smoker, the patient had smoked two packs of cigarettes per day since the age of 18.

The patient was principally admitted to the hospital for an evaluation of a 2 cm coin lesion that was discovered in chest films of the left lung. A bronchoscopic biopsy of the lesion showed the presence of adenocarcinoma, and after the ruling out of metastases, a left upper lobectomy was done. Clubbing of the fingers and toes resolved within three months after the operation.

Questions

I.   Fill in the Blank

Fill in the blank with the appropriate term.

1. Indicate the types of word elements in the term osteoarthropathy: osteo is a _____, arthro is a _____, and pathy is a _____.

2. Osteoarthropathy means _____.
3. Indicate the types of word elements in the term arthralgia: arth is a
   _____; algia is a _____.
4. Arthralgia means _____.

II.   Matching

Match the term to its meaning. (The same meaning may be used more than once.)
Insert the appropriate letter in the space next to the question number.

Choices:

_____ **1.** clubbing
_____ **2.** hypertrophic
_____ **3.** rheumatoid arthritis
_____ **4.** adenosarcoma
_____ **5.** periostitis
_____ **6.** lobectomy
_____ **7.** bronchoscopy

a. glandular and muscular tissue tumor
b. inflammation of bone covering
c. curving of the nails with finger en-largement
d. chronic form of crippling arthritis
e. increase in organ size
f. surgical removal of a lobe of an organ
g. procedure used to examine the respiratory passages

III.   Spell Check

Circle each incorrectly spelled term and write it correctly in the space provided.

1. roentgenogram   _____
2. hypertrofic   _____
3. periostitus   _____
4. diarrhea   _____
5. clubing   _____
6. lobectomy   _____

R. *Increasing Your Medical Terminology Word Power 3*

1. Read the following report.
2. Prepare to answer the questions at the end of the section.
3. Circle all unfamiliar terms with a red pencil.
4. Underline familiar terms with a blue pencil.
5. Use your knowledge of word elements, a medical dictionary, and the key terms to find the meaning of unfamiliar terms.

Sacral Fracture with Compression of Cauda Equina

Key Terms

cauda equina (KAW-da ē-KWIN-a)   the end portion of the spinal cord and the spinal nerve roots below the first lumbar nerve

compression (kom-PRESH-un)   squeezed together

dysesthesia (dis-es-THĒ-zē-a)   abnormal sensation or feeling on the skin, such as numbness, tingling, or burning

laminectomy (lam-i-NEK-tō-mē)   excision of a vertebral posterior arch

C ASE REPORT

A 26-year-old male roofer fell 30 feet, landing on his buttocks and outstretched left leg. Immediately on impact, he experienced severe sacral pain and numbness of his *genitalia* (jen-i-TAL-ē-a).

The accident victim had a transverse fracture of the sacrum between S2 and S3 levels. Computerized tomography (tō-MOG-ra-fē) of the sacrum also revealed longitudinal (lon-ji-TU-di-nal) fractures of the left side of the sacrum. The patient received appropriate medication every six hours beginning with admission and continuing for one week postoperatively.

Forty-eight hours after admission, the patient underwent a sacral *laminectomy* of S2 and S3. A simple cast was applied to the left *fibular* (FIB-ū-lar) fracture. Postoperatively, the patient's recovery was slow. A *dysesthetic* (dis-es-THES-tik) pain in the left foot gradually disappeared. Intensive physical therapy was required to enable the patient to walk.

The case reported here is one of a complex fracture of the sacrum with both transverse and longitudinal components to the fracture. Compression of the cauda equina is one condition observed in these types of situations.

Questions

I.   Fill in the Blank

Fill in the blank with the appropriate term.

1.   Where were longitudinal fractures found in the patient? _____
2.   The sacral *laminectomy* involved what parts of the spinal cord?

     _____

3.   *Dysesthesia* means _____
4.   One condition observed in cases of complex fractures of the sacrum involving both transverse and longitudinal components of the fracture is _____

II.   Spell Check

Circle each incorrectly spelled term and write it correctly in the space provided.

1.   compresion   _____
2.   dysesthestic   _____
3.   computerized   _____
4.   fibuler   _____
5.   genetalia   _____
6.   cauda equina   _____

Term Search Challenge

Locate 16 terms in the puzzle.

1.   Write the specific term next to its definition. Then find that term in the puzzle diagram and circle it.
2.   Terms may be read from left to right, backward, up, down, or diagonally.
3.   If a term appears more than once, circle it only once. (A term or abbreviation may be found inside others.)
4.   Check your answers.

Clues:

1. The study of bone _____

2. The structure that attaches muscles to bones

   _____

3. Bone also is known as this kind of tissue _____

4. The skeleton portion that contains the bones of the upper and lower extremities_____

5. The musculoskeletal component that binds bones to bones

   _____

6. A mature bone cell _____

7. The type of bone that is relatively solid _____

8. The five major types of bones _____, _____,

   _____, _____, _____.

9. U-shaped bone in a superior position of the larynx

   _____

10. Injury to a joint _____

11. Two terms for the location where bones meet _____,

    _____

Term Search Puzzle

S	P	R	A	I	N	C	T	I	T	O	J	R
E	O	C	O	M	P	A	C	T	N	S	O	A
S	S	L	S	H	O	R	T	L	E	T	I	C
A	T	U	T	E	N	D	O	N	M	E	N	T
M	E	N	E	L	I	G	A	M	E	N	T	U
O	O	L	O	N	G	A	T	A	G	F	S	R
I	C	L	L	T	F	C	E	N	I	L	I	E
D	Y	Y	O	S	T	E	O	C	L	A	S	T
G	T	G	G	H	Y	O	I	D	S	T	S	R
C	E	A	Y	I	R	R	E	G	U	L	A	R
A	A	P	P	E	N	D	I	C	U	L	A	R
N	E	E	N	O	S	S	E	O	U	S	S	R
A	N	O	I	T	A	L	U	C	I	T	R	A

Blood Components and Functions

"Of all the infectious diseases there is no doubt that malaria has caused the greatest harm to the greatest number."

—Laderman, 1975

INFORMATIONAL CHALLENGE

A. Blood Components and Functions

I.   Fill in the Blank

Fill in the blank with the appropriate term.

1. The liquid or fluid portion of blood is called _____.
2. The process for blood formation is hemato-_____.
3. The process of red blood cell formation is erythro-_____.
4. List two agranulocytes. _____ and _____
5. The process that separates plasma from the formed elements of blood is called _____.
6. The three types of globulins are _____, _____, and _____.

II.   Matching 1: Components and Functions of Blood

Match the term to its meaning. (The same meaning may be used more than once.) Insert the appropriate letter in the space next to the question number.

Choices:

_____ 1. plasma cells
_____ 2. erythrocytes
_____ 3. monocyte
_____ 4. platelets
_____ 5. neutrophil
_____ 6. hemoglobin
_____ 7. albumin
_____ 8. eosinophil
_____ 9. basophil

a. fragments of megakaryocytes
b. has kidney-shaped nucleus
c. example of a granulocyte
d. carries oxygen to body tissues
e. produce antibodies (immunoglobulins)
f. one type of protein found in plasma
g. oxygen-carrying pigment in red blood cells
h. largest leukocyte
i. contains blue- or basic-staining granules
j. most plentiful leukocyte

III.   Matching 2: Blood Coagulation

Match the term to its meaning. (The same meaning may be used more than once.)
Insert the appropriate letter in the space next to the question number.

Choices:

_____	**1.** fibrinogen	**a.** fluid from clotted blood
_____	**2.** heparin	**b.** insoluble threads of fibrinogen formed when blood clots
_____	**3.** serum	
_____	**4.** thrombin	**c.** an anticoagulant
_____	**5.** fibrin	**d.** source of fibrin
_____	**6.** hemostasis	**e.** converts fibrinogen into fibrin
_____	**7.** thrombus	**f.** stopping the bleeding from a damaged blood vessel
_____	**8.** prothrombin	**g.** blood clot
		h. plasma coagulation factor that is converted to thrombin by the combined actions of various factors and calcium

IV.   Spell Check

Circle each incorrectly spelled term and write it correctly in the space provided.

   1. capillarys   _____
   2. lookocyte   _____
   3. albumin   _____
   4. imuknoglobulin   _____
   5. hematopoesis   _____
   6. baseophil   _____
   7. polymorphonuclear _____
   8. nutrophil   _____
   9. anticoagulent   _____
  10. makrophaje   _____
  11. coegulation   _____
  12. fibrinogen   _____

V.   Word Analysis 1: Word Roots and Combining Forms

Table 14-11 lists a number of terms with their pronunciations and definitions.

TABLE 14-11   WORD ANALYSIS 1: WORD ROOTS AND COMBINING FORMS

Term and Pronunciation	Definition
agglutinophilic (a-gloo-tin-ō-FIL-ik)	attraction to rapid clumping
basophilic (bā'-sō-FIL-ik)	attraction to basic stains
hypochromia (hī-pō-KRŌ-mē-a)	reduced color (refers to hemoglobin content of red blood cells)

(Continued)

TABLE 14-11   (CONTINUED)

Term and Pronunciation	Definition
eosinophilic (ē-ō-sin-ō-FIL-ik)	attraction to eosin (stain)
erythopenia (e-rith-rō-PĒ-nē-a)	deficiency of red blood cells
granulocytopenia (gran-ū-lō-sī-tō-PĒ-nē-a)	granulocytes
hematology (hē-ma-TOL-ō-jē)	the study of blood (and blood-forming tissues)
hemolysis (hē-MOL-i-sis)	destruction of red blood cells
immunogenic (im-ū-nō-JEN-ik)	inducing protection
isochromatic (ī-sō-krō-MAT-ik)	having the same color
karyocyte (KAR-ē-ō-sīt)	nucleated (blood cell)
leukocytopoiesis (loo-kō-sī-tō-poy-Ē-sis)	formation of white blood cells
monocytosis (mon-ō-sī-TŌ-sis)	abnormal number of monocytes in the blood
polymorphonuclear (pol-ē-mor-fō-NŪ-klē-ar)	nucleus with several parts
myelocyte (MĪ-el-ō-sīt)	large cell in the bone marrow from which leukocytes develop
neutrophilia (nū-trō-FIL-ē-a)	increase in the number of neutrophils
nucleophilic (nū-klē-ō-FIL-ik)	attraction to nuclei
phagocytic (fag-ō-SIT-ik)	pertaining to phagocytes or phagocytosis
poikilocytosis (poy-kil-ō-sī-TŌ-sis)	variations in red-blood-cell shapes
reticulocytosis (rē-tik-ū-lō-sī-TŌ-sis)	increase in the number of reticulocytes (cells with a network of granules of filaments)
sideropenia (sid-er-ō-PĒ-nē-a)	iron deficiency
spherocytosis (sfē-rō-sī-TŌ-sis)	condition in which red blood cells assume a spherical shape
thrombosis (throm-BŌ-sis)	blood clot development

1. Analyze each term.
2. Circle all combining forms and word roots and label them **cf** and **wr**, respectively.
3. Check your answers (shown in Table 14-13).

VI. Word Analysis 2: Suffixes

Table 14-12 lists a number of terms with their pronunciations and definitions.

TABLE 14-12   WORD ANALYSIS 2: SUFFIXES

Term and Pronunciation	Definition
erythrocytic (e-rith'-rō-SIT-ik)	pertaining to red blood cells (erythrocytes)
leukapheresis (loo-ka-fe-RĒ-sis)	removal of leukocytes from blood, which is then transfused back into the patient
lymphoblast (LIM-fō-blast)	cell that gives rise to a lymphocyte
erythrocytosis (e-rith-rō-sī-TŌ-sis)	abnormal increase in the number of red blood cells
leukemia (loo-KĒ-mē-a)	abnormal increase in the number of leukocytes
hemoglobin (hē-mō-GLŌ-bin)	iron-carrying protein in red blood cells
immunoglobulin (im-ū-nō-GLOB-ū-lin)	protective proteins of the body; antibody
eosinophilia (ē-ō-sin-ō-FIL-ē-a)	tendency toward an increased number of eosinophils
electrophoresis (ē-lek-trō-for-ē-sis)	transport of particles in an electrical field
erythropoiesis (e-rith-rō-poy-Ē-sis)	formation of red blood cells
hemostasis (hē-MOS-tā-sis)	control of bleeding or circulation

1. Analyze each term.
2. Circle all suffixes and label them **s**.
3. Check your answers (shown in Table 14-14).

B. Word Elements Associated with Blood

I. Fill in the Blank

Fill in the blank with the appropriate term.

1. Two combining forms used to indicate *nucleus* are _____ and _____.
2. Two combining forms for *blood* are _____ and _____.
3. Two combining forms used for *red* are _____ and _____.
4. For the term *polymorphonuclear,* the prefix (p) is _____, combining form (cf) is _____, word root (wr) is _____, and suffix (s) is _____.
5. Two suffixes for *protein* are _____ and _____.

II. Matching: Combining Forms and/or Word Roots Associated with Blood

Match the term to its meaning. (The same meaning may be used more than once.) Insert the appropriate letter in the space next to the question number.

Choices:

_____ **1.** chrom/o	**a.** blood
_____ **2.** spher/o	**b.** nucleus
_____ **3.** neutr/o	**c.** equal, same
_____ **4.** hem/o	**d.** color
_____ **5.** granul/o	**e.** clot
_____ **6.** leuk/o	**f.** sphere
_____ **7.** is/o	**g.** granules
_____ **8.** kary/o	**h.** shape, form
_____ **9.** morph/o	**i.** white
_____ **10.** thromb/o	**j.** neutral

III. Spell Check

Circle each incorrectly spelled term and write it correctly in the space provided.

1. aglutinofilic _____

2. hypokromia _____

3. eocinophilic _____

4. hematology _____

5. imunogenic _____

6. kareocyte _____

7. polymorphonuclear _____

8. milocyte _____

9. nutrophilia _____

10. fagocytic _____

11. sideropenia _____

12. trombosis _____

13. lukaphiresis _____

14. erythrocytosis _____

15. erythropoesis _____

16. hemostasis _____

C. Bleeding Disorders/Diseases

I. Matching 1: Signs and Symptoms of Blood Diseases or Disorders

Match the term to its meaning. (The same meaning may be used more than once.) Insert the appropriate letter in the space next to the question number.

Choices:

_____ **1.** swelling of tissues	**a.** splenomegaly
_____ **2.** large hemorrhagic areas in the skin	**b.** edema
	c. petechiae
_____ **3.** enlarged spleen	**d.** ecchymoses
_____ **4.** yellowing	**e.** jaundice
_____ **5.** small hemorrhagic areas in the skin	**f.** lymphadenopathy
	g. macrocytic

_____ **6.** enlarged lymph nodes

_____ **7.** presence of bacteria in
blood

_____ **8.** presence of microorganisms in blood

_____ **9.** low white-blood-cell
count

_____ **10.** high white-blood-cell
count

_____ **11.** larger-than-normal sized
red blood cells

h. leukocytosis

i. septicemia

j. leukopenia

k. bacteremia

II.   Matching 2: Diseases and Disorders of the Blood and Lymphatic Systems

Match the term to its meaning. (The same meaning may be used more than once.)
Insert the appropriate letter in the space next to the question number.

Choices:

_____ **1.** myeloma

_____ **2.** acute lymphocytic
leukemia

_____ **3.** multiple myeloma

_____ **4.** chronic myelogenous
leukemia

_____ **5.** hemophilia

_____ **6.** hemochromatosis

_____ **7.** anemia

_____ **8.** sickle-cell anemia

_____ **9.** malaria

_____ **10.** HIV infection

a. deficiency in red blood cells or
hemoglobins

b. genetic deficiency of blood-factors
clotting

c. cancer with large number of immature granulocytes

d. malignancy with large number of
immature lymphocytes

e. sickle cells caused by an inherited
condition

f. malignant tumor of antibody-
producing cells

g. excessive deposits of iron in the body

h. infectious disease caused by a
protozoan

i. infectious disease that eventually results in AIDS

III.   Spell Check

Circle each incorrectly spelled term and write it correctly in the space provided.

1. borreliosis _____

2. discrasia _____

3. hemofilia _____

4. panocytopenia _____

5. polycythimea _____

6. thalasemia _____

7. granulocytosis _____

8. leukemia _____

9. lymfositic _____

10. myelogenous _____

11. myeloma _____

12. basophilia _____

D. Diagnostic Tests and Clinical Procedures

I.   Matching 1: Laboratory Tests and Clinical Procedures, Part 1

Match the term to its meaning. (The same meaning may be used more than once.) Insert the appropriate letter in the space next to the question number.

Choices:

_____ **1.** WBC count
_____ **2.** hematocrit
_____ **3.** prothrombin time
_____ **4.** WBC differential count
_____ **5.** partial thromboplastin time
_____ **6.** hemoglobin test
_____ **7.** complete blood count
_____ **8.** coagulation time
_____ **9.** erythrocyte sedimentation rate
_____ **10.** bleeding time

a. determines the percentage of different white blood cells
b. measurement of the hemoglobin content in specific volume of blood
c. determines the presence and action of blood-clotting factors
d. determines the time needed for a small wound to stop bleeding
e. determines the number of wbcs in volume of blood
f. determines time necessary for venous blood to clot
g. includes blood-cell counts and hemoglobin determination
h. detects clotting defects
i. measures volume of erythrocytes in volume of blood
j. measures speed at which rbcs settle out of plasma

II.   Matching 2: Laboratory Tests and Clinical Procedures, Part 2

Match the term to its meaning. (The same meaning may be used more than once.) Insert the appropriate letter in the space next to the question number.

Choices:

_____ **1.** provides bone marrow specimen
_____ **2.** identification of a pathogen
_____ **3.** used to follow the recovery from certain diseases
_____ **4.** determines numbers of platelets
_____ **5.** agglutination of blood cells with standard antibody preparations
_____ **6.** prevents transfusion reaction
_____ **7.** detects unusual antibodies on red blood cells

a. platelet count
b. sternal puncture
c. isolation and blood culture
d. blood typing
e. serologic tests
f. cross matching
g. Coomb's test

III.   Spell Check: Diagnostic Tests and Procedures

Circle each incorrectly spelled term and write it correctly in the space provided.

1. coagulation   _____
2. hemoglobin   _____

    3. thrombplastin   _____

    4. diferential   _____

    5. biopsy   _____

    6. prothombin   _____

    7. hematrocrit   _____

    8. sedementation   _____

E. Medical Vocabulary Building

I.   Matching: Medical Vocabulary Building

Match the term to its meaning. (The same meaning may be used more than once.)
Insert the appropriate letter in the space next to the question number.

Choices:

_____ **1.** allergy   **a.** immature red blood cell

_____ **2.** hyperglycemia   **b.** red blood cell stimulating hormone

_____ **3.** hematologist   **c.** excessive sugar in the blood

_____ **4.** erythropoietin   **d.** hypersensitivity to a substance

_____ **5.** erythroblast   **e.** white blood cell removal from the

_____ **6.** hyperlipemia   blood

_____ **7.** leukapheresis   **f.** excessive fat in the blood

_____ **8.** septicemia   **g.** heredity form of anemia

_____ **9.** stem cell   **h.** bone marrow cell that gives rise to

_____ **10.** thalassemia   various blood cell types

                                i. microorganisms in the blood

                                j. specialist in the study of blood

F. Abbreviations for Blood Cell Types, Physiologic Properties, Blood Diseases, and Diagnostic Tests

I.   Matching 1: Abbreviations for Blood Cell Types and Physiologic Properties

Match the term to its meaning. (The same meaning may be used more than once.)
Insert the appropriate letter in the space next to the question number.

Choices:

_____ **1.** B-lymphocyte   **a.** Ig

_____ **2.** polymorphonuclear   **b.** Hb

        leukocyte   **c.** wbc

_____ **3.** Rhesus factor   **d.** T-cell

_____ **4.** immunoglobulin   **e.** segs

_____ **5.** white blood cell   **f.** B-cell

_____ **6.** hemoglobin   **g.** PMNL

_____ **7.** T-lymphocyte   **h.** Rh

_____ **8.** segmented PMNLs   **i.** AHF

_____ **9.** monocyte   **j.** mono

_____ **10.** antihemophilic factor

II.   Matching 2: Abbreviations for Blood Diseases and Diagnostic Tests

Match the term to its meaning. (The same meaning may be used more than once.)
Insert the appropriate letter in the space next to the question number.

Choices:

_____ **1.** AIDS   **a.** complete blood count
_____ **2.** CBC   **b.** human immunodeficiency virus
_____ **3.** ALL   **c.** acute myelogenous leukemia
_____ **4.** diff   **d.** enzyme-linked immunoabsorbent
_____ **5.** HT   assay
_____ **6.** AML   **e.** acquired immune deficiency
_____ **7.** PPT   syndrome
_____ **8.** HIV   **f.** acute lymphocytic leukemia
_____ **9.** ELISA   **g.** differential white blood cell count
_____ **10.** PTT   **h.** hematocrit
_____ **11.** Wb   **i.** partial prothrombin time
                         j. partial thromboplastin time
                         k. Western blot assay

III.   Spell Check

Circle each incorrectly spelled term and write it correctly in the space provided.

1. platlet   _____
2. mylocyte   _____
3. macrophaje   _____
4. hepatitis   _____
5. Rhesus   _____
6. sedimentation   _____
7. immunoglobulinn   _____
8. corpuculer   _____

G. Increasing Your Medical Terminology Word Power 1

1. Read the following report.
2. Prepare to answer the questions at the end of the section.
3. Circle all unfamiliar terms with a red pencil.
4. Underline familiar terms with a blue pencil.
5. Use your knowledge of word elements, a medical dictionary, and the key terms to find the meanings of unfamiliar terms.

Thrombotic Thrombocytopenic Purpura (TTP)

Key Terms

hyaline (HĪ-a-lin)   not transparent but allowing the passage of light

intravascular   within blood cells

paresis (PAR-ē-sis)   partial paralysis

parethesia (par-es-THĒ-zē-a)   numbness

pathogenesis (path-ō-JEN-e-sis)   origin and development of a disease

plasma infusion   introduction of plasma through a blood vessel for therapeutic purposes

prognosis (prog-NŌ-sis)   prediction of the course and outcome

purpura (PUR-pū-ra)   hemorrhages into skin and other tissues

thrombi (THROM-bī)   blood clots

thrombocytopenia (throm-bō-sī-tō-PĒ-nē-a)   abnormal decrease in the number of platelets

thrombotic thrombocytopenic purpura (TTP)   a rare syndrome of unknown cause that typically exhibits a clinical picture of microangiopathic hemolytic anemia, thrombocytopenia, neurologic disorders, renal disease, and fever

B ACKGROUND

The pathogenesis of TTP is poorly understood. On histologic study, TTP is characterized by the presence of intravascular hyaline thrombi composed mainly of platelets with some fibrin in the arterioles and capillaries. Many treatment regimens have been employed with varying success, including splenectomy; administration of corticosteroids, antiplatelet agents, and heparin; whole-blood exchange transfusions; hemodialysis; and plasma infusions. Due to the rare nature of this disorder, clinical studies of treatment for TTP usually involve only a few patients.

R ESULTS OF STUDY

Of 40 patients with TTP, 17 were treated with plasma exchange, 15 with exchange transfusions, and 6 with both types of therapy. The replacement fluid used for plasma exchange was fresh-frozen plasma in all cases. The complete response rates for each type of treatment were as follows: 88 percent for plasma exchange (15 patients), 47 percent for exchange transfusions (7 patients), and 67 percent for exchange transfusions and plasma exchange (4 patients). Clinical and laboratory factors were examined for any statistically significant association with therapy response. Treatment with plasma exchange was most strongly associated with positive prognosis. Paresis, paresthesia, seizures, and mental status change showed no association with response to treatment. This study supports the view that plasma exchange has significantly improved the prognosis of patients with thrombotic thrombocytopenic purpura.

Questions

I.   Fill in the Blank

Fill in the blank with the appropriate term.

> **1.** How many patients with TTP received some type of treatment in this study? _____
>
> **2.** How many patients received treatment with the following?
>
> **a.** plasma exchange _____
>
> **b.** exchange transfusions _____
>
> **c.** both types of therapy _____ .
>
> **3.** The treatment that significantly improved the prognosis of TTP patients was _____ .

II.   Matching: Word Elements

Match the term to its meaning. (The same meaning may be used more than once.) Insert the appropriate letter in the space next to the question number.

Choices:

_____ **1.** thromb/o	**a.** within	
_____ **2.** cyt/o	**b.** cell	
_____ **3.** path/o	**c.** disease	
_____ **4.** -penia	**d.** small	

_____ **5.** micr/o
_____ **6.** angi/o
_____ **7.** intra-
_____ **8.** -ole
_____ **9.** -ic
_____ **10.** -ectomy

e. decreased number
f. pertaining to
g. suffix for small
h. vessel
i. clot
j. excision

III.   Spell Check

Circle each incorrectly spelled term and write it correctly in the space provided.

1. hyalene _____
2. microangiopathic _____
3. parisis _____
4. paresthezia _____
5. pathagenesis _____
6. infussion _____
7. progknowsis _____
8. purpura _____
9. thrombi _____
10. thrombositopenia _____

H. Increasing Your Medical Terminology Word Power 2

1. Read the following report.
2. Prepare to answer the questions at the end of the section.
3. Circle all unfamiliar terms with a red pencil.
4. Underline familiar terms with a blue pencil.
5. Use your knowledge of word elements, a medical dictionary, and the key terms to find the meanings of unfamiliar terms.

Retroperitoneal Hemorrhage

Key Terms

anticoagulant (an'-ti-kō-AG-ū-lant)   agent that prevents or delays blood coagulation

arteriography (ar'-tē-re-OG-ra-fē)   x-ray procedure involving injecting a radiopaque dye

coagulation (kō-ag'-ū-LĀ-shun)   clotting

embolism (EM-bō-liz-em)   blockage of a blood vessel by a clot or foreign material

hematoma (hem'-a-TŌ-ma)   swelling or mass of blood found in tissue

heparin (HEP-a-rin)   blood clotting inhibitor

hyperdensity   excessively dark area involving body areas as seen in a radiograph

hypotension   below normal systolic and diastolic blood pressure

retroperitoneal (ret'-rō-per-i-tō-NĒ-al)   behind the peritoneum and outside the peritoneal cavity

thrombosis (throm-BŌ-sis)   the formation or existence of a blood clot

transcatheter (trans-KATH-e-ter)   tube passed across or beyond the body surface for evacuating fluid from or injecting fluid into body cavities

warfarin (WAR-fer-in)   specific anticoagulant (named for the Wisconsin Alumni Research Foundation)

C ASE HISTORY

Left flank pain and hypotension developed in a 65-year-old female during the administration of intravenous heparin and warfarin for her deep venous thrombosis. Laboratory results showed a prothrombin time of 15.5 seconds, a partial thromboplastin time of 102 seconds, and a platelet count of 132,000 per cubic centimeter. Computed tomography (CT) showed a large mass in the left side of the abdomen, suggestive of a large retroperitoneal hematoma. The CT also showed an area of hypersensitivity, indicating ongoing hemorrhage. The patient's hematocrit continued to fall even when intravenous heparin was discontinued and two units of fresh-frozen plasma and six units of packed red cells were administered. Coagulation tests were repeated and were found to show a prothrombin time of 12.8 seconds, a partial thromboplastin time of 27 seconds, and a platelet count of 107,000 per cubic centimeter. Arteriography of the left lumbar arteries at the level of L2 and L3 clearly showed active bleeding. A transcatheter embolism blocked the bleeding vessels, and fortunately the bleeding stopped. The patient's condition quickly stabilized. Anticoagulant therapy was not resumed, and the patient was discharged 21 days later.

Questions

I.   Matching

Match the term to its meaning. (The same meaning may be used more than once.) Insert the appropriate letter in the space next to the question number.

Choices:

_____ **1.** arteriography	**a.** blocking of a blood vessel by a blood clot
_____ **2.** embolism	**b.** x-ray procedure involving the injection of a radiopaque dye
_____ **3.** hematoma	
_____ **4.** hypotension	**c.** decrease of systolic and diastolic blood pressures below normal
_____ **5.** retroperitoneal	
_____ **6.** thrombosis	**d.** swelling or blood mass in tissue
_____ **7.** transcatheter	**e.** located behind the peritoneum and outside the peritoneal cavity
_____ **8.** warfarin	
	f. blood clot formation within vascular system
	g. anticoagulant
	h. tube passed across or beyond body surface for removal or injecting fluids into body cavities

II.   Spell Check

Circle each incorrectly spelled term and write it correctly in the space provided.

1. hypotesion   _____

2. retroperitoneal   _____

3. transcatheiter   _____

4. heparin   _____

5. antecoagulent   _____

6. thrombosis   _____

7. artereography _____

8. embolization _____

I. Increasing Your Medical Terminology Word Power 3

1. Read the following report.
2. Prepare to answer the questions at the end of the section.
3. Circle all unfamiliar terms with a red pencil.
4. Underline familiar terms with a blue pencil.
5. Use your knowledge of word elements, a medical dictionary, and the key terms to find the meanings of unfamiliar terms.

Chronic Myelocytic Leukemia

Key Terms

adenopathy (ad-e-NOP-a-thē)   enlarged lymph nodes

erythematous (er-i-THĒM-a-tus)   reddened

leukemia (loo-KĒ-mē-a)   disease in which uncontrolled division of leukocytes and related cells occurs; also known as cancer of the blood

myelogenous (mī-e-LOJ-en-us)   originating in bone marrow

myelocytic (mī-el-ō-SIT-ik)   pertaining to myelocytes (large cells in red bone marrow from which leukocytes develop)

nodule (NOD-ūl)   small swelling

otitis media (ō-TĪ-tis, MĒ-dē-a)   middle ear infection

papule (PAP-ūl)   small elevated area on the skin

thrombocytopenia (throm-bō-sī-tō-PĒ-nē-a)   abnormal decrease in the number of platelets

*B*ACKGROUND INFORMATION

Chronic myelocytic leukemia is a rare malignancy occurring in childhood. It differs from the adult form in several respects, including a more rapid course and certain hematologic abnormalities, such as a lower overall white-blood-cell count with an obvious monocytosis, anemia, and thrombocytopenia.

*C*ASE HISTORY

A three-year-old female developed erythematous papules and nodules on her legs that slowly disappeared over a four-week period. Two months later she had a 48-hour episode of diarrhea and developed many erythematous papules on her legs. These skin lesions spread to her trunk and arms in two days' time. The patient's pediatrician noted extreme swelling of the feet and ankles, and shortly thereafter diagnosed the condition as otitis media. An appropriate antibiotic was prescribed.

The laboratory reported an elevated white blood cell count with 18% lymphocytes, 11% monocytes, 2% basophils, 3% myelocytes, and 15% immature leukocytes. Based on these results the patient was referred to the University Pediatrics Department for further study and treatment.

Two weeks later the patient exhibited cervical and inguinal adenopathy. Her liver and spleen also were enlarged and palpable. In addition, many new erythematous nodules appeared on the legs, buttocks, and upper arms. The patient's platelet count had also dropped significantly. At this point biopsies of an enlarged inguinal lymph node and selected papules and nodules were ordered. Examination of the biopsied material revealed a bone marrow disorder and a chronic myelogenous leukemia. These findings were confirmed by a second laboratory. The patient's condition continued to worsen. Her hemoglobin and platelets fell to significantly dangerous levels. She was given transfusions of platelets and erythrocytes, but this approach helped only temporarily.

Questions

I.   Fill in the Blank

Fill in the blank with the appropriate term.

1. What type of lesions developed on the patient's legs?
   _____

2. What is the medical term for a middle ear infection?
   _____

3. In which areas of the body was adenopathy observed?
   _____

4. Was the platelet count high or low as the patient's condition progressed? _____

II.   Spell Check

Circle each incorrectly spelled term and write it correctly in the space provided.

1. otitis media   _____
2. papul   _____
3. pediatrician   _____
4. myelogenous   _____
5. erithematous   _____
6. diarrhea   _____
7. adenopathy   _____
8. inquinal   _____

Term Search Challenge

Locate 14 terms in the puzzle.

1. Write the specific term next to its definition. Then find that term in the puzzle diagram and circle it.
2. Terms may be read from left to right, backward, up, down, or diagonally.
3. If a term appears more than once, circle it only once. (A term may be found inside others.)
4. Check your answers.

Clues:

1. Another term for red blood cells _____
2. The process of blood cell formation from specific bone marrow stem cells _____
3. The fluid portion of blood _____
4. The two types of proteins found in plasma _____ and
   _____

5. The iron-containing pigment found in hemoglobin

_____

6. The largest leukocyte, having a kidney or horseshoe-shaped nucleus

_____

7. T-lymphocytes are associated with which gland?

_____

8. The abbreviation used for acquired immune deficiency syndrome

_____

9. Another term for white blood cells _____

10. The term that refers to red blood cell formation is _____.

11. The clumping reaction that occurs when type A blood cells are mixed with antibodies against type A blood _____

12. The combining form for one or single _____

13. The condition resulting from hemoglobin-deficient cells

_____

Term Search Puzzle

```
H  E  M  A  T  O  P  O  I  E  S  I  S  A  H
T  F  D  P  G  M  E  T  Y  H  V  P  G  G  E
S  I  A  L  E  I  U  A  E  A  T  L  R  G  M
H  B  G  A  N  N  K  I  L  G  D  A  A  L  O
E  R  Y  T  H  R  O  C  Y  T  E  S  S  U  G
M  I  G  E  M  S  C  A  M  G  D  M  E  T  L
E  N  L  L  O  P  Y  Y  A  H  E  A  T  I  O
A  G  U  E  N  H  T  A  I  D  S  T  Y  N  B
A  T  I  T  O  E  E  O  S  I  N  O  C  A  I
A  P  L  S  R  R  S  E  L  D  T  P  O  T  N
N  G  L  O  B  U  L  I  N  S  H  H  K  I  P
E  H  E  M  O  P  H  I  L  I  Y  I  U  O  E
M  A  L  B  U  M  I  N  S  A  M  L  E  N  R
I  P  O  I  E  S  I  S  X  A  U  S  L  J  T
A  M  O  N  O  C  Y  T  E  T  S  T  P  C  L
```

CHAPTER 15

The Immune System and Immune Mechanisms

"The development of immunity (resistance) in its broadest sense is a process by which the body learns from experience of past infections to deal more efficiently with subsequent ones."

—Sir Macfarlane Burnet

INFORMATIONAL CHALLENGE

A. The Lymphatic System and Basic Immunologic Concepts

I.   Fill in the Blank

Fill in the blank with the appropriate term or phrase.

1. List four general components of the lymphatic system.

a. _____
b. _____
c. _____
d. _____

2. List three functions of immunological responses.

a. _____
b. _____
c. _____

3. List five factors contributing to an individual's nonspecific resistance.

a. _____
b. _____
c. _____
d. _____
e. _____

4. List five cardinal signs of inflammation.

a. _____
b. _____
c. _____
d. _____
e. _____

II.   Matching: Nonspecific Immune Mechanisms

Match the term to its meaning. (The same meaning may be used more than once.)
Insert the appropriate letter in the space next to the question number.

Choices:

_____ **1.** phagocytosis
_____ **2.** 37°C
_____ **3.** complement
_____ **4.** interferon
_____ **5.** fever
_____ **6.** 98.6°F

a. body chemical known to interfere with disease agent's actions

b. includes ingestion, digestion, and destruction of foreign cells and/or disease agents

c. elevation of body temperature

d. normal body temperature

e. body chemical normally produced in response to rival infections

III.   Spell Check

Circle each incorrectly spelled term and write it correctly in the space provided.

1. imune   _____
2. phagositosis   _____
3. interfearon   _____
4. makrophajes   _____
5. complement   _____
6. antigen   _____

B. General Immunity Mechanisms

I.   Fill in the Blank

Fill in the blank with the appropriate term or phrase.

1. List three properties of an immunogen.

    a. _____
    b. _____
    c. _____

2. List two chemicals known to be strongly antigenic.

    a. _____
    b. _____

3. In what part of a typical lymph node is the highest concentration of:

    a. B-lymphocytes? _____
    b. plasma cells? _____

4. List two materials that induce Ig production.

    a. _____
    b. _____

5. List the five immunoglobulin classes.

    a. _____
    b. _____
    c. _____
    d. _____
    e. _____

6. The first reaction to an antigen by the immune system is called
_____.

7. The secondary reaction of the immune system to a second exposure of an antigen is called the _____.

II.   Matching: Specific Immune Responses

Match the term to its meaning. (The same meaning may be used more than once.) Insert the appropriate letter in the space next to the question number.

Choices:

_____ **1.** antigen
_____ **2.** immunoglobulin
_____ **3.** plasma cell
_____ **4.** immunogen
_____ **5.** primary response
_____ **6.** secondary response
_____ **7.** T$_{DH}$-lymphocyte
_____ **8.** IgE
_____ **9.** cell-mediated immunity
_____ **10.** thymus
_____ **11.** lymphokine
_____ **12.** primary immunodeficiency disease

a. major factor in humoral immunity
b. the first exposure to an antigen, causing antibody formation
c. includes foreign cells that stimulate an immune response
d. anamnestic response
e. immunoglobulin-producing cell of the body
f. major factor in cell-mediated immunity
g. does not involve immunoglobulins in defending against foreign substances
h. immunoglobulin class responsible for allergies
i. gland involved with T-cell development
j. product of certain T-cells
k. inherited immune system defect

III.   Spell Check

Circle each incorrectly spelled term and write it correctly in the space provided.

1. macrophages   _____
2. humeral   _____
3. polysacharide   _____
4. haptenn   _____
5. glykoprotein   _____
6. interferon   _____
7. atenuated   _____
8. vacine   _____

C. Selected Immune Responses, T-Lymphocytes, and Ig Structure

I.   Fill in the Blank

Fill in the blank with the appropriate term.

1. Two specific immune responses found in humans are _____ and _____.

2. The specific components of T-cells that are used to interact with antigens are called _____.

3. Define the following abbreviations.

    a. CD: _____

    b. APC: _____

    c. HLA: _____

    d. MHC: _____

    e. TCR: _____

4. Give the general function of the T-lymphocyte populations listed.

    a. T_H: _____

    _____

    b. T_{DH}: _____

    _____

    c. T_C: _____

    _____

    d. T_S: _____

    _____

II.   Vision Quiz: Immunoglobulin (Ig) Structure and Functions

Figure 15-8 shows the general structure of a basic Ig molecule. Identify and write the name of the numbered parts in the spaces provided.

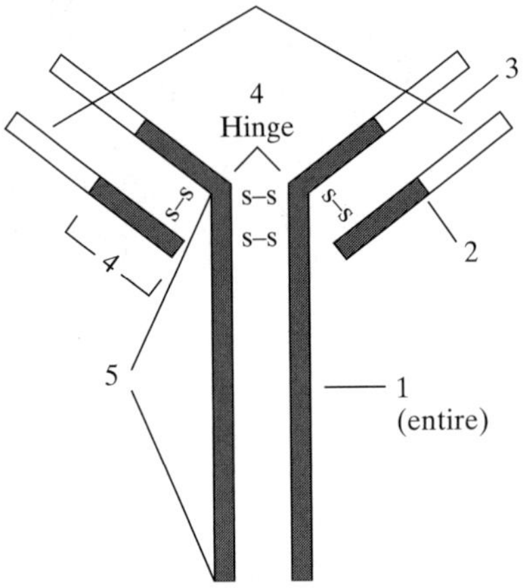

FIGURE 15-8   Vision Quiz. Immunoglobulin (Ig) Structure and Functions.

    1. _____

    2. _____

    3. _____

    4. _____

    5. _____

D. States of Immunity and Immunodeficiencies

I.   Matching

Match the term to its meaning. (The same meaning may be used more than once.) Insert the appropriate letter in the space next to the question number.

Choices:

_____ **1.** use of vaccines

_____ **2.** transfer of specific Igs obtained from immunized person to nonimmunized individual

    a. passive immunity

    b. active immunity

    c. adoptive immunity

    d. innate immunity

_____ **3.** transfer of immune T-cells to nonimmunized person

_____ **4.** type of immunity with which an individual is born

_____ **5.** type of immunity resulting from lifelong exposure to foreign materials

_____ **6.** acquired immune system defects during lifetime

_____ **7.** inherited immune system defects

_____ **8.** AIDS

e. acquired immunity
f. secondary immunodeficiency
g. primary immunodeficiency

II.   Spell Check

Circle each incorrectly spelled term and write it correctly in the space provided.

1. immunodeficiency _____
2. inate _____
3. akquired _____
4. pasive _____
5. phagsitik _____
6. immunozashun _____
7. adoptive _____

E. Word Elements Associated with the Lymphatic System and Immune Mechanisms

I.   Word Analysis: Lymphatics and Immune Mechanisms

Table 15-7 lists a number of terms with their pronunciations and definitions.

1. Analyze each term.
2. Circle all combining forms, word roots, prefixes, and suffixes and label them **cf**, **wr**, **p**, and **s**, respectively.
3. Check your answers (shown in Table 15-8).

TABLE 15-7   WORD ANALYSIS: LYMPHATICS AND IMMUNE MECHANISMS

Term and Pronunciation	Definition
agglutinophilic (a-gloo-tin-ō-FIL-ik)	attraction for rapid clumping
electrophoresis (ē-LEK-trō-for-ē-sis)	transport of particles in an electrical field medium
immunogenic (im-ū-nō-JEN-ik)	producing protection
immunoglobulin (im-ū-nō-GLOB-ū-lin)	protective protein of the body; antibody
leukapheresis (loo-ka-fe-RĒ-sis)	removal of white blood cells

(Continued)

TABLE 15-7   (CONTINUED)

Term and Pronunciation	Definition
monocytosis (mon-ō-sī-TŌ-sis)	abnormally high number of monocytes in the blood
neutrophilia (nū-trō-FIL-ē-a)	increase in the number of neutrophils
phagocytic (fag-ō-SIT-ik)	pertaining to phagocytes or phagocytosis
polymorphonuclear (pol-ē-mor-fō-NŪ-klē-ar)	nucleus with several nucleus parts

F. Medical Vocabulary Building

I.   Matching

Match the term to its meaning. (The same meaning may be used more than once.) Insert the appropriate letter in the space next to the question number.

Choices:

_____ **1.** attenuated
_____ **2.** autoantibody
_____ **3.** antigen-presenting cell
_____ **4.** immunodeficient
_____ **5.** hypersensitivity
_____ **6.** natural killer cell
_____ **7.** macrophage
_____ **8.** plasma
_____ **9.** serology
_____ **10.** tolerance
_____ **11.** vaccination

a. cell that primarily presents an antigen to a T-cell
b. weakened state
c. antibody to self-antigens
d. immune response resulting in host tissue damage, sometimes referred to as allergies
e. having a dysfunctional immune system
f. large leukocyte with phagocytic properties
g. lymphocyte known to recognize and kill foreign cells or infected host cells in a nonspecific manner
h. liquid portion of blood lacking cells but having deactivated blood-clotting proteins
i. study of antigen-antibody reactions *in vitro*
j. administration of inactive or weakened pathogens to stimulate protective immunity
k. inability to produce an immune response to specific antigens

II.   Spell Check

Circle each incorrectly spelled term and write it correctly in the space provided.

1. hypersensitivity _____
2. vacination _____
3. imunodeficient _____

    4. tolerence   _____

    5. attenuated   _____

    6. seralogy   _____

G. *Abbreviations*

I.   Matching

Match the term to its meaning. (The same meaning may be used more than once.) Insert the appropriate letter in the space next to the question number.

                             Choices:

_____ **1.** ABO	**a.**	monocyte
_____ **2.** B-cell	**b.**	Rhesus factor
_____ **3.** Ig	**c.**	human immunodeficiency virus
_____ **4.** mono	**d.**	B-lymphocyte
_____ **5.** Rh	**e.**	T-lymphocyte
_____ **6.** T-cell	**f.**	immunoglobulin
_____ **7.** HIV	**g.**	T helper cell
_____ **8.** T$_H$	**h.**	A, B, O, and AB blood-type system

H. *Increasing Your Medical Terminology Word Power 1*

    1. Read the following report.

    2. Prepare to answer the questions at the end of the section.

    3. Circle all unfamiliar terms with a red pencil.

    4. Underline familiar terms with a blue pencil.

    5. Use your knowledge of word elements, a medical dictionary, and the key terms to find the meaning of unfamiliar terms.

Chronic Urticaria and Angioedema

Key Terms

angioedema (an'-jē-ō-ē-DĒ-ma)   vascular skin reactions such as pale elevations (*urticaria*) in response to a sensitivity to certain foods, drugs, etc.

antinuclear antibody   a group of antibodies that react against normal cell's nuclear parts

arthralgia (ar-THRAL-jē-a)   joint pain

autoimmune (aw'-tō-im-MŪN) disorder   disease in which the body responds against itself

cholinergic (kō-lin-ER-jik)   nerve ending that releases *acetylcholine* (as'-se-til-KŌ-lēn), a substance important to nerve impulse transmission

dermatographism (der'ma-tō-GRAF-ism)   urticaria caused by sensitivity to physical agents such as cold and the sun

hives (hīvz)   eruption of itchy skin areas caused by contact with or ingestion of various allergy-causing foods

idiosyncratic (id'-ē-ō-sin-KRAT-ik)   characteristics by which one individual differs from another

periorbital (per'-ē-OR-bi-tal)   surrounding the eye socket

pruritus (proo-RĪ-tis)   severe itching

urticaria (ur-ti-KĀ-rē-a)   vascular reaction of the skin that is characterized by the brief appearance of pale, localized elevations of the skin and associated with severe itching

vasculopathy (vas'-kū-LŌP-a-thē)   any blood vessel disease

Introduction

Chronic urticaria was once considered to be a result of an anxiety disorder or an allergic or idiosyncratic reaction to foods, food additives, or food dyes. There are insufficient data to support these views. Sticking to a diet of rice, lamb, and water for five or more days has no effect on chronic urticaria or *angioedema*. In addition, an infectious cause is unlikely. An autoimmune mechanism, however, appears to be the most likely cause.

*P*ATHOGENS

Chronic urticaria appears to be an autoimmune disorder in a substantial number of patients. About 30 to 45 percent of patients have circulating IgGs directed against a particular subunit of the IgE receptor. In addition, approximately 10 percent have immunoglobulins against another specific subunit of IgE. These antibodies activate basophils and mast cells to release histamine. The associated lesions in patients typically exhibit a perivascular infiltration of lymphocytes, an increased number of monocytes, and a variable number of neutrophils and eosinophils, similar to the findings in a late-phase allergic reaction.

*D*IAGNOSIS

Chronic urticaria and angioedema are diagnosed when hives occur on a regular basis for more than six weeks. This interval is sufficient to rule out most identifiable causes of urticaria, such as drug reactions and food or contact allergies. Angioedema accompanies urticaria in about 30–40 percent of affected individuals. When present, the condition typically affects the lips, face, (particularly the periorbital area), hands, feet, penis, or scrotum. At times there may be a swelling of the tongue or throat, but the larynx never appears to be involved. Approximately 40 percent of patients experience hives alone, and about 25 percent have angioedema but not urticaria.

The most common alternative diagnosis is hives caused by dermatographism. In severe cases, patients experience hives every day for months or years. The lesions can be any shape, but most commonly linear. In dermatographism, individual hives last for 30 minutes to over 2 hours, as they do in most other types of physically caused hives. Exposure of a sensitive individual to the sun would be an example here. In contrast, hives associated with chronic urticaria would last about 4 to 36 hours.

A patient's history and findings on physical examination may suggest an underlying cause of urticaria. At times, chronic urticaria and angioedema are the result of an underlying connective-tissue disorder or a systemic vasculitis.

There are few, if any, diagnostic tests for chronic urticaria and angioedema. The results of a complete blood count and urinalysis are generally normal. A skin biopsy may be helpful in patients who have fever, arthralgias, and lesions lasting 36 hours or more.

*T*HERAPY

Non-sedating antihistamines help to reduce and eliminate the itching and the incidence of hives in patients with mild chronic urticaria. Unfortunately, individuals with more severe forms of the condition may not benefit from the usual doses of antihistamines. Relatively recent studies show promising results in some individuals with cyclosporine.

Questions

I.   Matching

Match the term to its meaning. (The same meaning may be used more than once.)
Insert the appropriate letter in the space next to the question number.

Choices:

_____ **1.** arthralgia   **a.** urticaria caused by sensitivity to
_____ **2.** hives   cold and the sun
_____ **3.** idiosyncratic   **b.** vascular skin reactions in response to
_____ **4.** periorbital   a food allergy
_____ **5.** pruritus   **c.** eruptions of itchy skin areas caused
_____ **6.** vasculopathy   by a food allergy
_____ **7.** dermatographism **d.** characteristics that differ among
_____ **8.** angioedema   individuals
                                e. surrounding the eye socket
                                f. severe itch
                                g. any blood vessel disease
                                h. painful joints

II.   Spell Check

Circle each incorrectly spelled term and write it correctly in the space provided.

1. angitis   _____
2. cholinergic   _____
3. vasulopathy   _____
4. perioorbital   _____
5. urticara   _____
6. puritites   _____
7. dermatographism _____
8. idiosyncratik   _____

I. Increasing Your Medical Terminology Word Power 2

1. Read the following report.
2. Prepare to answer the questions at the end of the section.
3. Circle all unfamiliar terms with a red pencil.
4. Underline familiar terms with a blue pencil.
5. Use your knowledge of word elements, a medical dictionary, and the
key terms to find the meaning of unfamiliar terms.

Celiac Sprue in Children

Key Terms

anemia (a-NĒ-mē-a)   decrease in red blood cells, hemoglobin, or red blood cell
volume

aphthous stomatitis (AF-thus stō-ma-TĪ-tis)   small ulcers on the mucous membrane of the mouth

constipation (kon'-sti-PĀ-shun)   difficulty in evacuation of the bowels

distention   swelling or expanding

edema (e-DĒ-ma)   excess body tissue fluid

enteropathy (en'-ter-OP-a-thē)   any intestinal disease

folate (FŌ-lāt)   member of the vitamin B complex

hypertransaminasemia (hī'-per-trans-AM-in-as-ē-mē-a)   absence of an enzyme responsible for the transfer of amino groups

malabsorption (mal-ab-SORP-shun)   inadequate take-up of nutrients from the intestinal tract

puberty (PŪ-ber-tē)   point at which individuals become functionally capable of reproduction

rickets (RIK-ets)   vitamin D deficiency in children causing abnormalities in bone shape and structure

Introduction

Celiac sprue is also known as *celiac disease* and *gluten-sensitive enteropathy*. The condition is characterized by malabsorption resulting from inflammation causing injury to the small intestine mucosa, following the ingestion of wheat gluten or related rye and barley proteins. Individuals show improvement when placed on a strict gluten-free diet and a relapse when there is a reintroduction of dietary gluten.

Until fairly recently, celiac sprue was considered an uncommon occurrence in the United States, with an estimated prevalence of about 1 case per 3,000. However, a greater awareness of cases and the availability of new, accurate blood tests have led to the realization that celiac sprue is much more common than previously thought.

$\mathcal{P}$ ATHOGENESIS

Celiac sprue results from an inappropriate T-lymphocyte-mediated immune response against ingested gluten in genetically predisposed individuals. Over 95 percent of patients with the condition express the pertinent HLA genes, which clearly have gluten-derived protein-like molecules known to stimulate intestinal mucosal T-cells and the corresponding T-cell immune response. The enzyme transglutaminase is one of the targets of the autoimmune response in celiac sprue.

$\mathcal{C}$ LINICAL FEATURES

Individuals with celiac sprue exhibit a wide variety of gastrointestinal and extraintestinal signs and symptoms. Classically, 4- to 24-month-old infants with the condition exhibit impaired growth, diarrhea, and abdominal distention. Vomiting, pallor, and edema are quite common. The onset of signs and symptoms is gradual and follows the introduction of cereals into the diet.

Individuals with severe, untreated celiac sprue may present with short stature, pubertal delay, iron and folate deficiency accompanied by anemia, and rickets. Other signs and symptoms that have been reported include recurrent abdominal pain, hypertransaminasemia, recurrent aphthous stomatitis, arthralgia, and defects in dental enamel. Children may also have behavioral disturbances such as depression and may have poor performance in school.

Questions

I.   Fill in the Blank

Fill in the blank with the appropriate term.

1. What substances are responsible for celiac sprue? _____
_____.

2. The term for any intestinal disease is _____.

3. Vitamin D deficiency is called _____.

II.   Matching

Match the term to its meaning. (The same meaning may be used more than once.)
Insert the appropriate letter in the space next to the question number.

Choices:

_____ **1.** constipation

_____ **2.** distention

_____ **3.** edema

_____ **4.** enteropathy

_____ **5.** malabsorption

_____ **6.** pallor

_____ **7.** puberty

a. localized swelling of body tissues

b. inadequate uptake of nutrients from the intestinal tract

c. point at which an individual becomes functionally capable of reproducing

d. swelling or expanding

e. any intestinal disease

f. lack of color

g. difficulty in evacuation of bowels

III.   Spell Check

Circle each incorrectly spelled term and write it correctly in the space provided.

1. afthous   _____

2. stomatitis   _____

3. paller   _____

4. ricketts   _____

5. hypertranaminacemia _____

6. diarhea   _____

7. sproo   _____

8. celiac   _____

J. Increasing Your Medical Terminology Word Power 3

1. Read the following report.

2. Prepare to answer the questions at the end of the section.

3. Circle all unfamiliar terms with a red pencil.

4. Underline familiar terms with a blue pencil.

5. Use your knowledge of word elements, a medical dictionary, and the key terms to find the meaning of unfamiliar terms.

The Guillain-Barré Syndrome and Vaccination

Key Terms

afebrile (a-FEB-ril)   without fever

areflexia (ā'-re-FLEK-sē-a)   absence of reflexes

axon (ĀK-son)   neuron part that conducts impulses away from the cell body

***Campylobacter jejuni* (KAM-pī-lō-BAK-ter je-JUN-ē)**   Gram-negative bacterium known to cause gastrointestinal infections

enteritis (en'-ter-Ī-tis)   inflammation of the intestines

epitope (EP-i-tōp)   any antigen component that functions as an antigenic determinant

ganglioside (GANG-lē-ō-sid)   lipid chemical group found in nerve tissue and in the spleen.

hyporeflexia (hi'-pō-rē-FLEX-sē-ā)   reduced reflex function

myelin sheath   fat-like covering around the axons of certain nerves

polyneuritis (pol'-ē-nū-RĪ-tis)   inflammation of several nerves

polyneuropathy (pol'-e-nū-ROP-a-thē)   any disorder or related condition affecting peripheral nerves

symmetric   balance between parts of the body as a whole or the relative position of parts on opposite sides of the body

toxoid (TOKS-oyd)   modified toxin used to stimulate antibody production against the toxin

Introduction

Guillain-Barré syndrome (GBS) is characterized by a loss of reflexes and symmetric paralysis, generally beginning in the legs, with eventual complete or near complete recovery in the majority of cases. The condition is controlled by an immune response that results in the direct destruction of either the myelin sheath surrounding the peripheral nerves or the axon itself. GBS may or may not follow triggering events, including immunizations (vaccinations). Among the vaccines reported to have an association with the onset of GBS are the swine influenza vaccine used in the years 1976–77, oral poliomyelitis vaccine, smallpox vaccine, and tetanus toxoid. In subsequent years, from 1978 through 1988, the risks for contracting GBS were relatively low. However, in the 1990–91 flu season, a slight elevated risk was found among individuals aged from 18 to 64.

The Vaccine Adverse Event Reporting System (**VAERS**) of the Centers for Disease Control and Prevention (**CDC**) and the Food and Drug Administration (**FDA**) monitor occurrences of vaccine-associated GBS.

C LINICAL FEATURES

In definite cases of GBS, patients may be afebrile and exhibit symmetric, progressive paralysis in more than one limb. *Areflexia* or *hyporeflexia* in the legs and arms and a cerebrospinal fluid protein level above 40 milligrams (mg) per deciliter (dL) with a mononuclear-cell count of less than 10 per milliliter (mL) occurring within four weeks of the onset of the condition are also clinically relevant.

P ATHOGENESIS

It is probably fair to say that influenza vaccines over the past 30 or more years have been associated with a minimal risk of causing GBS. The same is probably true for the use of other vaccines and certain infections that have been followed by sporadic cases of the syndrome. The vaccines responsible for causing GBS currently could include the ones used against hepatitis B, poliomyelitis, rubella, and rabies.

Previous infections linked to GBS include those caused by Epstein-Barr virus (a common cause of infectious mononucleosis), human immunodeficiency virus (HIV), mycoplasma, *Shigella*, and clostridia. The most compelling case for a direct relationship between GBS and preceding infections derives from experiences with the enteric pathogen *Campylobacter jejuni*. This bacterium has special relevance because of the frequency with which it precedes GBS and because of a lipopolysaccharide antigen on the cells of some strains that is similar, if not identical, to the ganglioside epitopes found on human peripheral nerves.

Ultimately, research studies may show that infectious disease agents and vaccines share specific antigens found on human peripheral nerves. In all likelihood the complexity of affected individuals will also be factors in uncovering the basic cause or causes of GBS.

Questions

I.   Fill in the Blank

Fill in the blank with the appropriate term.

1. Define the following abbreviations:

    a. GBS _____

    b. CDC _____

    c. FDA _____

    d. mg _____

    e. dL _____

    f. mL _____

2. List three types of immunizing preparations known to be associated with possible GBS occurrences.

    a. _____

    b. _____

    c. _____

3. List two agencies that monitor vaccine-associated GBS cases.

    a. _____

    b. _____

4. List four regularly found infectious agents preceding GBS

    a. _____

    b. _____

    c. _____

    d. _____

II.   Matching

Match the term to its meaning. (The same meaning may be used more than once.) Insert the appropriate letter in the space next to the question number.

Choices:

_____ **1.** axon
_____ **2.** afebrile
_____ **3.** enteritis
_____ **4.** hyporeflexia
_____ **5.** polyneuritis
_____ **6.** symmetric
_____ **7.** toxoid
_____ **8.** epitope

a. without fever
b. neuron part that conducts nerve impulses away from the cell body
c. inflammation of the intestines
d. an antigenic determinant
e. reduced reflex function
f. inflammation of many nerves
g. inactivated toxin
h. balance between parts of the entire body

III.   Spell Check

Circle each incorrectly spelled term and write it correctly in the space provided.

1. vaccine   _____
2. eptipoe   _____
3. symetric   _____
4. influensa   _____
5. toxoid   _____
6. areflexea   _____

Term Search Challenge

Locate 14 terms in the puzzle.

1. Write the specific term next to its definition. Then find that term in the puzzle and circle it.
2. Terms may be read from left to right, backward, up, down, or diagonally.

3. If a term appears more than once, circle it only once. (A term or abbreviation may be found inside others.)
4. Check your answers.

Clues:

1. The term for a stable internal environment within the human body

   _____

2. The fluid found within lymph vessels _____
3. Substances that stimulate an immune response _____
4. Redness, pain, swelling, heat, and the loss of normal function are all features of this nonspecific response _____
5. The immunoglobulin-producing cell _____
6. Another term for an immunoglobulin _____
7. T-lymphocytes are associated with the _____ gland.
8. The abbreviation for acquired immune deficiency syndrome

   _____

9. Another term for white blood cells _____
10. The term that refers to an immune response-causing agent

    _____

11. The clumping reaction that occurs when type A red blood cells are mixed with antibodies against type A blood _____
12. The combining form for *one* or *single* _____
13. The structures that filter lymph before its return to venous blood

    _____

14. The sudden, second increase in immunoglobulin levels by additional immunogen exposure is the _____ response.

Term Search Puzzle

```
L  Y  M  P  H  A  G  Q  U  A  L  P  R  S  H
J  L  K  L  M  I  M  M  U  N  O  G  E  N  O
O  T  T  J  K  D  A  N  T  I  B  O  D  Y  M
L  O  M  P  H  S  A  D  E  N  I  T  I  S  E
I  N  F  L  A  M  M  A  T  I  O  N  I  S  O
A  G  G  L  U  T  I  N  A  T  I  O  N  T  S
L  R  S  E  V  W  X  O  Y  Z  I  O  N  T  T
U  T  U  U  E  R  E  D  S  A  C  T  S  C  A
V  P  O  K  R  T  S  E  I  N  F  A  N  T  S
M  O  N  O  S  I  V  S  I  D  M  O  R  F  I
M  I  O  C  P  L  A  S  M  A  C  E  L  L  S
N  N  S  E  T  Y  C  O  K  U  E  L  S  S  T
O  P  A  T  H  O  G  E  N  L  G  O  N  Y  M
P  L  O  E  I  N  I  M  S  U  M  Y  H  T  S
O  B  I  S  A  N  A  M  N  E  S  T  I  C  T
```

The Cardiovascular System

"Day in, day out, the human heart endures—leaving physiologists, as well as poets, marveling at its dependability."

—Rick Weiss

INFORMATIONAL CHALLENGE

A. Structure and Functions of Blood Vessels

I. Fill in the Blank

Fill in the blank with the appropriate term.

1. Small arteries are called _____.
2. Small veins are called _____.
3. The layers of an arterial wall are generally called _____.
4. The major artery of the body is the _____.
5. The major veins returning oxygen-deficient blood to the right atrium are the _____.

II. Matching: Structure and Function of Blood Vessels

Match the term to its meaning. (The same meaning may be used more than once.) Insert the appropriate letter in the space next to each question number.

Choices:

_____ 1. usually carries blood away from the heart
_____ 2. prevent blood backflow
_____ 3. upper chamber of the heart
_____ 4. lower chamber of the heart
_____ 5. usually carries blood to the heart
_____ 6. carry oxygen-deficient blood to the lungs
_____ 7. allows for the exchange of gases
_____ 8. carry oxygen-rich blood back to the heart

a. artery
b. capillary
c. ventricle
d. vein
e. valves
f. atrium
g. pulmonary veins
h. pulmonary arteries

III.   Spell Check

Circle each incorrectly spelled term and write it correctly in the space provided.

1. thorasic _____
2. perikardium _____
3. epicardium _____
4. atrium _____
5. atria _____
6. tricupid _____
7. atrioventrical _____
8. semeluner _____
9. mitrel _____
10. aorta _____

IV.   Vision Quiz: The Heart and Blood Vessels

Figure 16-13 shows the heart and associated blood vessels. Identify and write the name of the numbered parts in the spaces provided.

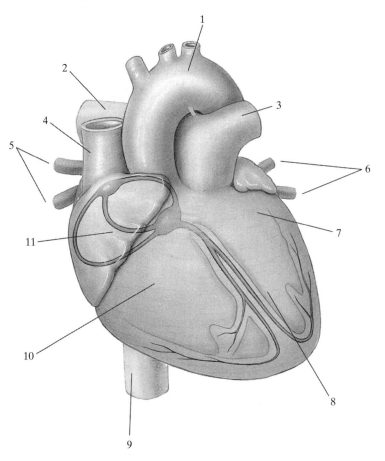

FIGURE 16-13   Vision Quiz. The human heart.

1. _____
2. _____
3. _____
4. _____
5. _____
6. _____

7. _____
8. _____
9. _____
10. _____
11. _____

B. Heart Structure and Function and Paths of Circulation

I.   Fill in the Blank

Fill in the blank with the appropriate term.

1. The right atrium receives oxygen-deficient blood by means of two large veins called the _____.
2. Air sacs of the lungs are called _____.
3. How many pulmonary veins are in the human body? _____
4. What is the largest artery in the body? _____
5. The heart is enclosed and protected by a loose-fitting sac called the _____.
6. The two upper chambers of the heart are the _____ (plural form).
7. Blood from the right atrium passes through the _____ valve to fill the right ventricle.
8. Oxygen-containing blood leaves the left ventricle through the ascending _____.
9. The part of the cardiac cycle in which a contraction of the ventricles occurs is called _____.
10. The part of the cardiac cycle in which a relaxation of the ventricles occurs is called _____.
11. What are the two major divisions (pathways) of blood flow in the body? _____ and _____.

II.   Matching 1: The Structures and Functions of the Heart

Match the term to its meaning. (The same meaning may be used more than once.)
Insert the appropriate letter in the space next to each question number.

Choices:

_____ **1.** myocardium
_____ **2.** heart valves
_____ **3.** pulmonary veins
_____ **4.** bicuspid or mitral valve
_____ **5.** coronary vessels
_____ **6.** right atrium
_____ **7.** ventricle
_____ **8.** atrioventricular valves
_____ **9.** electrocardiogram
_____ **10.** sinoatrial node

a. lower chamber of the heart
b. carry newly oxygenated blood to the left atrium
c. receives venous blood from the inferior vena cava and the superior vena cava
d. valves located between the atria and ventricles
e. pacemaker of the heart
f. separates the left atrium from the left ventricle
g. thick middle layer of the heart
h. maintain the flow of blood in one direction
i. provides a picture of electrical activity of the heart
j. supply blood to the heart

III.   Matching 2: Branches of the Aorta

Match the term to its meaning. (The same meaning may be used more than once.)
Insert the appropriate letter in the space next to each question number.

Choices:

_____ **1.** common carotid artery
_____ **2.** phrenic arteries
_____ **3.** superior mesenteric artery
_____ **4.** suprarenal arteries
_____ **5.** renal arteries
_____ **6.** celiac artery
_____ **7.** gonadal arteries
_____ **8.** lumbar arteries
_____ **9.** middle sacral artery

a. supplies blood to the spleen and liver
b. supplies blood to the small and large
   intestines
c. supplies blood to the neck and head
d. supply blood to the diaphragm
e. supply muscles of the skin
f. supply blood to the adrenal glands
g. supply blood to the testes or ovaries
h. provides blood to the coccyx

IV.   Matching 3: Selected Veins and Tissues Drained

Match the term to its meaning. (The same meaning may be used more than once.)
Insert the appropriate letter in the space next to each question number.

Choices:

_____ **1.** subclavian
_____ **2.** hepatic
_____ **3.** external iliac
_____ **4.** femoral
_____ **5.** great saphenous
_____ **6.** popiteal
_____ **7.** peroneal

a. foot
b. upper extremities
c. liver
d. lower limb
e. leg
f. thigh
g. lower leg

V.   Spell Check

Circle each incorrectly spelled term and write it correctly in the space provided.

1. venae cavae _____
2. alvoeli _____
3. pulmonary _____
4. caratid _____
5. iliac _____
6. seliac _____
7. gonadal _____
8. mesenteric _____
9. sacral _____
10. lumbar _____
11. safenous _____
12. popiteel _____
13. tibeal _____
14. peroneal _____

C. Conduction System of the Heart, the Electrocardiogram, and Blood Pressure

I.   Fill in the Blank

Fill in the blank with the appropriate term.

1. The period from the end of one contraction to the end of the next one is called _____.

2. List four specialized tissues that are involved with the electrical impulse generation to stimulate the cardiac muscle to contract.
   a. _____, b. _____,
   c. _____, d. _____

3. The cardiac cycle is started by the _____.

4. Ventricles contract as a result of the stimulation of _____.

5. The contraction of the heart caused by a change in electrical potential is referred to as _____ of muscle cells.

6. The recording of electrical changes that accompany the cardiac cycle is called an _____.

7. The three basic waves of an ECG are a. _____, b. _____, and c. _____.

8. The segments found between the basic waves are a. _____ and b. _____.

9. Which wave represents the electrical depolarization of both atria and indicates their contraction? _____

10. The repolarization of the ventricles following the delay between ventricular depolarization is represented by the _____ wave.

11. The segment representing the time period required for the blood flow from the atria into the ventricles is the _____.

12. The time required for the electrical impulse to pass through the specialized tissues of the conduction system is represented by the _____ interval.

13. The maximum pressure produced during ventricular contraction is called _____ pressure.

14. The lowest pressure left in the arteries before the next ventricular contraction is called _____ pressure.

15. The instrument used to measure an individual's blood pressure is called a _____.

II.   Spell Check

Circle each incorrectly spelled term and write it correctly in the space provided.

1. conduction   _____
2. sinoarial   _____
3. Perkinje   _____
4. node   _____
5. depolarization   _____
6. electrocardeograph _____
7. atrioventrikular   _____
8. stylus   _____

III.   Vision Quiz: The Electrocardiogram

Figure 16-14 shows an ECG. Identify and write the name of the numbered parts in the space provided.

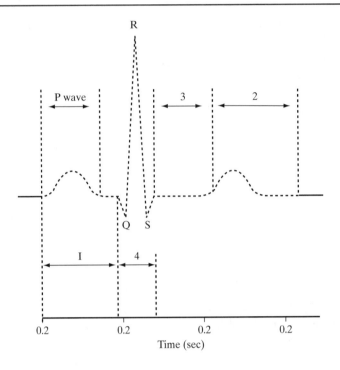

FIGURE 16-14   Vision Quiz. ECG.

1. _____
2. _____
3. _____
4. _____

D. Word Roots and/or Combining Forms for the Cardiovascular System

I.   Word Analysis: Prefixes, Word Roots, Combining Forms, and Suffixes
Table 16-12 lists a number of terms with their pronunciations and definitions.

TABLE 16-12   WORD ANALYSIS: PREFIXES, WORD ROOTS, COMBINING FORMS, AND SUFFIXES

Term and Pronunciation	Definition
aneurysmectomy (an-ū-riz-MEK-tō-mē)	surgical removal of the ballooning sac of an aneurysm
angiocardiopathy (an-jē-ō-kar-dē-OP-a-thē)	disease of the blood vessels of the heart
aortocoronary (ā-or'-tō-KOR-ō-nā-rē)	pertaining to both the aorta and coronary arteries
arteriosclerosis (ar-tē-rē-ō-skle-RŌ-sis)	hardening of the arteries
arteriolitis (ar-tēr-ē-ō-LĪ-tis)	inflammation of a small artery
atherosclerosis (ath-er-ō-skle-RŌ-sis)	a form of arteriosclerosis consisting of deposits of fats and other substances in arterial walls

(Continued)

TABLE 16-12   (CONTINUED)

Term and Pronunciation	Definition
atrioventricular (ā-trē-ō-ven-TRIK-ū-lar)	pertaining to both atrium and ventricle
cardiomegaly (kar-dē-ō-MEG-a-lē)	enlargement of the heart
coronary (KŌR-ō-na-rē)	pertaining to the heart
cyanosis (sī-a-NŌ-sis)	slight bluish to dark purplish discoloration of the skin caused by excess carbon dioxide in blood
phlebotomy (fle-BOT-ō-mē)	opening of a vein to obtain blood
sphygmomanometer (sfig-mō-man-OM-et-er)	an instrument used to measure the pulse; sphygmomanometer is also used to measure arterial blood pressure indirectly
stethomyositis (steth-ō-mī-ō-SĪ-tis)	inflammation of chest muscles
valvectomy (valv-EK-tō-mē)	surgical removal of a valve
valvular (VAL-vū-lar)	pertaining to a valve
vasal (VĀ-sal)	pertaining to a vessel
vasculopathy (vas-kū-LOP-a-thē)	any disease of blood vessels
venectasia (ve-nek-TĀ-zē-a)	stretching (dilation) of a vein
ventriculotomy (ven-trik-ū-LOT-ō-mē)	surgical incision of a ventricle
venulitis (ven-ū-LĪ-tis)	inflammation of a venule

1. Analyze each term.
2. Circle all prefixes, combining forms, word roots, and suffixes and label them **p**, **cf**, **wr**, and **s**, respectively.
3. Check your answers (shown in Table 16-13).

II.   Fill in the Blank

Fill in the blank with the appropriate term.

1. List one combining form and one word root for the heart. _____ and _____
2. List two word roots for vein. _____ and _____
3. In analyzing the term cardiomyopathy, cardi/o is a _____, my/o is a _____, and -pathy is a _____.

III.   Matching 1: Word Roots and Combining Forms Used with the Cardiovascular System

Match the term to its meaning. (The same meaning may be used more than once.) Insert the appropriate letter in the space next to each question number.

Choices:

_____ **1.** angi/o   **a.** chest
_____ **2.** steth/o   **b.** aorta
_____ **3.** venul/o   **c.** ventricle
_____ **4.** arti/o   **d.** vessel
_____ **5.** arteriol/o   **e.** pulse
_____ **6.** ather/o   **f.** small artery
_____ **7.** sphygm/o   **g.** yellowish plaque
_____ **8.** valv/o   **h.** valve
_____ **9.** aort/o   **i.** atrium
_____ **10.** ventricul/o   **j.** small vein

IV.   Matching 2: Suffix Applications

Match the suffix to its meaning. (The same suffix may be used more than once.) Enter the letter of your choice in the space provided. Insert the appropriate letter in the space next to the question.

     1. inflammation of a small artery, arteriol-_____

     2. x-ray record of a blood vessel, angio-_____

     3. pertaining to blood vessels of the heart, coron-_____

     4. arterial suture, arterio-_____

     5. study of the heart, cardio-_____

     6. enlargement of the heart, cardio-_____

     7. a bluish or purplish discoloration condition of the skin, cyan-

     _____

Choices:

     a. -itis   **e.** -megaly
     b. -rrhaphy   **f.** -osis
     c. -gram   **g.** -logy
     d. -ary

V.   Spell Check

Circle each incorrectly spelled term and write it correctly in the space provided.

     1. bradycarda   _____

     2. aortic   _____

     3. arteriosclrosis   _____

     4. stetomyositis   _____

     5. sphigmomanmetir   _____

     6. aneurysmectomy   _____

     7. ventriculotomy   _____

     8. stylus   _____

E. Cardiovascular Diseases and Disorders

I.   Matching 1: Disorders and Diseases of the Cardiovascular System

Match the term to its meaning. (The same meaning may be used more than once.) Insert the appropriate letter in the space next to the question number.

_____ **1.** a ballooning of a weak part of an artery
_____ **2.** any variation from normal rhythm
_____ **3.** fibrillation

_____ **4.** chest pain radiating to the left arm and jaw
_____ **5.** heart flutter
_____ **6.** inflammation of the blood vessels and the heart
_____ **7.** septal defect
_____ **8.** sudden stopping of cardiac output and circulation
_____ **9.** distended veins in the legs
_____ **10.** hardening of the arteries

Choices:

a. angina pectoris   **e.** congenital heart disease
b. arrhythmia   **f.** cardiac arrest
c. aneurysm   **g.** angiocarditis
d. arteriosclerosis   **h.** varicose veins

II.   Matching 2: Disorders and Diseases of the Cardiovascular System

Match the term to its meaning. (The same meaning may be used more than once.)
Insert the appropriate letter in the space next to the question number.

_____ **1.** myocardial infarction
_____ **2.** clot in a heart blood vessel
_____ **3.** arrhythmia
_____ **4.** thromboangitis obliterans
_____ **5.** atrioventricular defect
_____ **6.** varicose veins
_____ **7.** endocarditis
_____ **8.** coarctation of the aorta

Choices:

a. loss of rhythm (heart block)
b. distended veins in legs
c. inflammation of blood vessels in the legs
d. heart attack
e. inflammation of the heart's inner layer
f. Buerger's disease
g. congenital narrowing of the aorta
h. blood clot in coronary artery
i. defect pertaining to the atrium and ventricle
j. tetralogy of Fallot

III.   Spell Check

Circle each incorrectly spelled term and write it correctly in the space provided.

1. angeocarditis   _____
2. arhythamia   _____
3. aneurysm   _____
4. atrioventricular _____
5. occlusion   _____
6. atherosclerosis _____
7. thobosis   _____
8. infartion   _____
9. thromboangiitis _____
10. arteriosus   _____

F. Approaches to Treatment

I.   Matching 1: Approaches to Cardiovascular Treatment

Match the term to its meaning. (The same meaning may be used more than once.)
Insert the appropriate letter in the space next to each question number.

Choices:

_____ **1.** aneurysmectomy   **a.** excision of an aneurysm
_____ **2.** coronary bypass   **b.** repairs a stenosed mitral valve
_____ **3.** cardiac pacemaker   **c.** removal of hemorrhoids
_____ **4.** femoropoplitel bypass   **d.** used to regulate heart rate
_____ **5.** hemorrhoidectomy   **e.** brings new blood to heart muscles
_____ **6.** mitral commissurotomy   by detouring around blocked vessels
_____ **7.** vein ligation   **f.** diverts blood past a femoral artery
       g. tying off a vein

II.   Matching 2: Drug Treatment

Match the term to its meaning. (The same meaning may be used more than once.)
Insert the appropriate letter in the space next to the question number.

Choices:

_____ **1.** beta blocker   **a.** dissolves blood clots
_____ **2.** calcium blocker   **b.** blocks action of epinephrine
_____ **3.** digitalis   (adrenaline)
_____ **4.** nitroglycerin   **c.** relieves pain in angina pectoris
_____ **5.** streptokinase   **d.** blocks movement of calcium into
            muscle layers of blood vessels
       e. increases strength of heart muscle
            contraction and regularity

III.   Spell Check

Circle each incorrectly spelled term and write it correctly in the space provided.

1. anerysectomy   _____
2. femoropopliteel   _____
3. comisurotomy   _____
4. nitroglycerin   _____
5. plasminogen   _____
6. ligation   _____
7. hemorrhoidectomy   _____
8. angina   _____
9. thrombolytic   _____

G. Medical Vocabulary Building

I.   Matching

Match the term to its meaning. (The same meaning may be used more than once.)
Insert the appropriate letter in the space next to each question number.

Choices:

_____ **1.** angioblast   **a.** softening of aorta walls
_____ **2.** angionecrosis   **b.** pertaining to heart motion
_____ **3.** venoplasty   **c.** germ cell from which blood vessels
_____ **4.** cardiokinetic   develop

_____	**5.** cardioplegia	**d.**	paralysis of the heart
_____	**6.** cardioptosis	**e.**	a condition of blood vessel death
_____	**7.** dextrocardia	**f.**	blood vessel crushing to stop bleeding
_____	**8.** presystolic	**g.**	the condition of the heart being on the right side of the body
_____	**9.** vasotripsy	**h.**	pertaining to before systole
_____	**10.** venocyclosis	**i.**	injection of a drug or other material into a vein
		j.	downward displacement of the heart; heart prolapse

II.   Spell Check

Circle each incorrectly spelled term and write it correctly in the space provided.

1. angioblast   _____
2. dextrocardia   _____
3. aortamalashea   _____
4. presistolic   _____
5. cardiopleegia   _____
6. angionekrosis   _____

H. *Abbreviations*

I.   Matching 1: Cardiovascular Anatomy, Diagnosis, and Treatment

Match the term to its meaning. (The same meaning may be used more than once.)
Insert the appropriate letter in the space next to each question number.

Choices:

_____	**1.** CCU	**a.**	right atrium
_____	**2.** BP	**b.**	lactic dehydrogenase
_____	**3.** RA	**c.**	sinoatrial
_____	**4.** LD	**d.**	coronary care unit
_____	**5.** SA	**e.**	blood pressure
_____	**6.** HDL	**f.**	creatine kinase
_____	**7.** CK	**g.**	extracorporeal circulation
_____	**8.** VLDL	**h.**	very low-density lipoproteins
_____	**9.** ECC	**i.**	high-density lipoproteins
_____	**10.** EKG	**j.**	electrocardiogram

II.   Matching 2: Cardiovascular Diseases and Disorders

Match the term to its meaning. (The same meaning may be used more than once.)
Insert the appropriate letter in the space next to each question number.

Choices:

_____	**1.** premature ventricular contraction	**a.**	AI
		b.	PAT
_____	**2.** arteriosclerotic heart disease	**c.**	ASHD
		d.	PVC
_____	**3.** mitral stenosis	**e.**	MS

_____ **4.** paroxysmal atrial tachycardia

_____ **5.** coronary heart disease

_____ **6.** aortic insufficiency

_____ **7.** sudden cardiac death

_____ **8.** ventral septal defect

_____ **9.** aortic stenosis

_____ **10.** mitral valve prolapse

f. SCD

g. CHD

h. MVP

i. AS

j. VSD

III. Spell Check

Circle each incorrectly spelled term and write it correctly in the space provided.

1. atrioventirucular _____

2. kreatine _____

3. electrocardiogram _____

4. transaminase _____

5. asymmetrical _____

6. stensis _____

7. angioplasty _____

8. ventriculer _____

IV. Fill in the Blank

Write the meanings of the following abbreviations in the spaces provided.

1. CVP _____

2. CHD _____

3. CHF _____

4. MR _____

5. VPB _____

6. VT _____

7. CABG _____

I. Increasing Your Medical Terminology Word Power 1

1. Read the following report.

2. Prepare to answer the questions at the end of the section.

3. Circle all unfamiliar terms with a red pencil.

4. Underline familiar terms with a blue pencil.

5. Use your knowledge of word elements, a medical dictionary, and the key terms to find the meaning of unfamiliar terms.

Arrhythmias

Key Terms

anxiety a feeling of worry, uneasiness, and so on.

bradycardia (brad-ē-KAR-dē-a) a slow heart rate

contraction a shortening or tightening, as of a muscle

fibrillation (fib-bril-Ā-shun) quivering or spontaneous contraction of muscle

palpitation (pal-pi-TĀ-shun) rapid throbbing or beating

paroxysmal (par-ok-SIZ-mal) pertains to a sudden, periodic attack or recurrence of disease symptoms

premature contractions a tightening or shortening occurring before its normal time

tachycardia (tak-ē-KAR-dē-a) abnormally rapid heart rate

Introduction

Arrhythmias (a-RITH-mē-as), or abnormalities in heart rhythm, result from disturbances in the rhythm of the electrical impulses that trigger the heart's pumping. Just as a car may lose power when its timing is off, the arrhythmic heart may lose some of its capacity to pump blood effectively if its rhythm is abnormal. When pumping becomes ineffective, vital organs are deprived of their customary blood supply.

An arrhythmia is often signaled when a person complains of a racing or pounding heart, especially when the episode begins suddenly and in the absence of exercise or emotional stress. The medical term for the sensation of a racing heart is *palpitation*.

$\mathcal{T}$ YPES OF ARRHYTHMIAS

There are many types of arrhythmias. They include the following:

1. *Premature contractions:* The two major types—**atrial** or **ventricular**—depend on which of the heart's chambers is contracting prematurely. The involved chamber contracts earlier than normal, breaking step with regular heart rhythm. An individual with *premature ventricular contractions* (PVCs) might feel a thump in the chest. Infrequent contractions of this sort occur in many persons and do not require treatment. Too much coffee, too many cigarettes, or too much anxiety may bring on PVCs.

2. *Paroxysmal* (or sudden) *atrial tachycardia* (PAT): A person with this condition typically comes to an emergency room, anxiously describing the sudden onset of a very rapid heart rate. This fast, forceful, but regular heartbeat is due to abnormal conduction pathways in the atria.

3. *Ventricular tachycardia* (VT): The person with this condition experiences attacks of rapid heart rate, dizziness, and sometimes chest pain. This is a far more serious condition than atrial tachycardia because ventricular tachycardias represent electrical impulses originating in the ventricle, which can result in fatal ventricular fibrillation, or rapid and ineffective contractions of the ventricles.

4. *Atrial fibrillation* (AF): This arrhythmia is due to random, chaotic electrical impulses in the atria resulting in the loss of forceful contraction by these chambers.

5. *Ventricular fibrillation* (VF): When ventricular electrical activity becomes chaotic, the muscle tissue does not beat in a coordinated manner. Instead, a series of localized twitching, writhing movements occurs and there is no true pumping action. After a few minutes, all heart activity ceases. VF is frequently the cause of sudden death in patients with heart disease.

6. *Bradycardia:* here a heart beats at an abnormally slow rate. Although strictly defined as a rate below 60 beats a minute, problems generally do not occur until the rate falls below 40.

Questions

I.   Fill in the Blank

Fill in the blank with the appropriate term.

1. Give the prefixes for the following terms:
   a. slow _____
   b. rapid _____

2. What is the medical term for a rapid heartbeat? _____

3. What are the two major types of premature contractions?

    a. _____

    b. _____

4. The term for ineffective ventricular contractions is _____.

II.   Matching

Match the term to its meaning. (The same meaning may be used more than once.) Insert the appropriate letter in the space next to the question number.

Choices:

_____ **1.** anxiety	**a.**	abnormal, rapid heartbeat
_____ **2.** atrial	**b.**	a slow heartbeat
_____ **3.** fibrillation	**c.**	spontaneous contraction of muscle
_____ **4.** ventricular	**d.**	pertaining to ventricle
_____ **5.** contraction	**e.**	feeling of worry
_____ **6.** bradycardia	**f.**	rapid throbbing
_____ **7.** premature	**g.**	before normal time
_____ **8.** tachycardia	**h.**	sudden periodic attack
_____ **9.** paroxysmal	**i.**	a shortening or tightening of a muscle
_____ **10.** palpitation	**j.**	pertains to atrium

III.   Spell Check

Circle each incorrectly spelled term and write it correctly in the space provided.

1. arrhymias   _____

2. bradycarrdia   _____

3. fibrillation   _____

4. paroxymal   _____

5. palpitation   _____

6. ventricular   _____

7. atrial   _____

8. tackycardia   _____

J. Increasing Your Medical Terminology Word Power 2

1. Read the following report.

2. Prepare to answer the questions at the end of the section.

3. Circle all unfamiliar terms with a red pencil.

4. Underline familiar terms with a blue pencil.

5. Use your knowledge of word elements, a medical dictionary, and the key terms to find the meaning of unfamiliar terms.

Surgical Management of Atrial Fibrillation

Key Terms

dysrhythmia (dis-RITH-mē-a)   abnormal rhythm

fibrillation (fi-bril-Ā-shun)   as used here, an abnormal muscle fiber contraction

hemodynamics   the study of forces involved with the circulation of blood through the body

morbidity   the number of cases of a disease in relationship to a specific population

mortality death rate

sequelae (sē-KWE-lē) a condition following and resulting from a disease

thromboembolism blood vessel blockage by a blood clot detached from its site of formation

O VERVIEW

Atrial fibrillation is the most common dysrhythmia encountered in clinical practice. Although many patients tolerate it almost without problems, others may be troubled by the irregular heartbeat or by the medications required for its control. Satisfactory rate control is not possible by pharmacologic means with some patients. Some patients may suffer thromboembolic complications with drug therapy. In the absence of a satisfactory pharmacologic treatment for atrial fibrillation and its sequelae in many patients, a surgical approach to its cure can be used. Such procedures have led to a deeper understanding of the electrophysiologic basis of atrial fibrillation and to the development of surgical procedures that are highly effective in restoring sinus rhythm with an acceptable mortality and morbidity.

Although indications for cardiac arrhythmia surgery have narrowed during the last few years, surgery has evolved into an important therapeutic modality for the treatment of atrial fibrillation. The most common of arrhythmias is present in 0.4–2.0 percent of the general population, and in about 10 percent of the population over the age of 60 years. Frequently considered to be harmless, atrial fibrillation is associated with significant morbidity because of three harmful sequelae. These are (1) an irregularly appearing irregular heartbeat, which causes patient discomfort and anxiety; (2) loss of synchronous atrioventricular contraction, which compromises cardiac hemodynamics resulting in varying levels of congestive heart failure; and (3) stasis of blood flow in the left atrium, which increases the vulnerability to thromboembolism.

Surgical techniques have been designed either to eliminate the arrhythmia or to improve its attendant harmful sequelae. One such procedure can confine atrial fibrillation to the left atrium, while leaving the remainder of the heart in normal sinus rhythm. This type of surgical procedure can be successful in restoring a regular ventricular rhythm without the need for a permanent pacemaker. It also restores normal cardiac hemodynamics.

Questions

I. Fill in the Blank

Fill in the blank with the appropriate term.

1. What is the most common dysrhythmia found in clinical practice?
   _____

2. What percentage of the population over 60 years of age experiences atrial fibrillation? _____

3. List three harmful consequences of atrial fibrillation.

   a. _____
   b. _____
   c. _____

II. Matching

Match the term to its meaning. (The same meaning may be used more than once.) Insert the appropriate letter in the space next to the question number.

Choices:

_____ 1. hemodynamics
_____ 2. fibrillation
_____ 3. dysrhythmia
_____ 4. morbidity
_____ 5. mortality
_____ 6. sequela
_____ 7. thromboembolism

a. number of cases of diseases in relationship to a specific population
b. study of forces involved with blood circulation
c. abnormal rhythm
d. abnormal muscle-fiber contraction
e. death rate
f. a condition following and resulting from a disease
g. blood vessel blockage by a blood clot

III.   Spell Check

Circle each incorrectly spelled term and write it correctly in the space provided.

1. synchronous   _____
2. sequelae   _____
3. pharmacologic   _____
4. fibrillation   _____
5. dysrhythmia   _____
6. electrofisologic _____

K. Increasing Your Medical Terminology Word Power 3

1. Read the following report.
2. Prepare to answer the questions at the end of the section.
3. Circle all unfamiliar terms with a red pencil.
4. Underline familiar terms with a blue pencil.
5. Use your knowledge of word elements, a medical dictionary, and the key terms to find the meaning of unfamiliar terms.

Myocardial Ischemia in Men Undergoing Noncardiac Surgery

Key Terms

congestive heart failure   failure of the heart to maintain adequate circulation of blood, caused by an excessive amount of blood in the heart

coronary heart disease   sufficient narrowing of the coronary arteries to prevent an adequate blood supply to heart tissue

ischemia (is-KĒ-mē-a)   local and temporary deficiency of blood caused by blockage of circulation to a body part

myocardial infarction (mī-ō-KAR-dē-al in-FARK-shun)   heart attack caused by the blockage of one or more of the coronary arteries

postoperative   refers to the time period following a surgical operation

unstable angina (an-JĪ-na)   episodes of pain and constriction, around the heart, that become more frequent and severe

ventricular tachycardia (tak-ē-KAR-dē-a)   an abnormal, rapid beating of the ventricle

Introduction

Unfavorable cardiac events are a major cause of morbidity and mortality after noncardiac surgery. Of the 25 million patients who undergo noncardiac surgery in the United States each year, approximately 3 million have, or are at risk of having, coronary artery disease. Despite recent advances in the diagnosis and treatment of coronary artery disease, approximately 50,000 of these patients have a perioperative myocardial infarction, and more than half the 40,000 deaths after surgery are caused by cardiac events. Determining the risk factors for unfavorable postoperative cardiac outcomes would help in developing preventive and treatment strategies.

$\mathcal{R}$ ESULTS OF A STUDY

Four hundred and seventy-four men, who either had coronary artery disease or were at high risk for it and who were about to undergo elective noncardiac surgery, were studied. Historical, clinical, laboratory, and physiologic data about them was gathered during hospitalization and for 6 to 24 months after surgery. Myocardial ischemia was determined by continuous electrocardiographic monitoring that began two days before surgery and continued for two days after.

Eighty-three patients (18 percent) had postoperative cardiac events in the hospital that were classified as ischemic events (cardiac death, myocardial infarction, unstable angina, congestive heart failure, or ventricular tachycardia). All in all, postoperative myocardial ischemia occurred in 41 percent of the monitored patients. These findings show that early postoperative myocardial ischemia is an important consideration in high-risk patients undergoing noncardiac surgery.

Questions

I.   Matching: Myocardial Ischemia

Match the term to its meaning. (The same meaning may be used more than once.) Insert the appropriate letter in the space next to the question number.

Choices:

_____ **1.** ischemia
_____ **2.** unstable angina
_____ **3.** coronary heart disease
_____ **4.** myocardial infarction
_____ **5.** postoperative
_____ **6.** ventricular tachycardia

a. abnormal rapid ventricular beating
b. local and temporary blood deficiency caused by circulation blockage
c. after a surgical operation
d. narrowing of coronary arteries to prevent adequate blood flow
e. heart attack
f. periodic episodes of pain and constriction around the heart

II.   Spell Check

Circle each incorrectly spelled term and write it correctly in the space provided.

1. infarction   _____
2. tackycardia   _____
3. angina   _____
4. surgiry   _____
5. ishemia   _____
6. conjestive   _____

Term Search Challenge

Locate 18 terms in the puzzle.

1. Write the specific term next to its definition. Then find that term in the puzzle diagram and circle it.
2. Terms may be read from left to right, backward, up, down, or diagonally.
3. If a term appears more than once, circle it only once. (A term may be found inside others.)
4. Check your answers.

Clues:

1. The thinnest and most numerous blood vessels are the _____.
2. Blood vessels that return blood to the heart are the _____.
3. The number of chambers found in the human heart _____.
4. The inner layer of the heart is the _____.
5. The blood vessels that transport oxygenated blood to the left atrium are the _____ veins.
6. The region of the heart that functions as its pacemaker is the _____.
7. The term for a small artery is _____.
8. Blood vessels that carry blood away from the heart _____
9. The loose-fitting protective space that encloses the heart is the _____.
10. The heart valves located between the atria and ventricles are called _____.
11. Blood from the right atrium passes through the _____ valve to fill the right ventricle.
12. Another term used for bicuspid valve is the _____ valve.
13. The phase of contraction in the cardiac cycle is _____.
14. The phase of relaxation in the cardiac cycle is _____.
15. The blood vessels that supply the heart with blood are called the _____ arteries.
16. Abbreviation for an electrocardiogram is _____ or _____.
17. The major systemic artery from which all primary arteries arise is the _____.

Term Search Puzzle

```
A  T  R  I  O  V  E  C  T  R  S  S  A  M  C
H  E  M  O  A  E  N  O  R  O  I  Y  T  I  A
S  I  N  O  R  N  D  R  I  I  N  S  R  T  P
V  P  N  A  T  T  O  O  C  R  O  T  I  R  I
Y  H  R  T  E  R  C  N  U  E  A  O  V  A  L
R  E  I  R  R  I  A  A  S  P  T  L  C  L  L
A  L  N  I  I  C  R  R  P  U  R  E  N  T  A
N  B  F  A  O  U  D  Y  I  S  I  F  O  U  R
O  A  E  L  L  I  L  D  V  A  O  T  L  I
M  R  R  T  E  A  U  M  O  E  L  N  O  D  E
L  S  I  F  G  R  M  N  S  N  V  E  I  N  S
U  O  O  P  U  L  M  I  L  A  L  A  M  Y  O
P  E  R  I  C  A  R  D  I  U  M  T  R  A  E
D  I  A  S  T  O  L  E  A  O  R  T  A  A  K
A  R  T  E  R  I  E  S  H  I  J  K  E  C  G
```

The Respiratory System

"It was the fashion to suffer from the lungs; everybody was consumptive (infected with tuberculosis), poets especially; it was good form to spit blood after each emotion that was at all sensational, and to die before reaching the age of thirty."

—Anonymous

INFORMATIONAL CHALLENGE

A. Structure and Function of the Respiratory System

I.   Fill in the Blank

Fill in the blank with the appropriate term.

     1. The exchange of gases between the air and blood is called _____ respiration.

     2. Gas exchange between the blood and cells is known as _____ respiration.

     3. The units of the lung where gas exchange occurs are known as alveoli or _____.

     4. The region between the lungs in the chest cavity that contains body organs including the heart, trachea, esophagus, and the bronchi is called the _____.

II.   Matching: Structures and Functions of the Respiratory System

Match the term to its meaning. (The same meaning may be used more than once.) Insert the appropriate letter in the space next to the question number.

Choices:

_____ **1.** glottis	**a.** uppermost part of the lung
_____ **2.** tonsils	**b.** larynx
_____ **3.** apex	**c.** collections of lymph tissue in the throat
_____ **4.** oropharynx	
_____ **5.** paranasal sinuses	**d.** the opening or entrance to the larynx and trachea
_____ **6.** trachea	**e.** middle portion of the pharynx
_____ **7.** base	
_____ **8.** pleura	**f.** windpipe

_____ **9.** voice box
_____ **10.** pleural cavity

g. air spaces in certain bones of the skull
h. lower portion of the lung
i. space between the folds of the pleura
j. double-folded membrane surrounding the lungs

III.   Spell Check

Circle each incorrectly spelled term and write it correctly in the space provided.

1. fairnx   _____
2. epiglotis   _____
3. adenoyds   _____
4. bronchiole _____
5. mediastinum _____
6. diaphragm   _____
7. alvelus   _____
8. parietal   _____

IV.   Vision Quiz: The Human Respiratory System

Figure 17-7 shows the human respiratory tract. Identify and write the name of the numbered parts of the respiratory tract in the spaces provided.

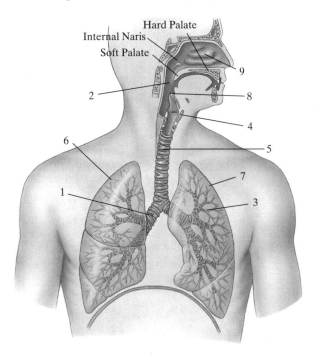

FIGURE 17-7   Vision Quiz. The basic anatomy of the human respiratory system.

1. _____
2. _____
3. _____
4. _____

     5. _____

     6. _____

     7. _____

     8. _____

     9. _____

B. *Word Elements Associated with the Respiratory System*

I.   Fill in the Blank

Fill in the blank with the appropriate term.

   1. Give two word roots used for the nose. _____ and
     _____

   2. Give the combining forms for the throat, _____, and the
     trachea, _____.

   3. List two combining forms for the chest. _____ and
     _____.

   4. Give the word roots used for the bronchial tube, _____,
     and bronchiole, _____.

   5. What are two word roots used for the lung? _____ and
     _____

   6. What is a combining form for the chest? _____

II.   Matching: Word Roots and/or Combining Forms Associated with the
      Respiratory System

Match the term to its meaning. (The same meaning may be used more than once.)
Insert the appropriate letter in the space next to the question number.

Choices:

_____	**1.** adenoid	**a.**	voice box
_____	**2.** laryng/o	**b.**	adenoids
_____	**3.** tonsill	**c.**	to breathe
_____	**4.** lob/o	**d.**	epiglottis
_____	**5.** phren/o	**e.**	sinus
_____	**6.** epiglott/o	**f.**	tonsils
_____	**7.** sinus/o	**g.**	alveolus
_____	**8.** pleur	**h.**	lobe
_____	**9.** alveol/o	**i.**	diaphragm
_____	**10.** spir/o	**j.**	pleura

III.   Spell Check

Circle each incorrectly spelled term and write it correctly in the space provided.

   1. epiglotitis   _____

   2. bronchiolectasis   _____

   3. pectoralgea   _____

   4. frenic   _____

5. rhinorhea   _____

6. pleurogenic   _____

IV.   Word Analysis: Word Elements Associated with the Respiratory System

Table 17-13 lists a number of terms with their pronunciations and definitions.

TABLE 17-13   WORD ANALYSIS: WORD ELEMENTS ASSOCIATED WITH THE RESPIRATORY SYSTEM

Term and Pronunciation	Definition
adenoidectomy (ad-e-noyd-EK-tō-mē)	removal or excision of the adenoids
alveolar (al-VĒ-ō-lar)	pertaining to air sac
bronchial (BRONG-kē-al)	pertaining to the bronchial tube (bronchi)
bronchiolectasis (brong-kē-ō-LEK-tā-sis)	dilation of the bronchioles
bronchitis (brong-KĪ-tis)	inflammation of the bronchial tubes
epiglottitis (ep-i-glot-Ī-tis)	inflammation of the epiglottis
laryngeal (lar-IN-jē-al)	pertaining to the larynx (voice box)
lobule (LOB-ūl)	small lobe pertaining to the nose
nasopharyngeal (nā-zō-far-IN-jē-al)	pertaining to the nose and pharynx (throat)
pectoralgia (pek-tō-RAL-jē-a)	pain in the chest
pharyngitis (far-in-JĪ-tis)	inflammation of the throat (sore throat)
phrenic (FREN-ik)	pertaining to the diaphragm
pleurogenic (ploo-rō-JEN-ik)	produced (arising) in the pleura
pneumogastric (nū-mō-GAS-trik)	pertaining to air in the stomach
pulmonary (PUL-mō-ne-rē)	concerning the lungs
rhinorrhea (ri-nō-RĒ-a)	discharge from the nose
sinusitis (sī-nus-Ī-tis)	inflammation of a sinus
spirometer (spī-ROM-et-er)	an instrument used to measure lung functions
thoracomyodynia (thō-ra-kō-mī-ō-DIN-ē-a)	pain in chest muscles
tonsillitis (ton-sil-Ī-tis)	inflammation of a tonsil
tracheolaryngeal (trā-kē-ō-lar-RIN-jē-al)	concerning the trachea and larynx

1. Analyze each term.
2. Circle all prefixes, suffixes, combining forms, and word roots and label them **p, s, cf,** and **wr,** respectively.
3. Check your answers (shown in Table 17-16).

C. *Respiratory System Diseases and Disorders*

I.   Matching 1: Respiratory System Diseases and Disorders

Match the term to its meaning. (The same meaning may be used more than once.) Insert the appropriate letter in the space next to the question number.

Choices:

_____ **1.** laryngitis	**a.** also known as pertussis
_____ **2.** whooping cough	**b.** infection of the nose, larynx, and bronchi
_____ **3.** URI	
_____ **4.** epistaxis	**c.** inflammation of the larynx
_____ **5.** tonsillitis	**d.** tonsil inflammation
_____ **6.** pharyngitis	**e.** sore throat
_____ **7.** pansinusitis	**f.** nosebleed
	g. inflammation of all sinuses

II.   Matching 2: Diseases and Disorders of Lower Respiratory Tract

Match the term to its meaning. (The same meaning may be used more than once.) Insert the appropriate letter in the space next to the question number.

Choices:

_____ **1.** anthracosis	**a.** diseases in which periodic attacks of wheezing, coughing, and shortness of breath occur
_____ **2.** atelectasis	
_____ **3.** byssinosis	
_____ **4.** empyema	**b.** brown-lung disease
_____ **5.** asthma	**c.** hereditary disorder in children and characterized by abnormal mucus production in respiratory tract
_____ **6.** respiratory distress syndrome	
_____ **7.** cystic fibrosis	**d.** atelectasis in the newborn
_____ **8.** hemothorax	**e.** blood in the pleural cavity
_____ **9.** pneumoconiosis	**f.** abnormal condition of dust in the lungs
	g. pus in the pleural cavity
	h. collapse of a normal lung area
	i. disease caused by coal dust

III.   Spell Check

Circle each incorrectly spelled term and write it correctly in the space provided.

1. edema   _____
2. diptheria   _____
3. pertusis   _____
4. nasofharyngitis   _____
5. absces   _____
6. rhonchi   _____
7. embulism   _____
8. tuberculosis   _____
9. pneumonia   _____

10. neumocystis _____

11. cocidiodomycosis _____

12. pulmonale _____

IV.   Word Analysis: Respiratory System Diseases and Disorders

Table 17-14 lists a number of terms with their pronunciations.

TABLE 17-14   WORD ANALYSIS: RESPIRATORY SYSTEM DISEASES AND DISORDERS

Term and Pronunciation

anthracosis (an-thra-KŌ-sis)

asbestosis (as-be-STŌ-sis)

bronchogenic (brong-kō-JEN-ik)

hemothorax (hē-mō-THŌ-raks)

laryngitis (lar-in-JĪ-tis)

nasopharyngitis (nā-zō-far-in-JĪ-tis)

pansinusitis (pan-sī-nus-Ī-tis)

pneumonia (nū-MŌ-nē-a)

pneumothorax (nū-mō-THŌ-raks)

tonsillitis (ton-sil-Ī-tis)

1. Analyze each term.

2. Circle all prefixes, suffixes, combining forms, and word roots and label them **p, s, cf,** and **wr,** respectively.

3. Check your answers (shown in Table 17-17).

D. Signs and Symptoms of Pulmonary Disease or Disorders

I.   Matching: Signs and Symptoms of Pulmonary Disease or Disorders

Match the term to its meaning. (The same meaning may be used more than once.) Insert the appropriate letter in the space next to the question number.

Choices:

_____ **1.** cyanosis
_____ **2.** tachypnea
_____ **3.** rales
_____ **4.** wheezing
_____ **5.** dyspnea
_____ **6.** hemoptysis
_____ **7.** dysphagia

a. abnormal rattling sounds heard on examination
b. bluish discoloration of the skin
c. whistling sounds during difficult breathing
d. increased rate of breathing
e. bloody septum
f. difficult breathing
g. difficulty in swallowing

II.   Spell Check

Circle each incorrectly spelled term and write it correctly in the space provided.

1. syanosis   _____

2. disphagia   _____

3. dyspnea   _____

4. hemoptisis   _____

5. rales   _____

6. ronchi   _____

7. tachypnea   _____

8. whezing   _____

E. Clinical and Diagnostic Procedures

I.   Matching 1: Clinical and Diagnostic Procedures

Match the term to its meaning. (The same meaning may be used more than once.)
Insert the appropriate letter in the space next to the question number.

Choices:

_____ **1.** laryngoscopy
_____ **2.** bronchoscopy
_____ **3.** bronchial washing
_____ **4.** lung scan
_____ **5.** tuberculin test
_____ **6.** tomogram
_____ **7.** angiogram
_____ **8.** pulmonary function tests

a. bronchi examination by means of a fiber optic tube

b. examination of voice box

c. test to detect susceptibility or active tuberculosis

d. the use of radioactive material to determine its distribution in the lungs

e. the use of radioactive material to examine the size and shape of blood vessels

f. an x-ray procedure used to obtain a detailed view of a selected tissue or organ

g. a procedure used to obtain bronchial secretions

h. test used to evaluate the functioning of the respiratory system

II.   Matching 2: Pulmonary Function

Match the term to its meaning. (The same meaning may be used more than once.)
Insert the appropriate letter in the space next to the question number.

Choices:

_____ **1.** respiratory rate
_____ **2.** tidal volume
_____ **3.** total lung capacity
_____ **4.** vital capacity
_____ **5.** residual air
_____ **6.** minute volume
_____ **7.** dead space

a. amount of air normally moved into and out of the lungs during the breathing

b. maximum quantity of air that can be moved into and out of the lungs

c. amount of air left in the lungs after maximum expiration

d. number of breaths per minute

e. quantity of air the lungs can hold

f. air not available for gas exchange

g. amount of air moved into and out of the lungs in one minute

III.   Spell Check

Circle each incorrectly spelled term and write it correctly in the space provided.

1. bronchiel   _____
2. tuberkulin   _____
3. laryngoscopy   _____
4. expiratory   _____
5. inspiratory   _____
6. residuel   _____
7. tidal   _____

IV.   Vision Quiz: Respiratory Volume and Capacity

Figure 17-8 shows a diagrammatic representation of respiratory volumes and their relationships to one another.

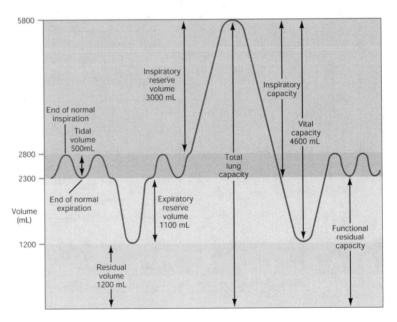

FIGURE 17-8

1. Locate and note the following respiratory volumes and capacities:
   a. Inspiratory Reserve Volume (IRV)
   b. Tidal Volume (TV)
   c. Expiratory Reserve Volume (EQV)
   d. Residual Volume (RV)

2. Using Figure 17-8, determine which of the respiratory volumes form the following respiratory capacities. (Capacity = Volume)
   a. Inspiratory Capacity (IC) = Inspiratory Reserve Volume (IRV) + _____
   b. Functional Residual Capacity (FRC) = _____ + _____
   c. Vital Capacity (VC) = _____ + _____ + _____
   d. Total Lung Capacity (TLC) = _____ + _____ + _____ + _____

F. Surgical Procedures

I. Matching: Surgical and Related Procedures

Match the term to its meaning. (The same meaning may be used more than once.)
Insert the appropriate letter in the space next to the question number.

Choices:

_____ **1.** laryngectomy

_____ **2.** endotracheal intubation

_____ **3.** thoracentesis

_____ **4.** pleurectomy

_____ **5.** rhinoplasty

_____ **6.** pneumonectomy

_____ **7.** septectomy

_____ **8.** lobectomy

_____ **9.** tracheostomy

a. plastic reconstruction of the nose

b. removal of the pleura

c. excision of the nasal septum

d. the insertion of a tube through the mouth, throat, and into the trachea

e. excision of the larynx

f. removal of the lobe

g. obtaining fluid from the pleural cavity with a needle puncture of the chest wall

h. excision of a lung

i. a surgical incision into the trachea to make a permanent airway

II. Spell Check

Circle each incorrectly spelled term and write it correctly in the space provided.

1. thorcentesis   _____

2. plerectomy   _____

3. rhinoplasty   _____

4. trachostomy   _____

5. pneumonectomy   _____

6. lobectomy   _____

III. Word Analysis: Surgical and Related Procedures

Table 17-15 lists a number of terms with their pronunciations.

TABLE 17-15   WORD ANALYSIS: SURGICAL AND RELATED PROCEDURES

Term and Pronunciation
endotracheal (en'-dō-TRĀ-kē-al)
laryngectomy (lar-in-JEK-tō-mē)
lobectomy (lō-BEK-tō-mē)
pleurectomy (ploo-REK-tō-mē)
pneumonectomy (nū-mō-NEK-tō-mē)

(Continued)

TABLE 17-15   (CONTINUED)

Term and Pronunciation

rhinoplasty (RĪ-nō-plas-tē)

septectomy (sep-TEK-tō-mē)

thoracentesis (thō-ra-sen-TĒ-sis)

tracheostomy (tra-kē-OS-tō-mē)

1. Analyze each term.
2. Circle all prefixes, suffixes, combining forms, and word roots and label them **p, s, cf,** and **wr,** respectively.
3. Check your answers (shown in Table 17-18).

G. Medical Vocabulary Building

I.   Matching: Medical Vocabulary Building

Match the term to its meaning. (The same meaning may be used more than once.) Insert the appropriate letter in the space next to the question number.

Choices:

_____ 1. aphonia

_____ 2. diaphragmalgia

_____ 3. aeropleura

_____ 4. orthopnea

_____ 5. eupnea

_____ 6. palatoplegia

_____ 7. rhinostenosis

_____ 8. pyothorax

_____ 9. Heimlich maneuver

_____ 10. pollinosis

a. hay fever
b. physical technique to remove a foreign body blocking the trachea
c. pus in the chest cavity
d. nasal passages narrowing
e. inability to breathe unless in an upright position
f. soft palate muscle paralysis
g. pain in the diaphragm
h. normal breathing
i. inability to produce vocal sounds
j. air in the pleural cavity

II.   Spell Check

Circle each incorrectly spelled term and write it correctly in the space provided.

1. ronchus   _____
2. asfixyia   _____
3. rhinostenosis   _____
4. diaframalgia   _____
5. polip   _____
6. pollinosis   _____
7. upnea   _____
8. aphonia   _____

H. *Abbreviations*

I.   Matching 1: Respiratory System Anatomy and Function Part-1

Match the term to its meaning. (The same meaning may be used more than once.)
Insert the appropriate letter in the space next to the question number.

Choices:

_____ **1.** ACD	**a.** expiratory volume
_____ **2.** FRC	**b.** forced expiratory flow
_____ **3.** FEF	**c.** functional residual capacity
_____ **4.** ERV	**d.** inspiratory capacity
_____ **5.** IC	**e.** anterior chest diameter
_____ **6.** FEV	**f.** inspiratory reserve volume
_____ **7.** MBC	**g.** forced expiratory volume
_____ **8.** IRV	**h.** left lower lobe
_____ **9.** LLL	**i.** midcostal line
_____ **10.** MCL	**j.** breathing capacity

II.   Matching 2: Respiratory System Anatomy and Function Part-2

Match the term to its meaning. (The same meaning may be used more than once.)
Insert the appropriate letter in the space next to the question number.

Choices:

_____ **1.** maximal expiratory flow rate	**a.** PA
	b. RLL
_____ **2.** midsternal line	**c.** MEFR
_____ **3.** posterior-anterior	**d.** MSL
_____ **4.** right lower lobe	**e.** RM
_____ **5.** respiratory movement	**f.** RV
_____ **6.** respiratory volume	**g.** TLA
_____ **7.** thoracic gas volume	**h.** TV
_____ **8.** vital capacity	**i.** TGV
_____ **9.** tidal volume	**j.** VC
_____ **10.** total lung volume	

III.   Matching 3: Respiratory System Diseases and Disorders

Match the term to its meaning. (The same meaning may be used more than once.)
Insert the appropriate letter in the space next to the question number.

Choices:

_____ **1.** AFB	**a.** acid-fast bacillus
_____ **2.** ARDS	**b.** respiratory disease
_____ **3.** ARD	**c.** acute respiratory disease
_____ **4.** INH	**d.** tuberculosis
_____ **5.** RD	**e.** isoniazid
_____ **6.** ARF	**f.** upper respiratory infection
_____ **7.** URI	**g.** sudden infant death syndrome
_____ **8.** tb	**h.** acute respiratory failure
_____ **9.** PND	**i.** paroxysmal nocturnal dyspnea
_____ **10.** SIDS	**j.** bacillus of Calmette and Guerín
_____ **11.** BCG	**k.** adult respiratory distress syndrome

IV.   Matching 4: Diagnostic Tests and Procedures

Match the term to its meaning. (The same meaning may be used more than once.)
Insert the appropriate letter in the space next to the question number.

Choices:

_____ **1.** anterior chest diameter   **a.** BS
_____ **2.** controlled mechanical   **b.** CXR
           ventilation   **c.** ACD
_____ **3.** chest x-ray   **d.** IMV
_____ **4.** continued positive airway   **e.** CMV
           pressure   **f.** IPPB
_____ **5.** breath sounds   **g.** CPAP
_____ **6.** intermittent mandatory   **h.** PAO_2
           pressure   **i.** TF
_____ **7.** intermittent positive-   **j.** SOB
           pressure breathing   **k.** PEEP
_____ **8.** tactile fremitus
_____ **9.** arterial oxygen tension
_____ **10.** positive end-expiratory
           pressure
_____ **11.** shortness of breath

V.   Spell Check

Circle each incorrectly spelled term and write it correctly in the space provided.

1. resuscitation   _____
2. residual   _____
3. thorasic   _____
4. bronchoscopy   _____
5. isoniazid   _____
6. fremitis   _____
7. intermitant   _____
8. distress   _____

VI.   Fill in the Blank

Fill in the blank with the appropriate term.

1. CPR _____
2. IC _____
3. TGV _____
4. PND _____
5. SIDS _____
6. AFB _____
7. TF _____
8. ARDS _____

I. Increasing Your Medical Terminology Word Power 1

1. Read the following report.
2. Prepare to answer the questions at the end of the section.
3. Circle all unfamiliar terms with a red pencil.
4. Underline familiar terms with a blue pencil.
5. Use your knowledge of word elements, a medical dictionary, and the
     key terms to find the meaning of unfamiliar terms.

Pneumothorax After Acupuncture

Key Terms

acupuncture (ak-ū-PUNGK-chur)   technique for treating a variety of conditions by passing thin needles through the skin to specific points; loss of sensation, usually in the form of pain, occurs

asthma (AZ-ma)   periodic or recurring difficulty in breathing accompanied by a spasm of the bronchial tubes or by swelling of their mucous membrane; usually caused by some form of allergy

bronchodilator therapy   treatment used to open bronchus to ease breathing

cannula (KAN-ū-la)   a tube containing a sharp instrument used to introduce or to remove substances such as fluids or gas

costovertebral (kos-tō-VER-tē-bral) pertains to a rib and a vertebra

cyanosis (sī-a-NŌ-sis)   slightly bluish or purple discoloration of the skin

dyspnea (DISP-nē-a)   difficulty in breathing

expiratory (eks-PĪ-ra-tōr-ē)   pertains to expelling air

hemithorax (hem-ē-THŌ-rax)   one-half of the chest

inspiratory (in-SPĪR-a-tōr-ē)   pertains to inhaling air

pleuritic (ploo-RIT-ik)   related to inflammation of the pleura

pneumothorax (nū-mō-THŌ-rax)   a collection of gas or air in the pleural cavity

tachypnea (tak'-ip-NĒ-a)   abnormal rapid breathing

thoracostomy (thō-rak-OS-tō-mē) tubes   tubes used to allow room for drainage of the chest

wheezing   a whistling sound resulting from a narrowing of the space of a respiratory passage

yin-yang   in Chinese philosophy and medicine, represents opposing concepts, forces, or other related factors, such as light–dark, sun–moon, male–female; the major goal of yin-yang is to have a proper balance of forces

Introduction

During the past twenty or so years, acupuncture has become an increasingly popular alternative treatment for a variety of illnesses. Although viewed by many as useful for musculoskeletal conditions, it is also used by some physicians for systemic illnesses, including asthma.

The principle of Chinese acupuncture is that inserting small needles along various channels restores the balance between yin and yang. The acupuncture needles are typically made of stainless steel and are small in size. The so-called lung channel runs from below the clavicle, down the median aspect of the arm, and ends in the thumb. Under usual circumstances, penetration of the skin along these points is harmless, although possibly associated with minor discomfort. Many physicians insert needles in other locations, however, including the upper back. Unfortunately, a pneumothorax can develop, particularly when the insertions are done during acute asthma attacks.

*C*ASE HISTORY

A twenty-nine-year-old woman underwent acupuncture for the treatment of asthma during her third pregnancy. She had a history of childhood asthma but was asymptomatic from age eleven until age twenty-seven. During her second pregnancy, asthma recurred. About two weeks before undergoing acupuncture, she had a worsening of her asthma despite the use of several medications.

On the day of admission, she visited an acupuncturist who inserted standard acupuncture needles bilaterally into the tissues of her upper back. At the time of the needle insertions, she experienced severe pleuritic chest pain that lasted until she left the acupuncturist's office three hours later. The severe dyspnea and tachypnea developed so rapidly that she could not talk comfortably. She was seen at a nearby emergency department where her x-ray film showed bilateral pneumothoraces, but the abnormality was not recognized until she was transferred to the medical center hospital for further evaluation.

She arrived at the hospital about nine hours after the initial acupuncture needle placement. She was in severe respiratory distress. Vital signs showed low blood pressure, a heart rate of 100 beats per minute, and respirations of 40 per minute. A physical examination revealed that she had bilateral costovertebral angle tenderness. Inspiratory and expiratory wheezing were also noted. There was no cyanosis or edema.

The patient was given oxygen by nasal cannula set at 6 liters per minute. Bilateral thoracostomy tubes were immediately placed, and there was a rush of escaping air from each hemithorax. Her condition rapidly improved, but she still required standard bronchodilator therapy and medication for asthma management. She was discharged after nine days and eventually bore a full-term infant.

Questions

I.   Matching

Match the term to its meaning. (The same meaning may be used more than once.) Insert the appropriate letter in the space next to the question number.

Choices:

_____ **1.** wheezing	**a.** abnormal rapid breathing
_____ **2.** hemithorax	**b.** collection of air in the pleural cavity
_____ **3.** cyanosis	**c.** pertains to inhaling
_____ **4.** pleuritic	**d.** bluish coloration of the skin
_____ **5.** inspiratory	**e.** pertains to exhaling
_____ **6.** expiratory	**f.** related to inflammation of the pleura
_____ **7.** acupuncture	**g.** one-half of the chest
_____ **8.** dyspnea	**h.** difficulty in breathing
_____ **9.** tachypnea	**i.** a whistling sound heard during abnormal breathing
_____ **10.** pneumothorax	**j.** use of thin needles to relieve pain

II.   Spell Check

Circle each incorrectly spelled term and write it correctly in the space provided.

1. neumothorax _____

2. tachepnea _____

3. costovertebral _____

4. pleuritic _____

5. canula _____

6. signosis _____

J. Increasing Your Medical Terminology Word Power 2

1. Read the following report.
2. Prepare to answer the questions at the end of the section.
3. Circle all unfamiliar terms with a red pencil.
4. Underline familiar terms with a blue pencil.
5. Use your knowledge of word elements, a medical dictionary, and the key terms to find the meaning of unfamiliar terms.

Spontaneous Pneumothorax

Key Terms

aspiration (as-pi-RĀ-shun)   drawing in or out as by suction

bulla (BUL-la)   a large blister filled with fluid

dyspnea (DISP-nē-a)   difficult breathing

hypoxemia (hī'-poks-Ē-mē-a)   insufficient oxygenation of the blood

iatrogenic (ī'-at-rō-JEN-ik)   pertains to any adverse condition induced in a patient caused by medical treatment

ipsilateral (ip'-si-LAT-er-al)   on the same side

pleuritic (ploo-RIT-ik)   related to, or like, pleurisy

pleurodesis (ploo'-rō-DĒ-sis)   production of a bond or bindings between the parietal and visceral pleura; usually done surgically

thoracotomy (thō'-rak-OT-ō-mē)   surgical incision of the chest wall

Introduction

Pneumothorax is classified as *spontaneous*, *traumatic*, or *iatrogenic*.

1. Primary spontaneous pneumothorax occurs in individuals without clinically apparent lung disease.
2. Secondary spontaneous pneumothorax is a complication of preexisting lung diseases.
3. Iatrogenic pneumothorax results from a complication of a diagnostic or therapeutic intervention.
4. Traumatic pneumothorax is caused by penetrating the chest or blunt injury (trauma) to the chest, with air entering the pleural space directly through the chest wall; visceral pleural penetration; or alveolar rupture caused by sudden chest compression.

*P*ATHOPHYSIOLOGY ASPECTS

Although patients with primary spontaneous pneumothorax do not have clinically apparent lung disease, subpleural bullae are found in 77 to 100 percent of patients during video-assisted thoracoscopic surgery. The mechanism of bulla formation remains unknown. A large, primary spontaneous pneumothorax results in a decrease in vital capacity that contributes to varying degrees of hypoxemia.

*C*LINICAL PRESENTATION

Most episodes of primary spontaneous pneumothorax occur while the patient is at rest. Virtually all patients have ipsilateral pleuritic chest pain or acute dyspnea. Chest pain may be minimal or severe and, at onset, has been described as "sharp" and later as a "steady ache." Signs and symptoms usually resolve within 24 hours, even if the pneumothorax remains untreated and does not resolve. Tachycardia is the most common physical finding.

𝒟 IAGNOSIS

The diagnosis of primary pneumothorax is suggested by the patient's history and is confirmed by the identification of a thin, visceral pleural line measuring less than 1 mm in width. This line is found to be displaced from the chest wall on a posterior-anterior chest radiograph taken with the patient in an upright position.

𝒯 REATMENT

The management of pneumothorax depends on the effective evacuation of air from the pleural space and in preventing recurrences. Therapeutic options that are available include

1. simple aspiration by means of a catheter, with immediate catheter removal after the pleural air is evacuated;
2. insertion of a chest tube;
3. pleurodesis;
4. thoracoscopy through a single insertion port into the chest;
5. video-assisted thoracoscopic surgery; or
6. thoracotomy.

Questions

I.   Fill in the Blank

Fill in the blank with the appropriate term.

1. When do symptoms of spontaneous pneumothorax resolve?
   _____
2. Which type of pneumothorax results from a complication of a diagnostic or therapeutic intervention? _____
3. What is the most common physical finding with primary pneumothorax? _____

II.   Matching: Spontaneous Pneumothorax

Match the term to its meaning. (The same meaning may be used more than once.) Insert the appropriate letter in the space next to the question number.

Choices:

_____ 1. bulla
_____ 2. dyspnea
_____ 3. aspiration
_____ 4. hypoxemia
_____ 5. pleuritic
_____ 6. iatrogenic
_____ 7. pleurodesis
_____ 8. thoractotomy

a. removal by suction
b. a large blister filled with fluid
c. difficult breathing
d. refers to condition caused by medical treatment
e. insufficient oxygen in the blood
f. related to pleurisy
g. surgical incision into the chest wall
h. bindings between the parietal and visceral pleura

III.   Spell Check

Circle each incorrectly spelled term and write it correctly in the space provided.

1. ipsilatyeral   _____
2. dyspnea   _____
3. asperation   _____
4. pleuritic   _____
5. neumothorax   _____
6. pleurodesis   _____

K. Increasing Your Medical Terminology Word Power 3

1. Read the following report.
2. Prepare to answer the questions at the end of the section.
3. Circle all unfamiliar terms with a red pencil.
4. Underline familiar terms with a blue pencil.
5. Use your knowledge of word elements, a medical dictionary, and the key terms to find the meaning of unfamiliar terms.

Folded Lung

Key Terms

asbestosis (as-be-STŌ-sis)   lung disease resulting from inhalation of asbestos

bronchogram (BRONG-kō-gram)   an x-ray (roentgenogram) of the lungs and bronchi

CT   computerized tomography

ipsilateral (ip'-si-LAT-er-al)   on the same side

lentiform (LENT-i-form)   lens-shaped

mesothelioma (mes'-ō-thē-lē-Ō-ma)   a rare form of cancer found within the lining of the pleura and membranous sac covering the heart

periphery (per-IF-e-rē)   outer part or surface

thoracotomy (thō'-rak-OT-ō-mē)   surgical incision into the chest wall

A REVIEW OF CASES

Nine individuals with folded lung examined by CT scans over a four-year period were identified from patient records. All of the patients were examined because of the presence of a mass or masses, visible on chest radiographs, that were regarded as suspicious of malignancy. One patient was examined because of increasing left basal pleural thickening together with a clinical suspicion of a mesothelioma.

Features seen in all lesions examined included a *peripheral location* (defined as a lesion with its outer edge not more than 2 cm from the pleura) and the presence of smoothly curved bronchi and vessels around the lesion.

In all patients there was at least a moderate degree of pleural thickening in the ipsilateral lung. Other features frequently, but not invariably, seen on air bronchograms included lesions within or next to the pleura and had at least two sharp margins.

The shape of the folded lung may be spherical, lentiform, or irregular. Some may calcify.

Six of the nine patients had an occupational history of asbestos exposure.

Questions

I.   Fill in the Blank

Fill in the blank with the appropriate term.

1. What feature was common in all patients? _____

_____

2. What two features were commonly found in all lesions?

_____ and _____

3. List three shapes found with folded-lung cases.

    a. _____

    b. _____

    c. _____

4. If a lesion occurs on the periphery of an organ, where is it located?

_____

II.   Spell Check

Circle each incorrectly spelled term and write it correctly in the space provided.

1. asbestos   _____
2. thoracotomy   _____
3. lentiform   _____
4. bronchgram   _____
5. peripheri   _____
6. mesothelioma   _____

Term Search Challenge

Locate 19 terms in the puzzle.

1. Write the specific term next to its definition. Then find that term in the puzzle diagram and circle it.
2. Terms may be read from left to right, backward, up, down, or diagonally.
3. If a term appears more than once, circle it only once. (A term may be found inside others.)
4. Check your answers.

Clues:

1. The exchange of gases between the air and blood is called _____ respiration.
2. The gas exchange between the blood and tissues is known as _____ respiration.
3. Another term for air sacs is _____.
4. The paired air spaces in certain bones of the skull are called paranasal _____.
5. The passageway for air into the voice box and for food into the esophagus is the _____ (throat).
6. The major organs containing the bronchial trees, air sacs and other pulmonary vessels are the _____.
7. The uppermost part of the lung is referred to as its _____.
8. The combining form for lung is _____.
9. A term for blood in the pleural cavity is _____-thorax.

10. Two combining forms for the nose are _____ and
    _____.

11. Another term for the voice box is _____.

12. The divisions of a lung are called _____.

13. The fold of cartilage that covers the voice box during swallowing is called _____.

14. The term used for an inflammation of the pleura is _____.

15. The examination procedure applied to the bronchi is _____.

16. The surgical procedure of cutting into the windpipe and the insertion of a tube for air exchange is called _____.

17. An instrument used to measure the air taken into and out of the lungs is a _____-meter.

18. The term for abnormal rattling sounds heard on auscultation (listening to sounds within the body) is _____.

Term Search Puzzle

```
A  L  V  E  O  L  I  T  R  A  C  S  E  G  E
L  O  B  E  S  P  U  L  M  P  B  P  P  T  X
E  M  P  A  P  N  A  S  O  E  R  I  I  N  T
M  A  X  I  L  L  A  R  Y  X  O  R  G  M  E
E  M  P  L  E  U  R  I  S  Y  N  O  L  O  R
P  H  R  L  U  N  G  S  T  I  C  P  O  I  N
F  H  E  P  R  R  H  I  N  O  H  N  T  D  A
R  V  N  N  A  R  A  L  E  S  O  E  T  A  L
O  M  O  N  E  M  P  H  Y  S  S  U  I  L  L
N  H  E  M  O  I  A  T  R  E  C  M  S  H  A
T  P  N  E  U  M  O  C  A  M  O  O  N  C  R
A  P  H  A  R  Y  N  X  H  A  P  N  I  A  Y
L  A  D  I  O  N  E  H  P  S  Y  O  R  B  N
T  R  A  C  H  E  O  S  T  O  M  Y  E  A  X
I  N  T  E  R  N  A  L  S  I  N  U  S  E  S
```

The Gastrointestinal System

It's a very odd thing
As odd as it can be
That whatever Ms. T. eats
Turns into Ms. T.

—Walter de la Mare, "Miss T."

INFORMATIONAL CHALLENGE

A. The Mouth and Associated Structures

I.   Fill in the Blank

Fill in the blank with the appropriate term.

1. List the three pairs of salivary glands of the mouth. _____, _____, and _____
2. Another term for swallowing is _____.
3. The process by which food is broken down mechanically into an absorbable form is called _____.

II.   Matching: The Mouth and Associated Structures

Match the term to its meaning. (The same meaning may be used more than once.) Insert the appropriate letter in the space next to the question number.

_____ **1.** cheeks   _____ **6.** papillae
_____ **2.** taste buds   _____ **7.** pharynx
_____ **3.** palate   _____ **8.** pulp
_____ **4.** gingiva   _____ **9.** crown
_____ **5.** tongue

Choices:

a. small elevations on the tongue giving it a rough surface
b. roof of the mouth
c. inner sides of the mouth
d. small projections on the tongue that are sensitive to the chemical nature of foods
e. the part of the tooth above the gums
f. functions to move food around the mouth during chewing and assists in swallowing

g. gums

h. central part of each tooth that contains blood vessels and nerves

i. passageway connecting the oral cavity to the esophagus and trachea

III.   Spell Check

Circle each incorrectly spelled term and write it correctly in the space provided.

    1. salivery   _____

    2. uvela   _____

    3. tonsills   _____

    4. palatine   _____

    5. tonsillectomy   _____

    6. paroted   _____

    7. sublingual   _____

    8. kuspids   _____

    9. decidious   _____

   10. incisor   _____

IV.   Vision Quiz: The Mouth

Figure 18-11 shows components of the mouth. Identify and write the name of the numbered components in the spaces provided.

    1. _____

    2. _____

    3. _____

    4. _____

    5. _____

    6. _____

    7. _____

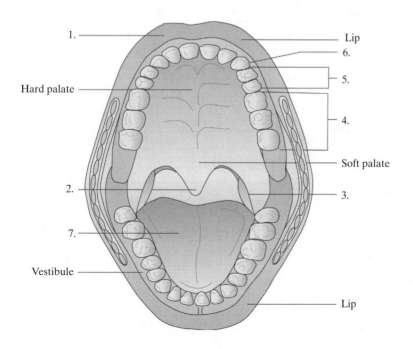

FIGURE 18-11   Vision Quiz. The Mouth.

B. Word Roots and/or Combining Forms Associated with the Mouth and Related Structures

I.   Fill in the Blank

Fill in the blank with the appropriate term.

1. List two combining forms for the *lips*. _____ and _____

2. Give two combining forms for the *tongue*. _____ and _____

II.   Matching

Match the term to its meaning. (The same meaning may be used more than once.) Insert the appropriate letter in the space next to the question number.

Choices:

_____ **1.** cheek	**a.** denti
_____ **2.** lip	**b.** gingiv
_____ **3.** gum	**c.** lingu
_____ **4.** tooth	**d.** bucc
_____ **5.** palate	**e.** palat/o
_____ **6.** tongue	**f.** cheil/o
_____ **7.** mouth	**g.** stomat/o
_____ **8.** salivary gland	**h.** or/o
_____ **9.** lower jaw	**i.** sialaden/o
_____ **10.** tonsil	**j.** submaxillary
	k. tonsill/o

III.   Spell Check

Circle each incorrectly spelled term and write it correctly in the space provided.

1. labiogingival _____

2. submaxilary _____

3. tonsiloscopy _____

4. orel _____

5. sialic _____

6. gingevitis _____

7. periodontitis _____

8. pharyngitis _____

9. cheilotomy _____

10. uvular _____

IV.   Word Analysis: Word Roots and Combining Forms for GI-Associated Organs, Glands, Products, and Substances

Table 18-16 lists a number of terms with their pronunciations and definitions.

1. Analyze each term.

2. Circle all combining forms and word roots and label them **cf** and **wr**, respectively.

3. Check your answers (shown in Table 18-19).

TABLE 18-16   WORD ANALYSIS: WORD ROOTS AND COMBINING FORMS FOR GI-ASSOCIATED ORGANS, GLANDS, PRODUCTS, AND SUBSTANCES

Term and Pronunciation	Brief Explanation
buccal (BUK-al)	pertaining to the cheek (or mouth)
cheilotomy (kī-LOT-ō-mē)	surgical excision (removal) of part of the lip
dentibuccal (den-ti-BUK-al)	pertaining to both the cheek and teeth
gingivitis (jin-ji-VĪ-tis)	inflammation of the gums
glossopharyngeal (glos-ō-fa-RIN-jē-al)	related to the tongue and throat
labiogingival (la-bē-ō-JIN-ji-val)	concerning or pertaining to the gums
lingual (LING-gwal)	pertaining to the tongue
periodontist (per'-ē-ō-DONT-ist)	dental specialist dealing with diseases and treatment of teeth, supporting tissue, and structures
oral (OR-al)	concerning the mouth
palatorrhaphy (pal-a-TOR-a-fē)	surgical operation for joining a cleft palate
pharyngitis (far'-in-JĪ-tis)	inflammation of the pharynx (throat); sore throat
sialic (sī-AL-ik)	concerning or resembling saliva
sialadenitis (sī-al-ad-e-NĪ-tis)	inflammation of a salivary gland
stomatopathy (stō-ma-TOP-a-thē)	(any) mouth disease
submaxillary (sub-MAK-si-ler-ē)	pertaining to the lower jaw
tonsilloscopy (ton-sil-LOS-kō-pē)	examination of the tonsils
uvular (Ū-vū-lar)	pertaining to the uvula

C. The Gastrointestinal System, Structure and Function

I.   Fill in the Blank

Fill in the blank with the appropriate term.

1. The rhythmic, wavelike movement of food through the digestive tract is called _____

2. The elimination of indigestible wastes (feces) from the body is called _____

3. List the three regions of the stomach. _____, _____, and _____

4. List the three anatomical regions of the large intestine.
_____, _____, and _____

5. List the four parts of the colon. _____, _____,
_____, and _____

II.   Matching: The Gastrointestinal System, Structure and Function

Match the term to its meaning. (The same meaning may be used more than once.)
Insert the appropriate letter in the space next to the question number.

Choices:

_____ 1. sphincters
_____ 2. gallbladder
_____ 3. emulsification
_____ 4. peristalsis
_____ 5. duodenum
_____ 6. lobule
_____ 7. sigmoid colon
_____ 8. hepatic portal system
_____ 9. bilirubin
_____ 10. villi

a. the involuntary wavelike contractions that move food along the GI tract
b. process in which fats are broken down into small forms
c. common bile duct and pancreatic duct empty into this part of the small intestines
d. blood vessels that bring blood to and from the liver
e. stores and concentrates bile
f. functional unit of the liver
g. portion of the large intestine shaped like an S
h. the rings of muscles that control the openings leading into and from the stomach
i. one type of bile pigment
j. microscopic projections in the small intestine that absorb nutrients such as amino acids and simple sugars

III.   Spell Check

Circle each incorrectly spelled term and write it correctly in the space provided

1. sigmoyd   _____
2. mastication   _____
3. degluton   _____
4. rugae   _____
5. viscera   _____
6. chime   _____
7. pharynx   _____
8. peristalsis   _____
9. gastrointestinal _____
10. sphincter   _____

IV.   Vision Quiz: The Gastrointestinal System

Figure 18-12 shows the GI system. Identify and write the name of the numbered parts of the system in the spaces provided.

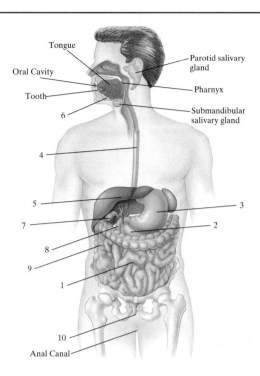

Tongue

Oral Cavity

Tooth

Parotid salivary gland

Pharnyx

Submandibular salivary gland

6

4

5

3

7

2

8

9

1

10

Anal Canal

FIGURE 18-12   Vision Quiz. The Gastrointestinal System.

1. _____

2. _____

3. _____

4. _____

5. _____

6. _____

7. _____

8. _____

9. _____

10. _____

D. *Word Roots and/or Combining Forms for the GI Tract and Related Areas*

I.   Fill in the Blank

Fill in the blank with the appropriate term.

1. Give two combining forms for the *appendix*. _____ and
_____.

2. List two combining forms for the *colon*. _____ and
_____.

II.   Matching 1: Word Roots and/or Combining Forms for the GI Tract and Related Areas

Match the term to its meaning. (The same meaning may be used more than once.)
Insert the appropriate letter in the space next to the question number.

Choices:

_____ **1.** an/o   **a.** duodenum

_____ **2.** duoden   **b.** stomach

_____ 3.	cec/o	c.	anus
_____ 4.	gastr	d.	small intestine
_____ 5.	enter/o	e.	cecum
_____ 6.	ileum	f.	peritoneo
_____ 7.	peritoneum	g.	proct/o
_____ 8.	anus and rectum	h.	pylor/o
_____ 9.	sigmoid colon	i.	ile/o
_____ 10.	pylorus	j.	sigmoid/o

III.   Matching 2: Word Roots and/or Combining Forms for Gastrointestinal-Associated Glands, Products, and Related Substances

Choices:

_____ 1.	starch	a.	bilirubin/o
_____ 2.	sugar	b.	amyl
_____ 3.	bile	c.	bili
_____ 4.	fat	d.	cholecyst/o
_____ 5.	pancreas	e.	gluc/o
_____ 6.	bilirubin	f.	chole
_____ 7.	gallbladder	g.	lip/o
_____ 8.	common bile duct	h.	choledoch/o
		i.	pancreat

IV.   Spell Check

Circle each incorrectly spelled term and write it correctly in the space provided.

1. apendix   _____
2. colonik   _____
3. enterorhexis   _____
4. celiak   _____
5. esofageal   _____
6. sialic   _____
7. peritoneal   _____
8. rectocolitis   _____
9. jejunoileitis _____
10. sigmoidoscopy _____

V.   Word Analysis: Word Roots and Combining Forms Associated with the GI Tract and Related Areas

Table 18-17 lists a number of terms with their pronunciations and definitions.

TABLE 18-17   WORD ANALYSIS: WORD ROOTS AND COMBINING FORMS ASSOCIATED WITH THE GI TRACT AND RELATED AREAS

Term and Pronunciation	Definition
abdominal (ab-DOM-i-nal)	pertaining to the abdomen
amyloid (AM-i-loyd)	resembling starch
anorectal (ā-nō-REK-tal)	pertaining to both the anus and the rectum

(Continued)

TABLE 18-17   (CONTINUED)

Term and Pronunciation	Definition
appendectomy (ap-en-DEK-tō-mē)	surgical removal of the appendix
appendicitis (a-pen-di-SĪ-tis)	inflammation of the appendix
biliuria (bil-i-Ū-rē-a)	presence of bile in urine
bilirubinemia (bil-i-roo-bin-Ē-mē-a)	presence of bilirubin in the blood
cecotomy (sē-KOT-ō-mē)	incision (cutting) into the cecum (the first part of the large intestine)
celiac (SĒ-lē-ak)	related to the abdomen or belly
choleic (kō-LĒ-ik)	pertaining to bile
cholecystectomy (kō-lē-sis-TEK-tō-mē)	surgical excision (removal) of the gallbladder
colostomy (kō-LOS-tō-mē)	surgical opening of the colon (usually through the abdominal wall)
colonic (kō-LON-ik)	pertaining to the colon
duodenoscopy (dū'-od-e-NOS-kō-pē)	examination of the duodenum (with an endoscope)
enterorrhexis (en-ter-ō-REKS-is)	rupture of the intestine
esophageal (ē-sof-a-JĒ-al)	pertaining to the esophagus
gastralgia (gas-TRAL-jē-a)	pain in the stomach
glycogenesis (glī'-kō-JEN-e-sis)	formation of glycogen (from glucose)
hepatitis (hep-a-TĪ-tis)	inflammation of the liver
hyperglycemia (hī-per-glī-SĒ-mē-a)	condition of excess sugar in the blood
ileorectal (il-ē-ō-REK-tal)	concerning the ileum and rectum
jejunoileitis (jē-jū-nō-il-ē-Ī-tis)	inflammation of the jejunum and ileum
lipolysis (lip-OL-i-sis)	breakdown of fat
pancreatitis (pan-krē-a-TĪ-tis)	inflammation of the pancreas
peritoneal (peri-tō-NĒ-al)	concerning the ileum and rectum
proctologist (prok-TOL-ō-jist)	a specialist in diseases of the rectum, anus, and colon

(Continued)

TABLE 18-17   (CONTINUED)

Term and Pronunciation	Definition
pyloralgia (pī-lō-RAL-jē-a)	pain around the pylorus sphincter
rectocolitis (rek-tō-kō-LĪ-tis)	inflammation of both the rectum and colon
sigmoidoscopy (sig-moy-DOS-kō-pē)	examination of the sigmoid colon with a sigmoidoscope (sig-MOY-dō-skōp)

1. Analyze each term.
2. Circle all combining forms and word roots and label them **wr** and **cf**, respectively.
3. Check your answers (shown in Table 18-20).

E. GI Diseases and Disorders

I.   Matching 1: Diseases and Disorders of the Oral Cavity

Match the term to its meaning. (The same meaning may be used more than once.) Insert the appropriate letter in the space next to the question number.

Choices:

_____ **1.** canker sores
_____ **2.** congenital opening of the roof of the mouth
_____ **3.** herpes virus infection
_____ **4.** destruction of teeth-supporting structures
_____ **5.** pyorrhea
_____ **6.** white patches on the sides of the tongue

a. aphthous stomatitis
b. periodontal disease
c. oral leukoplakia
d. fever blister
e. cleft palate

II.   Matching 2: GI Diseases and Disorders

Choices:

_____ **1.** appendicitis
_____ **2.** cholelithiasis
_____ **3.** hepatitis
_____ **4.** achlorhydria
_____ **5.** ileus
_____ **6.** colonic polyposis
_____ **7.** gastritis
_____ **8.** hemorrhoids
_____ **9.** intussusception
_____ **10.** inguinal hernia

a. absence of hydrochloric acid in the stomach
b. inflammation of the stomach
c. inflammation of the appendix
d. a mass of veins in the anorectum
e. intestinal blockage
f. inflammation of the liver
g. presence of gallstones in the gallbladder
h. slipping of intestinal part into another
i. presence of many polyps along intestine
j. small intestinal loop penetrating through the abdominal wall

III.   Matching 3: Signs and Symptoms Found with GI Diseases and Disorders

Choices:

_____ **1.** anorexia
_____ **2.** dysphagia
_____ **3.** borborygmus
_____ **4.** constipation
_____ **5.** melena
_____ **6.** flatus
_____ **7.** eructation
_____ **8.** hematochezia
_____ **9.** hematemesis
_____ **10.** regurgitation

a. belching
b. difficult elimination of feces
c. difficulty in swallowing
d. a gurgling in the large intestine
e. loss of appetite
f. vomiting of blood
g. passing of feces with blood
h. black stools
i. backup of fluids into the mouth from the stomach
j. expelling gas from the anus

IV.   Spell Check

Circle each incorrectly spelled term and write it correctly in the space provided.

1. dyspepsia   _____
2. diarhea   _____
3. jandice   _____
4. cholelithiasis _____
5. cirrhosis   _____
6. inflammatory   _____
7. angiectasis   _____
8. divertikulosis _____
9. hyatal   _____
10. intusception _____
11. colitis   _____
12. proctitic   _____

F. Suffixes for GI Diseases and Disorders

I.   Matching: Suffixes for GI Diseases and Disorders

Match the term to its meaning. (The same meaning may be used more than once.)
Insert the appropriate letter in the space next to the question number.

Choices:

_____ **1.** vomiting
_____ **2.** digestion
_____ **3.** stretching
_____ **4.** rupture
_____ **5.** swallowing
_____ **6.** spitting
_____ **7.** bursting forth
_____ **8.** violent contraction
_____ **9.** controlling

a. -pepsia
b. -emesis
c. -phagia
d. -rrhagia
e. -ectasia
f. -ptysis
g. -rrhexis
h. -stasis
i. -spasm

II.   Spell Check

Circle each incorrectly spelled term and write it correctly in the space provided.

1. gastroectesia   _____
2. angiectasis   _____

3. hemotemesis _____
4. dispepsia _____
5. gastrorhagia _____
6. gastrorrhea _____
7. pylorospasm _____
8. enterohexis _____
9. peristalsis _____
10. kolestasis _____

III.   Word Analysis: Suffixes Associated with GI Normal Activities, Diseases, and Disorders

Table 18-18 lists a number of terms with their pronunciations and definitions.

TABLE 18-18   WORD ANALYSIS: SUFFIXES ASSOCIATED WITH GI NORMAL ACTIVITIES, DISEASES, AND DISORDERS

Term and Pronunciation	Definition
gastroectasia (gas-trō-ek-TĀ-zē-a)	stretching of the stomach
angiectasis (an-jē-EK-tā-sis)	dilation of a blood vessel
hematemesis (hem-at-EM-ē-sis)	vomiting of blood
hemolysis (hē-MOL-i-sis)	destruction of red blood cells
dyspepsia (dis-PEP-sē-a)	painful digestion
dysphagia (dis-FĀ-jē-a)	painful or difficult swallowing
hemoptysis (hē-MOP-ti-sis)	spitting of blood
hemorrhage (HEM-e-rij)	abnormal discharge of blood
gastrorrhagia (gas-trō-RĀ-jē-a)	hemorrhage from the stomach
gastrorrhea (gas-trō-RĒ-a)	an excessive discharge of gastric juice (in stomach)
enterorrhexis (en-ter-ō-REKS-is)	rupture of the intestine
pylorospasm (pī-LOR-ō-spazm)	a sudden violent contraction of the opening of the pylorus
peristalsis (per-i-STAL-sis)	an involuntary wavelike movement that occurs in hollow body tubes such as the intestines
cholestasis (kō-lē-STĀ-sis)	controlling bile (the flow)

1. Analyze each term.
2. Circle all suffixes and label them **s**.
3. Check your answers (shown in Table 18-21).

G. GI Surgical Procedures and Clinical and Diagnostic Procedures

I.   Matching 1: GI Surgical Procedures

Match the term to its meaning. (The same meaning may be used more than once.)
Insert the appropriate letter in the space next to the question number.

Choices:

_____ **1.** appendectomy

_____ **2.** sigmoidoscopy

_____ **3.** vagotomy

_____ **4.** choledochotomy

_____ **5.** colostomy

_____ **6.** pyloroplasty

_____ **7.** cholecystectomy

a. removal of a portion of the common bile duct

b. removal of the appendix

c. opening of some portion of the colon

d. increasing size of the pyloric opening

e. surgical removal of the gallbladder

f. visual examination of the sigmoid colon

g. cutting the vagus nerve

II.   Matching 2: Clinical and Diagnostic Procedures

_____ **1.** ultrasonography

_____ **2.** upper GI series

_____ **3.** oral cholecystography

_____ **4.** liver scan

_____ **5.** liver biopsy

_____ **6.** percutaneous transhepatic cholangiography

_____ **7.** fiber-optic gastroscopy

_____ **8.** nasogastric intubation

_____ **9.** CT scan

Choices:

a. use of barium sulfate and following its path through the GI tract by x-ray

b. removal of liver tissue through the skin for microscopic exam

c. use of sound waves to obtain a record of internal organs

d. obtaining x-rays of the gallbladder with the use of dye taken orally

e. obtaining an image of the liver with the use of radioactive material and a special scanner

f. the removal of gastric or intestinal contents by a nasogastric tube inserted through the nose into the GI tract

g. the insertion of a flexible fiber-optic tube through the mouth or anus to examine the GI tract

h. the insertion of a needle through the skin and into the liver to obtain x-rays of the bile ducts

i. the use of an x-ray beam directed through a body plane to produce transverse views of body organs

III.   Matching 3: Laboratory Tests

Choices:

_____ **1.** alpha fetoprotein

_____ **2.** liver biopsy

_____ **3.** SGOT, SGPT

a. liver tumors

b. hepatitis

c. bile duct obstruction

_____ **4.** ALP   **d.** liver injury (necrosis)
_____ **5.** serum bilirubin   **e.** ulcer
_____ **6.** stool culture   **f.** colon cancer
_____ **7.** occult fecal blood test   **g.** amebic dysentery, tapeworms, bacterial infections, etc.

IV.   Spell Check

Circle each incorrectly spelled term and write it correctly in the space provided.

       1. bareum   _____
       2. ultrasonography   _____
       3. ocult   _____
       4. cholecystectomy   _____
       5. cholangiopancretography   _____
       6. bilirubin   _____

H. Medical Vocabulary Building

I.   Matching: Medical Vocabulary Building

Match the term to its meaning. (The same meaning may be used more than once.) Insert the appropriate letter in the space next to the question number.

Choices:

_____ **1.** anoscope   **a.** surgical incision of the common bile duct
_____ **2.** choledochotomy   **b.** an instrument used to examine the anus
_____ **3.** glycogenesis
_____ **4.** enteroclysis   **c.** glycogen formation from glucose
_____ **5.** glossotomy   **d.** solution injection into the intestine
_____ **6.** ascites   **e.** surgical incision into the tongue
_____ **7.** gastric esophageal reflux disorder   **f.** serious fluid accumulation in the peritoneal cavity
_____ **8.** eructation   **g.** gingival tumor
_____ **9.** epulis   **h.** belching
_____ **10.** halitosis   **i.** backward flow of gastric contents into the esophagus
_____ **11.** melena   **j.** bad breath
_____ **12.** paralytic ileus   **k.** black feces resulting from blood destruction by intestinal secretions
      l. intestinal paralysis causing distention and acute obstruction

II.   Spell Check

Circle each incorrectly spelled term and write it correctly in the space provided.

       1. eructation   _____
       2. asites   _____
       3. choldochotomy   _____
       4. haletosis   _____
       5. glossotomy   _____
       6. anoscope   _____

I. Abbreviations Used with GI-Tract Anatomy, Function, Medications, and Diagnostic or Laboratory Tests

I.   Matching 1: Abbreviations Used with GI-Tract Anatomy, Function, and Medications

Match the term to its meaning. (The same meaning may be used more than once.) Insert the appropriate letter in the space next to the question number.

Choices:

_____ **1.** LGI
_____ **2.** SBFT
_____ **3.** NG
_____ **4.** GB
_____ **5.** UGI
_____ **6.** TPN
_____ **7.** PO
_____ **8.** a.c.
_____ **9.** p.c.
_____**10.** p.o.
_____**11.** NPO

a. upper gastrointestinal
b. small bowel follow-through
c. gallbladder
d. lower gastrointestinal
e. before meals
f. nasogastric tube
g. given orally
h. after meals
i. total parenteral nutrition
j. nothing by mouth
k. by mouth

II.   Matching 2: Abbreviations Used with GI Diagnostic or Laboratory Tests

Choices:

_____ **1.** ALP
_____ **2.** BaE
_____ **3.** ALT
_____ **4.** IVC
_____ **5.** SGOT
_____ **6.** Ba
_____ **7.** AST
_____ **8.** SGPT
_____ **9.** CT
_____**10.** OCG

a. alanine transaminase
b. barium
c. intravenous cholangiograph
d. alkaline phosphatase
e. barium enema
f. serum glutamic oxalacetic transaminase
g. aspartic acid transaminase
h. serum glutamic pyruvic transaminase
i. computerized tomography
j. oral cholecystography

J. Increasing Your Medical Terminology Word Power 1

1. Read the following report.
2. Prepare to answer the questions at the end of the section.
3. Circle all unfamiliar terms with a red pencil.
4. Underline familiar terms with a blue pencil.
5. Use your knowledge of word elements, a medical dictionary, and the key terms to find the meaning of unfamiliar terms.

A Case of an Impacted Common Duct Stone

Key Terms

calculus (KAL-kū-lus)   commonly referred to as a stone; usually any abnormal accumulation within an animal body; plural form, calculi (KAL-kū-lī)

catheter (KATH-e-ter)   a tube device passed through the body for the removal or injection of fluids into body cavities

cholangiogram (kō-LAN-jē-ō-gram) a record (x-ray) of the bile ducts

cholecystectomy (kō-le-sis-TEK-tō-mē) surgical removal of the gallbladder

cholelithiasis (kō-lē-li-THĪ-a-sis) the formation or presence of calculi or gallstones in the gallbladder or common bile duct

contrast medium a substance used in x-ray examinations to provide a degree of blackness or density between the tissue or organ being filmed and the surrounding areas

extracorporeal (eks-tra-kor-POR-ē-al) outside the body

fogarty balloon a device used to expand a tube such as the common bile duct

impacted immovable or wedged in place

in situ (in SĪ-tū) in position or place

junction (JUNK-shun) the place where two parts come together or close to one another

lithotripsy (LITH-ō-trip-sē) a procedure used to crush a calculus

pancreatitis (pan-krē-a-TĪ-tis) an inflammation of the pancreas

sphincterotomy (sfink-ter-OT-ō-mē) surgical incision of any sphincter (SFINK-ter) muscle

t-tube a device inserted into the bile duct after removal of the gallbladder to allow for drainage and the introduction of a contrast medium for x-ray examinations

General Background

Common bile-duct calculi produce complications in more than 50 percent of patients and so must be removed. Effective removal requires a major surgical procedure, even though nonsurgical techniques are preferred. Surgical approaches used include calculus removal with the aid of a *T-tube*, or *sphincterotomy* followed by stone removal. *Extracorporeal* shockwave *lithotripsy* has been reported to be useful when surgical removal proves difficult.

A Case History

A seventy-nine-year-old white male with cholelithiasis was admitted to the medical center for an emergency cholecystectomy. A cholangiogram showed a calculus wedged in the lower end of the common bile duct with no drainage of the contrast medium occurring into the duodenum (dū-ō-DĒ-num). Six weeks after surgery, an unsuccessful attempt was made to remove the impacted stone through the T-tube. A large catheter was left *in situ*, and the patient was referred to another medical facility. A cholangiogram showed complete blockage of the distal portion of the common bile duct. The blockage by a gallstone was located beneath the junction of the common bile duct and the pancreatic duct. No contrast medium entered the duodenum and a diagnosis of an impacted common duct stone was made. Simple manipulations failed to dislodge the stone, and no further attempt was made to remove it. Instead, a series of smaller catheters were used and some drainage space alongside the stone eventually developed. Antibiotics were prescribed as a precautionary measure because pancreatitis could result as a complication.

A Fogarty balloon catheter was inserted through a movable catheter. The balloon was inflated beneath the gallstones, and then the gallstones were crushed with the use of a wire basket. Only small fragments of the stones were found to be left after this procedure. A final cholangiogram two days later showed that the ducts were clear. The patient was subsequently discharged.

Questions

I.   Fill in the Blank

Fill in the blank with the appropriate term.

1. Cholecystectomy means _____.
2. What do the following terms mean?
   a. extracorporeal: _____
   b. *in situ*: _____
   c. junction: _____

II.   Matching

Match the term to its meaning. (The same meaning may be used more than once.)
Insert the appropriate letter in the space next to the question number.

Choices:

_____ 1. lithotripsy   a. common term for stone
_____ 2. calculus   b. immovable
_____ 3. impacted   c. inflammation of pancreas
_____ 4. cholelithiasis   d. gallstone formation
_____ 5. cholangiogram   e. calculus crushing
_____ 6. pancreas inflammation   f. x-ray of bile ducts

III.   Spell Check

Circle each incorrectly spelled term and write it correctly in the space provided.

1. kalculus _____
2. catheter _____
3. extracorporal _____
4. pancreas _____
5. sfhincterotomy _____
6. gallbladde _____
7. calculi _____
8. sphincter _____

K. Increasing Your Medical Terminology Word Power 2

1. Read the following report.
2. Prepare to answer the questions at the end of the section.
3. Circle all unfamiliar terms with a red pencil.
4. Underline familiar terms with a blue pencil.
5. Use your knowledge of word elements, a medical dictionary, and the key terms to find the meaning of unfamiliar terms.

Infant Botulism: A Brief Consideration

Key Terms

blepharoptosis (blef-a-rōp-TŌ-sis)   drooping of the upper eyelid

flaccid (FLAK-sid)   relaxed; having defective or absent muscular tone

hypercapnia (hī-per-KAP-nē-a)   increased amount of carbon dioxide in blood

hypoxemia (hī-poks-Ē-mē-a)   insufficient oxygenation of the blood

morbidity   the number of sick persons in relation to a specific population

mortality rate   the death rate in relation to a specific population

neurotoxin   a poison that attacks the nervous system

sequela (sē-KWĒ-la)   a condition following and resulting from a disease

spore (bacterial)   a resting but highly resistant stage in the life cycle of certain bacteria

INTRODUCTION

In the United States during 1966, laboratory-confirmed infant botulism cases were diagnosed in 80 infants, or 3 per 100,000 live births. Early, nonspecific symptoms such as impaired feeding and listlessness, are often misinterpreted. Most infants diagnosed with infant botulism, unlike with other cases of acute flaccid paralysis, will survive and regain full motor function without sequelae. The case mortality rate for infants hospitalized in the U.S. from 1984 to 1996 was 0.3 percent.

Despite these more benign features, the disease has its impact on its victims, their families, and society. Recovery from infant botulism can be prolonged and dangerous. From 1976 to 1992, the average stay in California was more than 1 month, with maximal stays of greater than 6 months. Infants hospitalized in California, the location of about half of the cases recognized in the U.S., cost over $3,000,000 per year in direct hospital charges. During hospitalization, affected infants are subject to persistent risk of additional morbidity or death from complications. After hospital discharge, patients require extended recuperation at home lasting several weeks to months. Evidence also exists of infants who have died at home of sudden, severe infant botulism prior to diagnosis.

CAUSE

Infant botulism results when spores of *Clostridium botulinum* colonize in the large intestine and become active cells producing powerful botulism neurotoxin. Humans are most vulnerable between 2 and 32 weeks of age, with an average of cases occurring under 6 months.

The environmental source of clostridial spores leading to a case of infant botulism is usually identified. It is generally presumed that many cases begin by occult (concealed) ingestion of spores carried on aerosolized environment-associated dust particles. The current ability to prevent the disease is limited. Laboratory and epidemiological evidence implicate the consumption of honey as a cause.

SIGNS AND SYMPTOMS

The signs and symptoms of infant botulism are subtle and easily misinterpreted, thus leading to frustrating delays in diagnosis. An early obvious sign is an inability to feed because of weakness to suck and swallow. Until sufficiently dehydrated, many affected infants drool, which may be taken as a sign of teething. Other signs and symptoms may include a pathetic faint cry, repetitive moans, head lag, blepharoptosis, and flattened facial expression. With additional nerve damage, dehydration and starvation progress, and the arms and legs become progressively limp and weak. In about half the cases, there is respiratory failure due to upper airway flaccidity and obstruction, aspiration, or respiratory paralysis; the hypoxemia of obstruction usually precedes the hypercapnia of paralysis. In the severest cases, infants become completely immobile and flaccid, with fixed pupils.

*C*OMPLICATIONS

The most common complications of infant botulism are secondary infections, especially lower respiratory tract infections, otitis media, or urinary tract infections due to bladder paralysis.

*T*REATMENT

Treatment for infant botulism previously has been limited to weeks or months of supportive care, including nasoenteral tube feedings, respiratory support, and the recognition and treatment of complications. Currently, botulism immune globulin, a human-derived antitoxin (antibody) preparation, is available throughout the U.S. for the treatment of infant botulism.

Questions

I.   Fill in the Blank

Fill in the blank with the appropriate term.

1. What type of food appears to be the source of disease agents in the cases of infant botulism? _____

2. What is the bacterial cause of infant botulism? _____
_____

3. What type of toxin is produced by the causative agent?
_____

4. What does blepharoptosis mean? _____

5. What is the current treatment for the disease? _____
_____

II.   Matching

Match the term to its meaning. (The same meaning may be used more than once.) Insert the appropriate letter in the space next to the question number.

                              Choices:

_____ 1. sequela   **a.** death rate
_____ 2. mortality rate   **b.** absence of muscle tone
_____ 3. flaccid   **c.** insufficient oxygen in the blood
_____ 4. hypoxemia   **d.** too much carbon dioxide in blood
_____ 5. hypercapnia   **e.** a condition following a disease

L. Increasing Your Medical Terminology Word Power 3

1. Read the following report.
2. Prepare to answer the questions at the end of the section.
3. Circle all unfamiliar terms with a red pencil.

4. Underline familiar terms with a blue pencil.
5. Use your knowledge of word elements, a medical dictionary, and the key terms to find the meaning of unfamiliar terms.

Expandable Metal Stents as Treatments for Cancerous GI Tract Obstructions

Key Terms

benign   opposite of malignant (cancerous)

dysphagia (dis-FĀ-jē-a)   inability to swallow or difficulty in swallowing

fistula (FIS-tū-la)   an abnormal tube-like passage from a normal cavity to a tube, a free surface, or to another cavity

fluoroscopy (FLOO-or-ō-skōp-ē)   the use of a fluoroscope for medical diagnosis or other medical procedures

palliation (pal-ē-Ā-shun)   an easing or reducing of the effect or intensity of a disease sign or symptom

pruritus (proo-RĪ-tus)   severe itching

resection (rē-SEK-shun)   partial excision of a body structure

stent   any material used to hold or support a graft or connection throughout healing

stricture (STRIK-chur)   a narrowing or constriction of the lumen of a hollow organ or tube

G ENERAL BACKGROUND: HOW STENTS WORK

The use of expandable metal stents are approved as treatments for gastrointestinal obstructions caused by cancerous processes. Gastrointestinal stents are placed by gastroenterologists under endoscopic guidance with the aid of fluoroscopy or by interventional radiologists using fluoroscopic guidance alone. Expandable metal stents are made of metal alloys and have varying shapes and sizes. Such stents are mounted in a preloaded constrained position on a delivery catheter. A guide wire is passed through the lumen of the catheter, and when the wire has been advanced beyond the obstruction, the stent is passed over it and positioned across the stricture. The holding part of the mechanism is released, which causes the length of the stent to decrease and its diameter (width) to increase.

E SOPHAGEAL STENTS

Esophageal carcinoma accounts for most cases of dysphagia resulting from cancer, and usually the tumor is unresectable. Dysphagia may also result from extrinsic compression due to lung cancer or malignant lymphadenopathy. Expandable metal stents are one of the treatment alternatives for palliation of dysphagia due to cancer.

Esophageal expandable metal stents are also used to treat tracheoesophageal fistulas due to cancer. Such fistulas develop in patients with advanced esophageal and lung cancer and lead to continuous aspiration of saliva. Tracheoesophageal fistula is the only condition in which covered expandable metal stents may increase survival as compared with other therapies.

*B*ILIARY STENTS

Treatment of obstructive jaundice due to cancer relieves pruritus, improves appetite, and reduces fat malabsorption. Surgical palliation of this condition involves the creation of an anastomosis between the bile duct and the duodenum or jejunum to bypass the obstructed biliary tree. Nonsurgical palliation is achieved by placing stents endoscopically across the cancerous stricture to restore biliary continuity.

*G*ASTRODUODENAL STENTS

Successful placement of expandable metal stents for palliation of cancerous obstruction of the upper gastrointestinal tract has been reported in several series, with clinical success rates similar to those of surgical palliative bypass. Approximately 90 percent of patients with gastrointestinal stents improve clinically.

Complications after placement of expandable stents in the upper gastrointestinal tract include perforation, bleeding, stent migration, stent malpositioning, and occlusion of the stent by tumor overgrowth or growth or by food impaction.

*C*OLORECTAL STENTS

Placement of a colorectal stent is a consideration for preoperative decompression and for palliation of cancerous large-bowel obstruction. Up to 30 percent of patients with primary colorectal carcinoma present with large-bowel obstruction. The traditional method of managing complete or subtotal colonic obstruction due to cancer, particularly left-sided obstruction, involves the creation of a diverting colostomy.

Candidates for placement of a colorectal stent for palliation include patients with colorectal carcinoma and obstruction who have extensive local or metastatic disease or who are poor candidates for surgical resection, and patients with colonic obstruction secondary to noncolonic pelvic cancers, such as bladder or ovarian carcinoma, or metastatic cancers such as breast carcinoma.

*F*UTURE POSSIBILITIES

Biodegradable and bioabsorbable expandable stents are being considered for benign disease treatments.

Questions

I.   Fill in the blank

Fill in the blank with the appropriate term.

    1. What type of cancer accounts for most cases of dysphagia?

       _____

    2. List two other causes of dysphagia.
        a. _____
        b. _____

3. List three conditions that are relieved by treatment of cancer-caused obstructive jaundice.
   a. _____
   b. _____
   c. _____

4. What is the traditional approach to managing complete colonic obstruction caused by cancer? _____
_____

II.   Spell Check

Circle each incorrectly spelled term and write it correctly in the space provided.

1. stent   _____
2. colorectal   _____
3. fluoroscopy _____
4. palliation   _____
5. anastomosis _____
6. esophageal   _____

Term Search Challenge

Locate 17 terms in the puzzle.

1. Write the specific term next to its definition. Then find that term in the puzzle diagram and circle it.
2. Terms may be read from left to right, backward, up, down, or diagonally. Unrelated words occasionally appear in the diagram.
3. If a term appears more than once, circle it only once. (A term may be found inside others.)
4. Check your answers.

Clues:

1. Proteins that speed up chemical reactions and/or aid digestion _____
2. Part of the tooth found above the gums _____
3. Main portion of the tooth found below the gums _____
4. The three pairs of exocrine glands found in the oral cavity are the _____ glands.
5. The flap of tissue that covers the larynx (voice box) during the swallowing of food _____
6. Another term for the large intestine is the _____.
7. The _____ colon is shaped like an **S**.
8. The _____ stores bile.
9. The combining form for the gum is _____.
10. A word root for tooth _____
11. A combining form for the lip _____
12. The combining form for the throat is _____.
13. The term for lack of appetite is a(n) _____.
14. A sore of the mucous membrane or skin is a(n) _____.

15. The two types of teeth that are used for the crushing and grinding of food are _____ and _____.

16. The tough outer surface covering of a tooth's crown is the

_____.

Term Search Puzzle

```
E  P  H  A  R  Y  N  G  O  T  A  P  E  H  S
A  N  O  R  E  X  I  A  F  L  A  T  U  S  I
P  R  Z  F  S  P  H  I  N  T  E  R  S  D  G
T  A  G  Y  L  D  E  N  T  N  C  B  P  I  M
O  L  N  L  M  L  A  B  I  O  I  I  I  G  O
L  O  H  C  F  E  C  E  S  D  D  C  L  E  I
I  M  I  T  R  O  S  T  A  O  N  U  E  S  D
E  K  P  J  G  E  S  L  L  E  U  S  T  T  G
H  J  I  E  L  U  A  T  I  N  A  P  U  I  I
C  O  L  O  N  L  R  S  V  A  J  I  V  O  N
O  O  E  M  U  C  O  S  A  M  J  D  U  N  G
L  T  S  U  T  E  G  U  R  E  V  I  L  T  I
T  O  T  Q  R  R  U  E  Y  L  H  I  A  U  V
L  O  N  G  A  L  L  B  L  A  D  D  E  R  O
C  R  O  W  N  E  P  I  G  L  O  T  T  I  S
```

CHAPTER 19

The Urinary System

"Insults and injuries to the human organism have always challenged the ingenuity of human individuals and groups to devise means and forms toward their prevention, control, and treatment."

—David Landy

A. Kidney Structure and Function

I.   Fill in the Blank

Fill in the blank with the appropriate term.

1. The medical specialty that deals with the structure, function, and diseases of the male and female urinary systems, and the male reproductive system, is known as _____.
2. Another term for urination is _____.
3. The basic functional unit of the kidney is the
_____.
4. List three steps involved with urine formation.
_____, _____, and
_____

II.   Matching: Kidney Structure and Function

Match the term to its meaning. (The same meaning may be used more than once.) Insert the appropriate letter in the space next to the question number.

Choices:

_____ **1.** urethra
_____ **2.** trigone
_____ **3.** ureter
_____ **4.** glomerulus
_____ **5.** urinary bladder
_____ **6.** urea
_____ **7.** calyx

a. major nitrogen-containing waste product in urine
b. one of two tubes leading from the kidneys to the urinary bladder
c. sac that holds urine
d. small ball of capillaries in cortex in kidney
e. tube leading from the urinary bladder to the outside of the body
f. cuplike collecting region of the renal pelvis
g. triangular area in the urinary bladder where the ureters enter and the urethra exits

III.   Spell Check

Circle each incorrectly spelled term and write it correctly in the space provided.

1. calx   _____

2. helum   _____

3. creatinine _____

4. electrolight _____

5. uric   _____

6. uretra   _____

IV.   Vision Quiz 1: The Kidney

Figure 19-8 shows the components of the human kidney. Identify and write the name of the numbered parts in the spaces provided.

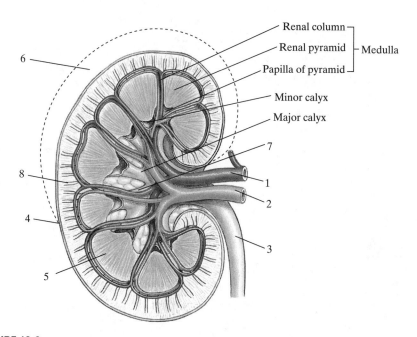

FIGURE 19-8   Vision Quiz. The kidney.

1. _____

2. _____

3. _____

4. _____

5. _____

6. _____

7. _____

8. _____

V.   Vision Quiz 2: The Nephron

Figure 19-9 shows the parts of a human nephron. Identify and write the name of the numbered structures in the spaces provided.

1. _____

2. _____

3. _____

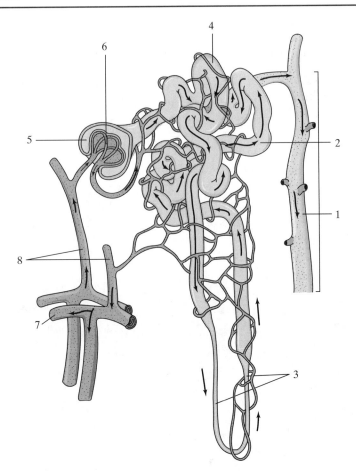

FIGURE 19-9   Vision Quiz. The nephron.

4. _____

5. _____

6. _____

7. _____

8. _____

B. Word Roots and/or Combining Forms for the Structures of the Urinary Tract

I.   Fill in the Blank

Fill in the blank with the appropriate term.

1. Give two combining forms for the *kidney*. _____ and _____

2. What is the combining form for the *urethra*? _____

3. Give the word root for ureter. _____

II.   Matching: Word Roots and/or Combining Forms for Renal Anatomy and Function

Match the term to its meaning. (The same meaning may be used more than once.) Insert the appropriate letter in the space next to the question number.

Choices:

_____ **1.** calyx	**a.** cortic/o
_____ **2.** glomerulus	**b.** cali
_____ **3.** renal pelvis	**c.** cyst/o
_____ **4.** meatus	**d.** pyel/o
_____ **5.** urinary tract	**e.** meat/o
_____ **6.** urea	**f.** gloerul
_____ **7.** cartex	**g.** ur/o
_____ **8.** medulla	**h.** vesic/o
_____ **9.** trigone	**i.** trigon/o
_____ **10.** urinary bladder	

III.   Spell Check

Circle each incorrectly spelled term and write it correctly in the space provided.

1. calectasis _____

2. cistitis _____

3. glomerular _____

4. medulary _____

5. urethritis _____

6. ureterolithotomy _____

IV.   Word Analysis: Word Elements Associated With The Urinary Tract

Table 19-11 lists a number of terms with their pronunciations and definitions.

TABLE 19-11   WORD ANALYSIS: THE URINARY TRACT

Term and Pronunciation	Definition
caliectasis (kal-ē-EK-ta-sis)	stretching (dilation) of a calyx
cortical (KOR-ti-kal)	pertaining to the cortex
cystitis (sis-TĪ-tis)	inflammation of urinary bladder
glomerular (glō-MER-ū-lar)	pertaining to glomerulus, a collection of small blood vessels (capillaries)
meatal (mē-Ā-tal)	pertaining to the meatus
medullary (MED-ū-lar-ē)	pertaining to the medulla
nephrectomy (ne-FREK-tō-mē)	removal of the kidney
pyelogram (PĪ-e-lō-gram)	an x-ray (record) of the renal pelvis
renopathy (rē-NOP-a-thē)	any disease of the kidney
trigonectomy (trī-gon-EK-tō-mē)	surgical removal of the triangular base of urinary bladder (trigone)

(Continued)

TABLE 19-11   (CONTINED)

Term and Pronunciation	Definition
urogram (Ū-rō-gram)	an x-ray of any portion of the urinary tract
ureterolithotomy (ū-rē-ter-ō-lith-OT-ō-mē)	surgical removal of calculus (kidney stone) from ureter
urethritis (ū-rē-THRĪ-tis)	inflammation of the urethra
vesicospinal (ves-i-kō-SPĪ-nal)	pertaining to the urinary bladder and spinal cord

1. Analyze each term.
2. Circle all combining forms, word roots, prefixes, and suffixes, and label them **cf, wr, p,** and **s,** respectively.
3. Check your answers (shown in Table 19-13).

C. Signs and Symptoms Associated with Urinary System Diseases and Disorders

I.   Matching: Disorders and Diseases of the Kidney

Match the term to its meaning. (The same meaning may be used more than once.) Insert the appropriate letter in the space next to the question number.

Choices:

_____ 1. glomerulonephritis
_____ 2. nephritis
_____ 3. pyelonephritis
_____ 4. nephrolithiasis
_____ 5. renal hypertension
_____ 6. Wilms' tumor
_____ 7. cystitis
_____ 8. arterial nephrosclerosis
_____ 9. diabetes insipidus
_____ 10. hypernephroma
_____ 11. polycystic kidney

a. childhood malignant kidney tumor
b. urinary-bladder infection
c. kidney stones
d. inflammation of kidney
e. inflammation of kidney glomeruli
f. inflammation of renal pelvis
g. high blood pressure resulting from kidney disease
h. hardening of kidney arteries
i. renal carcinoma in the adult
j. inadequate secretion of antidiuretic hormone
k. many fluid-filled cysts within and on the kidney

II.   Matching: Signs and Symptoms of Urinary System Diseases and Disorders

Choices:

_____ 1. albuminuria
_____ 2. enuresis
_____ 3. dysuria
_____ 4. urinary retention
_____ 5. nocturia

a. painful urination
b. frequent voiding of urine during the night
c. excessive urine production
d. greater than normal times of voiding

_____ **6.** ureteral colic
_____ **7.** frequency
_____ **8.** vesicoureteral reflux
_____ **9.** polyuria
_____ **10.** oliguria

e. backflow of urine into the kidney
f. albumin in urine
g. reduced urine production
h. involuntary urinating during sleep
i. inability to urinate
j. extreme pain caused by passage of a stone in the ureter

III.   Spell Check

Circle each incorrectly spelled term and write it correctly in the space provided.

1. trauma   _____

2. disuria   _____

3. albuminuria   _____

4. enuresis   _____

5. vesicourtereal _____

6. hydronefrosis   _____

7. insipidis   _____

8. nephrolithiasis _____

9. pyelonephritis _____

IV.   Word Analysis: Urinary System Diseases and Disorders

Table 19-12 lists a number of terms with their pronunciations and definitions.

TABLE 19-12   WORD ANALYSIS: URINARY SYSTEM DISEASES AND DISORDERS

Term and Pronunciation	Brief Explanation
albuminuria (al-bū-mi-NŪ-rē-a)	presence of albumin in urine
azotemia (az-ō-TĒ-mē-a)	presence of urea and related substances in blood
bacteriuria (bak-tē-rē-Ū-rē-a)	bacteria in urine
polydipsia (pol-ē-DIP-sē-a)	excess thirst
ketoplasia (kē-tō-PLĀ-sē-a)	formation of ketones
nocturia (nok-TŪ-rē-a)	urination during the night
oliguria (ol-ig-Ū-rē-a)	small amount of urine (formation)
pyuria (pī-Ū-rē-a)	pus in the urine

1. Analyze each term.
2. Circle all combining forms, word roots, prefixes, and suffixes, and label them **cf, wr, p,** and **s,** respectively.
3. Check your answers (shown in Table 9-14).

D. Clinical and Diagnostic Procedures and Laboratory Tests

I.   Matching 1: Clinical Procedures for Diagnosis or Treatment

Match the term to its meaning. (The same meaning may be used more than once.)
Insert the appropriate letter in the space next to the question number.

Choices:

_____ **1.** intravenous pyelogram
_____ **2.** hemodialysis
_____ **3.** renal biopsy
_____ **4.** retrograde pyelogram
_____ **5.** ultrasonography
_____ **6.** dialysis
_____ **7.** renal scan
_____ **8.** renogram
_____ **9.** renal transplant
_____ **10.** angiography
_____ **11.** CT scans
_____ **12.** voiding cystourethrogram

a. obtaining kidney tissue for micro-scopic examination

b. the use of an artificial kidney system to filter an individual's blood

c. the introduction of contrast material directly through the bladder and ureters into the kidneys to detect stones or blockage

d. the use of sound waves to diagnose renal-system diseases or disorders

e. receiving a donor kidney

f. the use of IV-injected dye to follow the filling capacity of the urinary system

g. the use of IV injected contrast material to examine kidney veins and arteries

h. use of radioactive substances to show kidney size and shape

i. the use of radioactive substances to follow kidney function

j. procedure to separate wastes from the blood

k. following, with the aid of x-rays, the flow of urine containing contrast material

l. transverse x-ray view of the body

II.   Matching 2: Urine Analysis

Match the term to its meaning. (The same meaning may be used more than once.)
Insert the appropriate letter in the space provided next to the question number.

Choices:

_____ **1.** casts
_____ **2.** pH
_____ **3.** hematuria
_____ **4.** specific gravity
_____ **5.** ketosis
_____ **6.** phenylketonuria

a. refers to a comparison of the density of urine with that of water

b. refers to acid level

c. fiber-like or fatty solids

d. blood in the urine

e. ketone bodies in urine

f. abnormal amount of phenylalanine in the body

III.   Spell Check

Circle each incorrectly spelled term and write it correctly in the space provided.

1. dyalysis   _____

2. peritoneal   _____

  3. thromboemboli   _____

  4. hemodialysis   _____

  5. reenogram   _____

  6. catherterization   _____

  7. gluecose   _____

  8. hematuria   _____

  9. albumon   _____

10. bilirubin   _____

E. Medical Vocabulary Building

I.   Matching

Match the term to its meaning. (The same meaning may be used more than once.)
Insert the appropriate letter in the space next to the question number.

_____ **1.** dilation of the urinary bladder

_____ **2.** bladder and renal pelvis inflammation

_____ **3.** blood oozing from the mucous membrane into the bladder

_____ **4.** kidney congested with blood

_____ **5.** urine collection in the renal pelvis caused by a blocked outflow

_____ **6.** glandular tumor of the kidney

_____ **7.** inflammation of the trigone of the bladder

_____ **8.** pertaining to a connection between the ureter and the bladder

_____ **9.** pigment that gives urine a normal yellow color

_____ **10.** an acute pain occurring in the kidney caused by blockage during the passing of a stone

Choices:

a. urochrome	**f.** nephremia
b. renal colic	**g.** hydronephrosis
c. ureterovesical	**h.** cystopyelitis
d. trigonitis	**i.** cystistaxis
e. nephradenoma	**j.** cystectasy

II.   Spell Check

Circle each incorrectly spelled term and write it correctly in the space provided.

  1. cystitaxia   _____

  2. hydroneforsis   _____.

  3. trigonitis   _____

  4. cystopielitis   _____

  5. nephremia   _____

  6. uretreovesical   _____

F. Abbreviations

I.   Matching 1: Urinary System Anatomy and Function

Match the term to its meaning. (The same meaning may be used more than once.) Insert the appropriate letter in the space next to the question number.

Choices:

1. Cl^-		**a.**	potassium ion
2. ADH		**b.**	kidney, ureter, and bladder
3. KUB		**c.**	sodium ion
4. Na^+		**d.**	chloride ion
5. HCO_3^-		**e.**	antidiuretic hormone
6. pH		**f.**	bicarbonate
7. K^+		**g.**	degree of acidity or alkalinity

II.   Matching 2: Diseases, Disorders, and Procedures Used in Diagnosis and Treatment, Part 1

Match the term to its meaning. (The same meaning may be used more than once.) Insert the appropriate letter in the space next to the question number.

Choices:

_____ **1.** UTI

_____ **2.** U/A

_____ **3.** CAPD

_____ **4.** NGU

_____ **5.** HD

_____ **6.** BUN

_____ **7.** CRF

_____ **8.** Cysto

a. continuous ambulatory peritoneal dialysis

b. urinalysis

c. hemodialysis

d. urinary tract infection

e. cystoscopic examination

f. chronic renal failure

g. blood urea nitrogen

h. nongonococcal urethritis

III.   Matching 3: Diseases, Disorders, and Procedures Used in Diagnosis and Treatment, Part 2

Match the term to its meaning. (The same meaning may be used more than once.) Insert the appropriate letter in the space next to the question number.

Choices:

_____ **1.** urinalysis

_____ **2.** phenylketonuria

_____ **3.** intravenous pyelogram

_____ **4.** voiding cystourethrogram

_____ **5.** intermittent peritoneal dialysis

_____ **6.** cystometrogram

_____ **7.** peritoneal dialysis

a. VCU

b. PD

c. IPD

d. CMG

e. PKU

f. U/A

g. IVP

IV.   Spell Check

Circle each incorrectly spelled term and write it correctly in the space provided.

1. pheniketonuria _____

2. dialysis   _____

3. pielogram   _____

4. urinalysis   _____

5. potasiumion   _____

6. nongonococcal   _____

G. *Increasing Your Medical Terminology Word Power 1*

1. Read the following report.
2. Prepare to answer the questions at the end of the section.
3. Circle all unfamiliar terms with a red pencil.
4. Underline familiar terms with a blue pencil.
5. Use your knowledge of word elements, a medical dictionary, and the key terms to find the meaning of unfamiliar terms.

Recovery of Function in a Single Kidney after Intraarterial Thrombolytic Therapy

Key Terms

angiography (an-jē-OG-ra-fē)   x-ray of blood vessels after the injection of a substance that is not penetrated by x-rays

anuria (an-Ū-rē-a)   an absence of urine formation

calculous (KAL-kū-los)   like a calculus (stone)

calculus (KAL-kū-lus)   a (kidney) stone

cystoscopy (sis-TOS-kō-pē)   urinary-bladder examination

dialysis (dī-AL-i-sis)   the passage of a fluid through a membrane; used in cases of kidney disorders to remove toxic substances and maintain normal functioning of the organ

infusion (in-FŪ-zhun)   introducing a liquid into the body, through a vein, for treatment

nephrectomy (ne-FREK-tō-mē)   removal of a kidney

perfusion (per-FŪ-zhun)   passing a fluid through a structure or spaces

pyelogram (PĪ-e-lō-gram)   an x-ray of the ureter and renal pelvis

pyonephrosis (pī-ō-nef-RŌ-sis)   pus accumulation in the pelvis of the kidney

retrograde pyelography   x-ray procedure involving the injection of a dye that is not penetrated by x-rays into the kidneys from below

streptokinase (strep-tō-KĪ-nās)   a bacterial enzyme that is capable of dissolving blood clots

thromboembolism (throm-bō-EM-bō-lizm)   blockage of a blood vessel by a blood clot (throm-bus)

$\mathcal{T}$HE CASE

An eighty-one-year-old man had acute right abdominal pain and anuria. His medical history included a left nephrectomy for calculous pyonephrosis.

At cystoscopy, no blockage of urine was noted, and the right retrograde pyelogram was normal. However, the presence of several renal artery thromboemboli (throm-bō-EM-bō-lī) were confirmed by angiography. Laboratory studies showed certain abnormalities, including an elevated white-blood-cell count.

An arterial catheter was inserted into the right renal artery and the infusion of streptokinase was begun approximately 18 hours after the onset of the symptoms. Repeated angiography of 24 and 48 hours showed progressive dissolving of the blood clots. Systemic anticoagulation treatment was started and the streptokinase infusion was discontinued after 48 hours. No adverse effects from the infusion were observed.

Dialysis was also started. Initially, the patient required dialysis three times per week. Within the next four weeks, urine output increased and all laboratory tests were normal. Dialysis was discontinued.

Ten weeks after treatment was started, the patient was released with his renal function restored to normal.

Questions

I.   Matching

Match the term to its meaning. (The same meaning may be used more than once.) Insert the letter of your choice in the space provided next to the question number.

Choices:

_____ **1.** anuria	**a.** pus in the kidney pelvis
_____ **2.** pyelogram	**b.** blood clot
_____ **3.** calculus	**c.** absence of urine formation
_____ **4.** pyonephrosis	**d.** kidney stone
_____ **5.** thrombus	**e.** urinary-bladder examination
_____ **6.** streptokinase	**f.** an x-ray of the ureter and renal pelvis
_____ **7.** perfusion	**g.** removal of a kidney
_____ **8.** thromboembolism	**h.** blockage of blood vessels by a clot
_____ **9.** cystoscopy	**i.** passing fluid through spaces
_____ **10.** nephrectomy	**j.** enzyme capable of dissolving blood clots

H.   *Increasing Your Medical Terminology Word Power 2*

    1. Read the following report.
    2. Prepare to answer the questions at the end of the section.
    3. Circle all unfamiliar terms with a red pencil.
    4. Underline familiar terms with a blue pencil.
    5. Use your knowledge of word elements, a medical dictionary, and the key terms to find the meaning of unfamiliar terms.

Renal-Cell Carcinoma

Key Terms

chromophilic (krō-mō-FIL-ik)   easily stained

chromophobic (krō-mō-FŌ-bik)   stains poorly

contralateral (kon-tra-LAT-er-al)   originating or affecting the opposite side of the body

flank   the part of the body between the ribs and the upper border of the ileum

hematuria (hēm-a-TŪ-rē-a)   blood in the urine

hypertension   refers to higher-than-normal blood pressure

nephrectomy (ne-FREK-tō-mē)   removal of a kidney

nephroblastoma (nef-rō-blas-TŌ-ma)   a rapidly developing tumor in children; also called Wilms' tumor

oncocytic (ON-kō-sit-ik)   pertains to tumor development

palpable (PAL-pa-bl)   detectable by touch

varicocele (VAR-i-kō-sēl)   spermatic cord vein enlargement

I NTRODUCTION

Renal-cell carcinoma typically does not present early warning signs. In addition, the condition exhibits diverse clinical signs and symptoms, and resistance to radiotherapy and chemotherapy.

E PIDEMIOLOGY

Renal-cell carcinoma accounts for 2 percent of all cancers. Its incidence varies among countries by a factor of 20 among men and by a factor of 10 among women. The highest rates occur in North Americans and Scandinavians.

Renal-cell carcinoma originates in the renal cortex and accounts for 80 to 85 percent of malignant kidney tumors. Other histologic types of the disease include transitional-cell carcinoma of the renal pelvis, making up 15 to 20 percent of kidney cancers in adults, and nephroblastoma (*Wilms' tumor*) in children.

Renal-cell carcinoma occurs nearly twice as often in men as in women, and in the United States its incidence is equivalent among whites and blacks. Patients are generally more than 40 years of age at diagnosis, and disease occurs mainly in the seventh and eighth decades of life.

Results of recent international case-control studies have provided new insight into the causative role of environmental factors. Such factors include cigarette smoking—which doubles the likelihood of renal-cell carcinoma—and obesity, particularly in women, in whom there is a linear relationship between increasing body weight and the increased risk of renal-cell carcinoma. Other factors found to be associated with the development of the disease include hypertension, treatment for hypertension, and occupational exposure to petroleum products, heavy metals, or asbestos. Heredity may also play a role in increasing the risk of disease development.

P ATHOLOGICAL CLASSIFICATION

A new histopathological classification of renal tumor was proposed in 1986, based on morphologic, histochemical, and electron-microscopic information. The five types of carcinomas currently recognized are: (1) *clear-cell*, (2) *chromophilic*, (3) *chromophobic*, (4) *oncocytic*, and (5) *collecting-duct tumors*.

D IAGNOSIS

Because of its diverse presentation of signs and symptoms, renal-cell carcinoma has been referred to as the "internist's tumor." Small, localized tumors rarely produce signs of the disease. Diagnosis is therefore often delayed until after the disease is advanced. The most common presentations are hematuria, abdominal pain, and a palpable mass in the flank or abdomen. Other signs and symptoms are relatively nonspecific and include fever, night sweats, malaise, and weight loss. Two percent of males present with a varicocele, usually on the left side of the body due to an obstruction of the testicular vein.

In recent years, the widespread use of computerized tomography and ultrasonography for other conditions has led to an increased detection of renal-cell carcinoma as an incidental finding.

SURGERY

Surgical resection remains the cornerstone of treatment for renal-cell carcinoma. The radical nephrectomy procedure used includes a resection of the kidney, perirenal fat, and the ipsilateral adrenal gland. Partial nephrectomy, also referred to as nephron-sparing surgery, should be attempted in patients with bilateral tumors of a functionally solitary kidney. This approach should also be a consideration in selected patients in whom the contralateral kidney is threatened by associated diseases such as hypertension or diabetes mellitus.

Questions

I.   Fill in the Blank

Fill in the blank with the appropriate term.

1. In what part of the kidney do renal-cell carcinomas originate?
    _____

2. Does renal-cell carcinoma occur more frequently in men or women?
    _____

3. At what age would renal-cell carcinoma likely occur?
    _____

4. List two main factors contributing to renal-cell carcinoma development.
    a. _____
    b. _____

5. List the five currently recognized types of renal-cell carcinomas.
    a. _____
    b. _____
    c. _____
    d. _____
    e. _____

6. What are the common signs and symptoms of renal-cell carcinoma?
    a. _____
    b. _____
    c. _____

7. What causes the varicocele in males with renal-cell carcinoma?
    _____

8. When should nephron-sparing surgery be a consideration in dealing with renal-cell tumors? _____
    _____
    _____

II.   Matching

Match the term to its meaning. (The same meaning may be used more than once.) Insert the appropriate letter in the space next to the question number.

Choices:

_____ 1. nephroblastoma   a. higher than normal blood pressure
_____ 2. hypertension   b. spermatic cord vein enlargement
_____ 3. chromophilic   c. easily stained
_____ 4. chromophobic   d. detectable by touch

_____	**5.** palpable	**e.**	stains poorly
_____	**6.** hematuria	**f.**	blood in the urine
_____	**7.** varicocele	**g.**	rapidly developing tumor in children
_____	**8.** contralateral	**h.**	affecting the opposite side of the body

III.   Spell Check

Circle each incorrectly spelled term and write it correctly in the space provided.

    1. nefroblastoma   _____

    2. palapable   _____

    3. varicoseal   _____

    4. hematuria   _____

    5. chromofilic   _____

    6. ipsilateral   _____

I. Increasing Your Medical Terminology Word Power 3

    1. Read the following report.

    2. Prepare to answer the questions at the end of the section.

    3. Circle all unfamiliar terms with a red pencil.

    4. Underline familiar terms with a blue pencil.

    5. Use your knowledge of word elements, a medical dictionary, and the key terms to find the meaning of unfamiliar terms.

Condyloma of the Bladder

Key Terms

apoplexy (AP-ō-plek-sē)   sudden hemorrhage in an organ

catheterization (kath-e-ter-i-ZĀ-shun)   the use of a tube-like device to remove fluids from or inject fluids into body cavities

condyloma (kon'-di-LŌ-ma)   wartlike growth

meningitis (men-in-JĪ-tis)   inflammation of the membranes covering the brain and spinal cord

polyp (POL-ip)   a tumor with a stem

CASE STUDY

An eighty-year-old man, who had suffered mental disturbances due to meningitis from the age of three years, died of massive bleeding from duodenal and gastric ulcers. He had been hospitalized for nine years because of cerebral apoplexy and renal failure. Fifteen months and four days before his death, his bladder was catheterized for two different time periods, twelve weeks and two weeks, respectively. At autopsy, two whitish polyp-like tumors were uncovered in the neck of the urinary bladder. Laboratory investigation showed the presence of human papilloma (pap-i-LŌ-ma) virus.

Questions

I.   Fill in the Blank

Fill in the blank with the appropriate term.

    1. What was the cause of death in the described case?

    _____

2. What were the conditions responsible for the patient's hospitalization?

_____

3. In what body area were polyp-like tumors found?

_____

4. What virus was found in the polyp-like tumors of the patient?

_____

II.   Spell Check

Circle each incorrectly spelled term and write it correctly in the space provided.

1. menijitis   _____
2. apoplixy   _____
3. papiloma   _____
4. polip   _____
5. condiloma   _____
6. catherization   _____

Term Search Challenge

Locate 17 terms in the puzzle.

1. Write the specific term next to its definition. Then find that term in the puzzle diagram and circle it.
2. Terms may be read from left to right, backward, up, down, or diagonally.
3. If a term appears more than once, circle it only once. (A term may be found inside others.)
4. Check your answers.

Clues:

1. The urinary system consists of two_____, two _____, a urinary _____, and the _____

2. The outer region of a kidney is called the _____.

3. The inner region of a kidney is called the _____.

4. Two combining forms for kidney are _____ and _____.

5. Two combining forms for urinary bladder are _____ and _____.

6. The term for albumin in the urine _____

7. The cup-like collecting region of the renal pelvis (plural form) _____

8. The term for an inflammation of the urinary bladder _____

9. Tiny ball of capillaries in the kidney cortex _____

10. The term to indicate an increase in acidity of the blood _____

11. The abbreviation for phenylketonuria _____

12. Pyelonephritis is an inflammation of the renal _____.

Term Search Puzzle

```
K U R E T H R A T P K U N C X
I U R E A L P E L V I S E Y E
D L N E N O G I R T T S P S T
N N O I T I R U T C I M H T R
E G L O M E R U L U S P R I O
Y E F I L T R A T I O N O T C
S P H R O V E S I C O O M I T
S C A L I O D I A L Y S L S U
I I A L B U M I N U R I A O R
N T A L A C I D O S I S L I E
A I L P Y E D D I A L Y J E T
M S B U M C P Y U R I A T T E
W C Y S T O E O T E I N P I R
O T R I G O N S R R E N O N S
B L A D D E R P M E D U L L A
```

The Endocrines

"[P]ersons who are fed and sheltered will suffer from a variety of chronic disorders . . . that do not destroy life but often ruin it. . . ."

— Rene Dubois

INFORMATIONAL CHALLENGE

A. Endocrine Glands Structure and Function

I.   Fill in the Blank

Fill in the blank with the appropriate term.

1. The specific chemical messengers of endocrine glands are called
_____.

2. Hormones attach to specific _____ as target tissues.

3. _____ glands secrete their products directly into ducts.

4. _____ glands secrete their products directly into the bloodstream.

5. List five actions of prostaglandins.

a. _____

b. _____

c. _____

d. _____

e. _____

II.   Matching 1: Sources of Hormones

Match the term to its meaning. (The same meaning may be used more than once.)
Insert the appropriate letter in the space next to the question number.

Choices:

_____ **1.** calcitonin

_____ **2.** epinephrine

_____ **3.** cortisol

_____ **4.** triiodothyronine

_____ **5.** aldosterone

_____ **6.** parathyroid hormone

_____ **7.** estradiol

_____ **8.** progesterone

_____ **9.** thyroxine

_____ **10.** estrogens

a. parathyroid glands

b. adrenal cortex

c. adrenal medulla

d. thyroid gland

e. ovaries

f. testes

III.   Matching 2: Hormone Production Sites

Match the term to its meaning. (The same meaning may be used more than once.)
Insert the appropriate letter in the space next to the question number.

                                    Choices:

_____ **1.** ACTH   **a.** pancreas
_____ **2.** insulin   **b.** pituitary (anterior lobe)
_____ **3.** ADH   **c.** pituitary (posterior lobe)
_____ **4.** glucagon   **d.** hypothalamus
_____ **5.** prolactin
_____ **6.** TSH
_____ **7.** oxytocin

IV.   Matching 3: Hormone Functions

Match the term to its meaning. (The same meaning may be used more than once.)
Insert the appropriate letter in the space next to the question number.

                                    Choices:

_____ **1.** growth hormone   **a.** stimulates red-blood-cell production
_____ **2.** FSH   by bone marrow
_____ **3.** erythropoietin   **b.** regulates transport of glucose to
_____ **4.** glucagons   body cells
_____ **5.** ADH   **c.** regulates calcium levels in blood
_____ **6.** insulin   **d.** increases bone growth
_____ **7.** calcitonin   **e.** stimulates passage of calcium into
_____ **8.** parathyroid hormone   bones from the blood
_____ **9.** MSH   **f.** stimulates egg growth in the ovaries
                                 g. stimulates reabsorption of water by
                                      the kidney
                                 h. increases skin pigmentation
                                 i. increases blood sugar through con-
                                      version of glycogen to glucose

V.   Spell Check

Circle each incorrectly spelled term and write it correctly in the space provided.

1. prolactin   _____
2. epenephrine   _____
3. pituitary   _____
4. calcitonin   _____
5. pancreas   _____
6. luteenizing   _____
7. antidiuretic   _____
8. testosterone   _____
9. thighroxine   _____
10. oxytocin   _____

VI.   Vision Quiz: The Endocrine System

Figure 20-9 shows the components of the human endocrine system. Identify and
write the names of the numbered glands or related parts of the endocrine system in
the spaces provided.

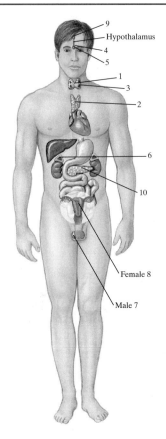

9
— Hypothalamus
4
5
1
3
2
6
10
Female 8
Male 7

FIGURE 20-9   Vision Quiz. The locations of endocrine glands.

Choices:

1. _____   **a.** anterior pituitary gland
2. _____   **b.** pineal gland
3. _____   **c.** parathyroid gland
4. _____   **d.** thyroid gland
5. _____   **e.** adrenal gland
6. _____   **f.** pancreas
7. _____   **g.** source of estrogen
8. _____   **h.** source of testosterone
9. _____   **i.** thymus gland
10. _____   **j.** posterior pituitary gland

B. Other Tissue Hormones

I.   Matching 1: Production Sites for Other Tissue Hormones

Match the term to its meaning. (The same meaning may be used more than once.)
Insert the appropriate letter in the space next to the question number.

Choices:

_____ **1.** prostaglandins   **a.** local tissues and/or cells
_____ **2.** epidermal growth factor   **b.** stomach
_____ **3.** secretin   **c.** salivary glands
_____ **4.** platelet-derived growth   **d.** blood platelets
       factor   **e.** small intestine

_____ **5.** lymphokines
_____ **6.** gastrin
_____ **7.** cholecystokinin
_____ **8.** human chorionic
gonadotropin
_____ **9.** human placental lactogen

f. placenta
g. lymphocytes

II.   Matching 2: Hormone Functions

Match the term to its meaning. (The same meaning may be used more than once.)
Insert the appropriate letter in the space next to the question number.

Choices:

_____ **1.** prostaglandins
_____ **2.** secretin
_____ **3.** gastrin
_____ **4.** cholecystokinin
_____ **5.** human chorionic
gonadotropin
_____ **6.** placental lactogen
_____ **7.** epidermal growth factor
_____ **8.** platelet-derived growth
factor
_____ **9.** lymphokines

a. stimulates gastric juice secretion
b. influences blood flow and pancreatic endocrine function
c. inhibits gastric juice secretion and causes ejection of bile from the gall-bladder
d. stimulates progesterone production
e. stimulates increases in epithelial-cell growth
f. stimulates breast tissue for lactation
g. stimulates smooth muscle fibers
h. involved in immune responses of the body
i. inhibits gastric juice secretion and increases pancreatic juice secretion

III.   Spell Check

Circle each incorrectly spelled term and write it correctly in the space provided.

1. gastren   _____
2. cholecystokinin   _____
3. secretin   _____
4. korionic   _____
5. gonadotropin   _____
6. lymphokine   _____
7. prastoglandins   _____
8. lactogen   _____

C. Combining Forms and/or Word Roots for the Endocrine System and Related Products

I.   Fill in the Blank

Fill in the blank with the appropriate term.

1. List two combining forms for milk. _____ and
_____

2. Give two word roots for sugar. _____ and
_____

3. Give two word roots for adrenal glands. _____
and _____

II.   Matching 1: Combining Forms and/or Word Roots for the Endocrine System and Related Products Part, 1

Match the term to its meaning. (The same meaning may be used more than once.) Insert the appropriate letter in the space next to the question number.

Choices:

_____ **1.** thyroid/o
_____ **2.** kal/i
_____ **3.** calc/o
_____ **4.** pineal/o
_____ **5.** parathyroid/o
_____ **6.** adren/o
_____ **7.** cortic/o
_____ **8.** thym/o
_____ **9.** natr/o
_____ **10.** gonad/o

a. parathyroid gland
b. thyroid gland
c. adrenal gland
d. cortex
e. calcium
f. potassium
g. pineal gland
h. sodium
i. thymus gland
j. sex glands

III.   Matching 2: Combining Forms and/or Word Roots for the Endocrine System and Related Products Part, 2

Match the term to its meaning. (The same meaning may be used more than once.) Insert the appropriate letter in the space next to the question number.

Choices:

_____ **1.** male
_____ **2.** pancreas
_____ **3.** female
_____ **4.** testes
_____ **5.** adrenal glands
_____ **6.** body

a. test/o
b. estr/o
c. andr/o
d. pancreat/o
e. adrenal/o
f. somat/o

IV.   Spell Check

Circle each incorrectly spelled term and write it correctly in the space provided.

1. pancreatektomy _____
2. testostirone _____
3. adrenomegale _____
4. andropathy _____
5. hypokalcemia _____
6. gonadotropin _____
7. prolactin _____
8. thyroiditis _____
9. gynekomasia _____
10. lactorhea _____

V.   Word Analysis: The Endocrine System

Table 20-12 lists a number of terms with their pronunciations and definitions.

TABLE 20-12   WORD ANALYSIS: THE ENDOCRINE SYSTEM

Term and Pronunciation	Brief Explanation
adrenalectomy (ad-rē-nal-EK-tō-mē)	surgical excision of an adrenal gland
adrenomegaly (ad-ren-ō-MEG-a-lē)	enlargement of the adrenal glands
andropathy (an-DROP-a-thē)	any disease mainly involving the male
cortical (KOR-ti-kal)	pertaining to the cortex
estrogenic (es-trō -JEN-ik)	producing the effects of the female hormone, estrogen
galactischia (gal-ak-TISK-ē-a)	holding back of milk flow
glucogenesis (gloo-kō-JEN-e-sis)	formation of glucose from glycogen
gonadectomy (gon-a-DEK-tō-mē)	excision of sex glands (ovary or testes)
gynecomastia (gī-nē-kō-MAS-tē-a)	abnormaly large mammary gland in the male
hyperglycemia (hī-per-glī-SĒ-mē-a)	deficient level (below normal) of sugar in the blood
hypocalcemia (hī-pō-kal-SE-mē-a)	abnormally low blood calcium concentration
hyponatremia (hī-pō-na-TRĒ-mē-a)	decreased concentration or level of sodium in the blood (less than normal)
kaliemia (kā-lē-Ē-mē-a)	potassium in the blood
lactorrhea (lak-tō-RĒ-a)	flow of breast milk between nursings and after weaning of offspring
pancreatitis (pan-krē-a-TĪ-tis)	inflammation of the pancreas
parathyroidectomy (par-a-thī-royd-EK-tō-mē)	excision of a parathyroid gland
pinealoma (pin-ē-a-LŌ-ma)	tumor of the pineal gland
polydipsia (pol-ē-DIP-sē-a)	condition of great thirst
somatic (so-MAT-ik)	pertaining to body cells
testalgia (tes-TAL-jē-a)	pain in the testicle
thymoma (thī-MŌ-ma)	tumor of the thymus gland
thyrocele (THĪ-rō-sēl)	hernia of the thyroid gland
thyroiditis (thī-royd-Ī-tis)	inflammation of the thyroid gland

1. Analyze each term.
2. Circle all word roots, combining forms, prefixes, and suffixes, and label them **wr**, **cf**, **p**, and **s** respectively.
3. Check your answers (shown in Table 20-13).

D. Endocrine Disorders and Diseases

I.   Matching 1: Endocrine Disorders Caused by Hypo- or Hyperactivity

Match the term to its meaning. (The same meaning may be used more than once.) Insert the appropriate letter in the space next to the question number.

		Choices:
_____	**1.** Cushing's syndrome	**a.** hyperactivity
_____	**2.** Addison's disease	**b.** hypoactivity
_____	**3.** diabetes mellitus	
_____	**4.** hyperinsulinism	
_____	**5.** tetany	
_____	**6.** acromegaly	
_____	**7.** gigantism	
_____	**8.** dwarfism	
_____	**9.** diabetes insipidus	
_____	**10.** cretinism	
_____	**11.** exophthalmic goiter	

II.   Matching 2: Endocrine Disorders and Diseases

Match the term to its meaning. (The same meaning may be used more than once.) Insert the appropriate letter in the space next to the question number.

Choices:

_____ **1.** myxedema

_____ **2.** hyperparathyroidism

_____ **3.** tetany

_____ **4.** cretinism

_____ **5.** endemic goiter

_____ **6.** pheochromocytoma

_____ **7.** diabetes mellitus (type 1)

_____ **8.** Addison's disease

_____ **9.** gigantism

_____ **10.** panhypopituitarism

a. enlarged thyroid gland due to iodine deficiency

b. hypothyroidism in the adult

c. increased calcium in the blood

d. decreased levels of parathyroid hormone

e. decreased production of glucocorticoid hormones

f. extreme hypothyroidism during childhood

g. lack of insulin production in children

h. excessive growth-hormone production in childhood

i. excess catecholamine production

j. deficiency in all pituitary hormones

III.   Spell Check

Circle each incorrectly spelled term and write it correctly in the space provided.

1. acromgaly   _____

2. Adison's   _____

3. mxydema   _____

4. goiter   _____

5. insipidus   _____

6. panhypopituitarism _____

7. pheochromacytoma _____

8. tetani   _____

IV.   Vision Quiz: Endocrine Diseases or Disorders

Figure 20-10 diagrammatically concerns diseases and/or disorders resulting from the hypo- and hyperactivities of selected endocrine glands. **Hyperactivity conditions** are indicated by dotted lines and **hypoactivities** are indicated by solid lines. Complete this quiz by selecting the disease or disorder associated with hyper- or hypoactivity of the endocrine glands shown. Insert the letter of the appropriate condition in the space provided next to the question number.

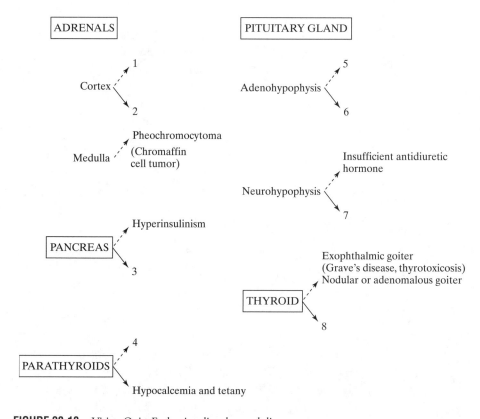

FIGURE 20-10   Vision Quiz. Endocrine disorders and diseases.

Choices:

1. _____   **a.** adrenal virilism

2. _____   **b.** diabetes insipidus

3. _____   **c.** myxedema

4. _____   **d.** diabetes mellitus

5. _____   **e.** dwarfism

6. _____   **f.** acromegaly

7. _____   **g.** hyperparathyroidism

8. _____   **h.** Addison's disease

E. Diagnostic and Surgical Procedures

I.   Matching 1: Clinical Procedures

Match the term to its meaning. (The same meaning may be used more than once.) Insert the appropriate letter in the space next to the question number.

Choices:

_____ 1. human chorionic gonadotropism

_____ 2. thyroid chemistries

_____ 3. glucose tolerance test

_____ 4. fasting blood sugar (FBS)

_____ 5. CAT scan

_____ 6. MRI

_____ 7. ultrasonography

_____ 8. thyroid scan

_____ 9. estradiol assay

_____ 10. immunoassay

a. blood or urine test to detect diabetes mellitus or hypoglycemia

b. used as pregnancy detection or uncovering testicular tumors

c. measures levels of thyroid hormones

d. the use of magnetic waves to create an image of body structures

e. procedure that uses x-rays to show body in cross-sections (slices)

f. procedure used to produce images by beaming sound waves into the body and capturing the echoes bouncing back from organs

g. blood or urine tests to determine female hormone concentrations

h. the use of immunological reactions to determine hormone levels

i. intravenous(IV) injection of radioactive iodine to evaluate size, position, and function of thyroid gland

II.   Matching 2: Surgical Procedures

Match the term to its meaning. (The same meaning may be used more than once.) Insert the appropriate letter in the space next to the question number.

Choices:

_____ 1. adrenalectomy

_____ 2. cryohypophysectomy

_____ 3. pinealectomy

_____ 4. parathyroidectomy

_____ 5. partial thyroidectomy

_____ 6. thyroid lobectomy

a. procedure to remove hypophysis with the use of a probe

b. removal of adrenal gland(s)

c. removal of fibrous nodular thyroid

d. surgical removal of the pineal body

e. removal of parathyroid gland

f. removal of thyroid gland isthmus and specific lobe for a solitary nodule

III.   Spell Check

Circle each incorrectly spelled term and write it correctly in the space provided.

1. exopthalmometry   _____

2. crohypophysectomy   _____

3. pinealectomy   _____

4. lobectomy   _____

5. thymectomy   _____

6. parathyroidectomy   _____

F. Medical Vocabulary Building

I.   Matching

Match the term to its meaning. (The same meaning may be used more than once.)
Insert the appropriate letter in the space next to the question number.

Choices:

_____ **1.** acidosis
_____ **2.** adenalgia
_____ **3.** adrenotropic
_____ **4.** euthyroid
_____ **5.** hirsutism
_____ **6.** hypocrinism
_____ **7.** hypogonadism
_____ **8.** insuloma
_____ **9.** progeria
_____ **10.** thyroptosis
_____ **11.** thyrotome
_____ **12.** thyrotoxicosis

a. pain in the gland
b. a condition of excessive acidity of body fluids
c. pertaining to adrenal gland nourishment
d. excessive growth of body hair
e. normal activity of the thyroid gland
f. a condition resulting from a deficient internal secretion of the glands
g. a condition resulting from deficient secretions of any gland
h. islets of Langerhans tumor
i. a condition characterized by premature aging during childhood
j. downward drooping of the thyroid gland into the thorax
k. an instrument used to cut thyroid cartilage
l. a toxic (poisonous) condition of the thyroid gland resulting from hyperactivity

II.   Spell Check

Circle each incorrectly spelled term and write it correctly in the space provided.

1. thyrotoxikosis _____
2. insuloma _____
3. hersutism _____
4. adrinotropic _____
5. projeria _____
6. hypocrinism _____
7. euthyroid _____
8. acidosis _____

G. Abbreviations

I.   Matching 1: Specific Hormones and Activities or Functions, Part 1

Match the term to its meaning. (The same meaning may be used more than once.)
Insert the appropriate letter in the space next to the question number

Choices:

_____ **1.** MSH
_____ **2.** hGH
_____ **3.** LH

a. low-density lipoprotein
b. melanocyte-stimulating hormone
c. follicle-stimulating hormone

_____	**4.** ATP	**d.** luteinizing hormone
_____	**5.** CRF	**e.** adenosine triphosphate
_____	**6.** FSH	**f.** human growth hormone
_____	**7.** LDL	**g.** interstitial cell-stimulating hormone
_____	**8.** DOC	**h.** antidiuretic hormone
_____	**9.** PGH	**i.** desoxycorticosterone
_____	**10.** ADH	**j.** corticotropin-releasing factor
_____	**11.** ICSH	**k.** pituitary growth hormone

II.   Matching 2: Specific Hormones and Activities or Functions, Part 2

Match the term to its meaning. (The same meaning may be used more than once.)
Insert the appropriate letter in the space next to the question number

Choices:

_____	**1.** 17-ketosteroids	**a.** TTH
_____	**2.** prolactin	**b.** T3
_____	**3.** parathyroid hormone	**c.** PRL
_____	**4.** thyrotropic hormone	**d.** PTH
_____	**5.** thyroxine	**e.** T4
_____	**6.** triiodothyronine	**f.** 17KS
_____	**7.** thyroid-stimulating hormone	**g.** TSH
_____	**8.** 17-hydroxycorticosteroids	**h.** 17-OH

III.   Matching 3: Procedures and Materials Used in Diagnosis or Treatment of Endocrine Disorders or Diseases

Match the term to its meaning. (The same meaning may be used more than once.)
Insert the appropriate letter in the space next to the question number

Choices:

_____	**1.** VLDL	**a.** protamine zinc insulin
_____	**2.** PZI	**b.** crystalline zinc insulin
_____	**3.** NPH	**c.** fasting blood sugar
_____	**4.** CZI	**d.** very low-density lipoprotein
_____	**5.** GTT	**e.** neutral protein Hagedorn (insulin)
_____	**6.** FBS	**f.** glucose tolerance test

IV.   Matching 4: Endocrine Diseases or Disorders

Match the term to its meaning. (The same meaning may be used more than once.)
Insert the appropriate letter in the space next to the question number

Choices:

_____	**1.** medullary carcinoma of the thyroid	**a.** DI
_____	**2.** diabetic ketoacidosis	**b.** DM
_____	**3.** diabetes insipidus	**c.** MCT
_____	**4.** insulin-dependent diabetes mellitus	**d.** NIDDM
_____	**5.** diabetes mellitus	**e.** DKA
_____	**6.** non-insulin-dependent diabetes mellitus	**f.** IDDM

H. Increasing Your Medical Terminology Word Power 1

1. Read the following report.
2. Prepare to answer the questions at the end of the section.
3. Circle all unfamiliar terms with a red pencil.
4. Underline familiar terms with a blue pencil.
5. Use your knowledge of word elements, a medical dictionary, and the key terms to find the meaning of unfamiliar terms.

A Pituitary Dwarfism Study

Key Terms

asphyxia (as-FIK-sē-a)   choking caused by an insufficient intake of oxygen

breech presentation   abnormality during delivery in which the fetal buttocks appear first rather than the head

dentition (den-TISH-un)   refers to the number, type, and arrangement of the teeth in the arch formed by the cutting and chewing surfaces of the mouth

genital hypoplasia (hī-pō-PLĀ-zē-a)   underdevelopment of the genitals

ischemia (is-KĒ-mē-a)   a temporary and local deficiency of blood caused by a blockage of the circulation to a body part

perinatal   period beginning after the twenty-eighth week of pregnancy through twenty-eight days after birth.

Individuals with pituitary dwarfism due to persistent growth-hormone (GH) deficiency in childhood are short, immature in appearance, have delayed dentition and muscular development, and genital hypoplasia. From an endocrinological standpoint, pituitary dwarfism is divided into complete GH deficiency and partial GH deficiency. Until several years ago, only dwarfs with severe or complete GH deficiency were treated with human GH because of its limited supply. However, because of the advances in gene technology, the effectiveness and safety of recombinant human GH (r-GH) therapy is now used for both complete GH deficiency and for partial GH deficiency. One group of patients under study had complete GH deficiency and pituitary-hormone deficiencies in luteinzing hormone, follicle-stimulating hormone, thyroid-stimulating hormone, adrenocorticotropic hormone, and so on. In addition, permanent—or secondary—dentition were absent.

The cause of pituitary dwarfism is not clear, but some investigators propose that perinatal abnormalities such as asphyxia or breech presentation may cause pituitary ischemia, resulting in pituitary dwarfism.

Questions

I.   Fill in the Blank

Fill in the blank with the appropriate term.

1. Give four physical features of individuals with pituitary dwarfism caused by persistent growth-hormone deficiency in childhood.

    a. _____

    b. _____

    c. _____

    d. _____

2. From an endocrinological standpoint, what is the basis of the categories of pituitary dwarfism? _____

3. What material is used for pituitary dwarfism treatment?

    _____

4. Give two possible causes of pituitary ischemia.

    a. _____
    b. _____

II.   Spell Check

Circle each incorrectly spelled term and write it correctly in the space provided.

1. dentishun   _____
2. ischemia   _____
3. lutenizing   _____
4. dwarfism   _____
5. breech   _____
6. hypoplazia   _____
7. deficiency   _____
8. pituitary   _____

I. Increasing Your Medical Terminology Word Power 2

1. Read the following report.
2. Prepare to answer the questions at the end of the section.
3. Circle all unfamiliar terms with a red pencil.
4. Underline familiar terms with a blue pencil.
5. Use your knowledge of word elements, a medical dictionary, and the key terms to find the meaning of unfamiliar terms.

An Unusual Case of Gigantism in Infancy

Key Terms

acromegaly (ak-rō-MEG-a-lē)   an elongation of the hands, feet, and certain head bones caused by an excess of growth hormone

café au lait (kaf-Ā-oh-lay)   patchy pigmented spots on the skin

cm   an abbreviation for centimeter; one-hundredth part of a meter, or 2.53 cm to the inch

CT   a computerized analysis of x-ray information that produces a cross-sectional view of the body being studied.

g   the abbreviation for gram

galactorrhea (ga-lak-tō-RĒ-a)   excessive flow of breast milk

genitalia (jen-i-TĀL-ē-a)   the reproductive organs

gigantism (JĪ-gan-tizm)   excessive development of body parts such as the hands, feet, and certain facial bones caused by the overproduction of growth hormone

hypophysectomy (hī-pof-i-SEK-tō-mē)   surgical removal of the pituitary gland

kg   abbreviation for kilogram; 1000 grams or 2.2 pounds

prepubertal (prē-PŪ-ber-tal)   before puberty

serum   the watery or fluid portion of blood that forms after clotting; serves as material for laboratory diagnosis tests

ultrasonogram   an image of an organ or tissue produced by ultrasound

G ENERAL BACKGROUND

Overproduction of human growth hormone (hGH) during childhood causes an excessive increase in body length, or *gigantism*. Children with gigantism may also develop *acromegalic* physical characteristics such as the thickening of soft tissue, enlargement of the hands and feet, and coarse facial features. Laboratory findings in children with excess hGH are similar to those found with adults.

C ASE REPORT

A 3,460-g baby girl measuring 51 cm in length was born after a normal pregnancy period. Her growth increased greatly during the first month of life and was quite dramatic by nine months. At eighteen months of age, her height, which measured 94 cm, was comparable to that of a thirty-three-month-old child. Her body weight, which was 15.2 kg, was comparable to that of a forty-two-month-old child. The child's facial features were coarse. She also had a wide nasal bridge, an enlarged forehead and jaw, and disproportionately large hands and feet. The genitalia were prepubertal. A 1-by-2-cm *café au lait* spot was also found on her abdomen. CT scans and ultrasonograms of the chest, abdomen, and pelvis were normal. The one exception noted was that the ovaries were slightly enlarged for the child's age. Other analytical procedures showed an enlargement of the pituitary gland. In addition, laboratory determinations of the serum levels of growth hormone and prolactin were found to be above normal. On the basis of these and related findings, the patient was given appropriate therapy to reduce the serum levels of both of these hormones.

At thirty-three months of age, the child's serum levels of growth hormone and prolactin were again found to be elevated significantly. In addition, CT scans still showed an enlarged pituitary gland. At this point it was considered advisable for the patient to undergo a partial *hypophysectomy*. One month after the operation, hormonal levels were still abnormally high. A total hypophysectomy was performed. After the operation, the patient was placed on long-term hormonal therapy, which included the administration of thyroxine and hydrocortisone. Examination of the removed tissue showed the presence of a tumor composed of cells that produced both growth hormone and prolactin.

One year later, the patient, who was now almost four years old, had normal serum levels of growth hormone and prolactin. In addition, her facial features softened and appeared less husky.

Questions

I.   Matching

Match the term to its meaning. (The same meaning may be used more than once.) Insert the appropriate letter in the space next to the question number.

Choices:

_____ **1.** hypophysectomy
_____ **2.** prepubertal
_____ **3.** ultrasonogram
_____ **4.** gigantism
_____ **5.** genitalia
_____ **6.** café au lait

a. before puberty
b. ultrasound record
c. surgical removal of pituitary gland
d. reproductive organs
e. condition caused by excess growth
       hormone production

_____ **7.** acromegaly   **f.** pigment spots on the skin

_____ **8.** galactorrhea   **g.** excess flow of breast milk

_____ **9.** prolactin   **h.** hormone associated with breast-milk production

II.   Spell Check

Circle each incorrectly spelled term and write it correctly in the space provided.

1. facial   _____
2. prepubertel   _____
3. gigantism   _____
4. ultrasonogram   _____
5. akromegaly   _____
6. galactorhea   _____
7. prolactin   _____
8. hypophsectomy   _____

J. Increasing Your Medical Terminology Word Power 3

1. Read the following report.
2. Prepare to answer the questions at the end of the section.
3. Circle all unfamiliar terms with a red pencil.
4. Underline familiar terms with a blue pencil.
5. Use your knowledge of word elements, a medical dictionary, and the key terms to find the meaning of unfamiliar terms.

Acromegaly Resulting from the Secretion of Growth Hormone by a Non-Hodgkin's Lymphoma

Key Terms

adenoma (ad'-e-NŌ-ma)   a neoplasm of glandular tissue

carpal tunnel syndrome   a condition characterized by soreness, tenderness, and weakness of the muscles of the thumb; results from pressure on the median nerve at the point at which it goes through the carpal tunnel of the wrist

cyclophosphamide (sī'-klō-FOS-fa-mīd)   an antineoplastic agent that also has been used to suppress the immune system responses

decompression (dē-com-PRESH-un)   the lowering of a body part

doxorubicin (dok'-sō-RŪ-bi-sin)   an antineoplastic agent

ectopic (ek-TOP-ik)   in an abnormal position

follicular (fō-LIK-ū-lar)   pertaining to follicles

hGH   human growth hormone

hodgkin's (HOJ-kins) lymphoma   a disease of unknown cause producing liver, spleen, and lymphoid tissue enlargement, and invasion of other body tissues

lymphadenopathy (lim-fad'-ē-NOP-a-thē)   disease of the lymph nodes

prednisolone (pred-NIS-ō-lōn)   a glucocorticosteroid drug

remission (ri-MISH-un)   lessening the severity of signs and symptoms of a disorder or disease

vincristine (vin-KRIS-tēn)   a plant extract used in the treatment of certain types of malignant tumors

visceromegaly (vis-er-ō-MEG-a-lē)   generalized enlargement of the abdominal visceral organs

G ENERAL BACKGROUND

Acromegaly is a systemic endocrine disorder caused by sustained hypersecretion of growth hormone. Typical signs and symptoms include skin thickening; enlargement of the hands, feet and mandible; and visceromegaly. An active disease state is indicated by the presence of excessive sweating and soft-tissue swelling. Most patients with the condition have a growth-secreting adenoma. The case report described here concerns a patient with recurrent non-Hodgkin's lymphoma and acromegaly resulting from the ectopic production of growth hormone by the lymphoma.

C ASE REPORT

In November, 1998, a 47-year-old woman was referred to the medical center for evaluation of malignant lymphoma. The patient had a six-month history of excessive sweating, bone pain, and weight loss of 6 kg, followed by a weight gain of 7 kg. In the following January, she underwent bilateral compression of the median nerve because of carpal tunnel syndrome. Abdominal lymphadenopathy was detected by ultrasonography and verified by abdominal computed tomography. The latter finding suggested the presence of a malignant lymphoma. A subsequent lymph-node biopsy revealed follicular non-Hodgkin's lymphoma.

The patient was treated with four cycles of cyclophosphamide, doxorubicin, etoposide, prednisolone, and vincristine. The lymphoma responded well to the treatment. The patient was well until the end of 1999, when excessive sweating and swelling of her hands and feet gradually reappeared. Nose, lips, and jaw enlargement were also noted by the patient. She was subsequently hospitalized in December, 1999, and evaluated for growth hormone excess.

Physical examination was normal except for the features of acromegaly and axillary and inguinal lymphadenopathy. Laboratory results of hormonal levels revealed elevated growth hormone concentrations. The results of magnetic resonance imaging of the pituitary gland were normal. However, abdominal computed tomography revealed liver and spleen enlargement, and multiple lymph nodes in the para-aortic region, compressing the vena cava. Inguinal lymph-node biopsy revealed follicular non-Hodgkin's lymphoma.

One cycle of treatment with the previously used drugs did not correct her condition. The clinical and biochemical signs of acromegaly persisted. The patient was therefore treated with another group of medications, which resulted in a rapid clinical improvement and a remarkable decrease in the serum concentration of hGH. The patient has since remained in remission.

Questions

I.   Fill in the Blank

Fill in the blank with the appropriate term.

   1. What were the signs and symptoms initially experienced by the patient? _____

2. List two clinical procedures that suggested the presence of a malignant lymphoma in the patient.

   a. _____

   b. _____

3. What were the physical findings on admission of the patient in December, 1999? _____

_____

4. What did abdominal computed tomography reveal in the patient?

_____

II.   Spell Check

Circle each incorrectly spelled term and write it correctly in the space provided.

   1. viseromegaly   _____

   2. carpal   _____

   3. follicular   _____

   4. Hogdkin's   _____

   5. adinoma   _____

   6. prednisolone   _____

   7. remission   _____

   8. ectopik   _____

Term Search Challenge

Locate 21 terms in the puzzle.

   1. Write the specific term next to its definition. Then find that term in the puzzle diagram and circle it.

   2. Terms may be read from left to right, backward, up, down, or diagonally.

   3. If a term appears more than once, circle it only once. (A term may be found inside others.)

   4. Check your answers.

Clues:

   1. The outer portion of the adrenal gland _____

   2. The inner part of the adrenal gland _____

   3. The substance from which thyroid hormones are made

   _____

   4. The specialized hormone-producing cells of the pancreas are the islets of _____

   5. TSH _____ -stimulating hormone

   6. The hormone secreted by the parathyroid gland _____ and _____

   7. The specific male hormone produced by the testes

   _____

   8. Two combining forms for the thyroid gland and

   _____

   9. Combining form for sex glands _____

   10. Combining form for male _____

   11. Combining form for female _____

   12. The condition in which there is a lack of insulin, diabetes

   _____

13. The group of hormones secreted by the testes and the adrenal cortex
    _____

14. Glands that secrete hormones directly into the bloodstream
    _____

15. The mineral substance for proper functioning of bones
    _____

16. Glands that secrete chemicals through channels or ducts
    _____

17. The chemical produced by an endocrine gland
    _____

18. Condition of an enlarged thyroid gland _____

19. Enlargement of arms and legs due to activity of pituitary gland after
    puberty _____

20. Abbreviation for antidiuretic hormone _____

Term Search Puzzle

```
C  O  R  T  E  X  C  A  L  C  I  U  M  M  I
H  N  G  H  L  T  T  G  O  I  T  E  R  E  O
O  A  E  S  T  R  O  H  O  T  S  I  N  G  D
R  R  L  U  S  T  V  R  Y  N  Y  M  O  A  I
M  I  O  A  N  D  R  O  O  R  A  R  O  L  N
O  E  X  O  C  R  I  N  E  L  O  D  H  Y  E
N  S  T  H  Y  R  O  I  D  O  M  R  O  O  H
E  T  T  E  S  T  O  S  T  E  R  O  N  E  T
S  T  O  M  E  L  L  I  T  U  S  L  O  N  E
D  O  C  P  A  R  A  T  H  O  R  M  O  N  E
A  D  H  O  L  A  N  G  E  R  H  A  N  S  S
G  O  N  A  D  O  E  U  V  X  A  C  E  T  H
R  S  T  T  H  Y  R  O  I  D  L  T  N  J  X
E  N  I  R  C  O  D  N  E  Y  T  H  H  R  U
M  E  D  U  L  L  A  A  N  D  R  O  G  E  N
```

CHAPTER 21

The Male Reproductive System

"What geography is to history, such is anatomy to medicine—it describes the theater."

—J. Fernel

INFORMATIONAL CHALLENGE

A. The Male Reproductive System

I.   Fill in the Blank

Fill in the blank with the appropriate term.

1. List the primary accessory glands of the male reproductive system.
   a. _____
   b. _____
   c. _____
   d. _____
   e. _____

2. List the supporting structure and accessory sex organs of the male reproductive system.
   a. _____
   b. _____

3. The sperm production process is known as _____-genesis.

4. The male hormone responsible for sperm production and secondary sex characteristics is _____.

5. The male sex hormone that inhibits sperm production is _____.

6. Give two functions of the epididymis.
   a. _____
   b. _____

7. What is the function of the seminal vesicles?
   _____

8. Name the two small glands located below the prostate and on either side of the urethra. _____
   _____

9. List the three sections of the male urethra.
   a. _____
   b. _____
   c. _____

10. The surgical procedure by which the foreskin is removed from the tip of the penis is _____.

11. List the three accessory sex glands of the male.

    a. _____

    b. _____

    c. _____

12. List two combining forms used for the testis:

    a. _____

    b. _____

13. What is the combining form used for vesicle?

    _____

II.   Matching 1: Structures and Functions of the Male Reproductive System

Match the term to its meaning. (The same meaning may be used more than once.) Insert the appropriate letter in the space next to the question number.

Choices:

_____ **1.** testes	**a.** male hormones
_____ **2.** seminiferous tubules	**b.** long tube located at top of each testis
_____ **3.** androgens	**c.** major male reproductive organs
_____ **4.** scrotum	**d.** transport sperm from epididymis
_____ **5.** ejaculatory ducts	**e.** site of sperm production
_____ **6.** vas deferens	**f.** soft tip of penis
_____ **7.** epididymis	**g.** expel sperm into urethra
_____ **8.** glans penis	**h.** tube used to expel both urine and sperm
_____ **9.** urethra	**i.** secretion neutralizes urine remaining in urethra
_____ **10.** bulbourethral glands	**j.** contains the testes

III.   Matching 2: Combining Forms for the Male Reproductive System

Match the term to its meaning. (The same meaning may be used more than once.) Insert the appropriate letter in the space next to the question number.

Choices:

_____ **1.** prostat/o	**a.** glans penis
_____ **2.** orchid/o	**b.** duct
_____ **3.** balan/o	**c.** testis
_____ **4.** vas/o	**d.** prostate
_____ **5.** vesicul/o	**e.** male
_____ **6.** andr/o	**f.** vesicle
_____ **7.** spermat/o	**g.** spermatozoa

IV.   Vision Quiz: The Male Reproductive System

Figure 21-5 shows the components of the male reproductive system. Identify and write the name of the numbered parts in the spaces provided.

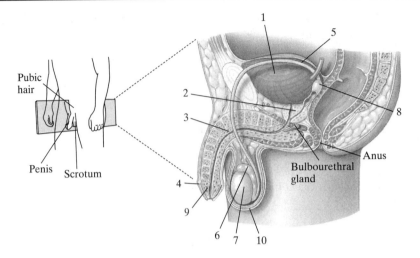

FIGURE 21-5   Vision Quiz. The Male Reproduction System

Choices:

_____ 1.   **a.** urinary bladder

_____ 2.   **b.** vas deferens (ductus deferens)

_____ 3.   **c.** urethra

_____ 4.   **d.** prostate gland

_____ 5.   **e.** seminal vesicle

_____ 6.   **f.** epididymis

_____ 7.   **g.** prepuce (foreskin)

_____ 8.   **h.** scrotum

_____ 9.   **i.** glans

_____ 10.   **j.** testes

V.   Spell Check

Circle each incorrectly spelled term and write it correctly in the space provided.

1. glanz   _____

2. prostate   _____

3. prepus   _____

4. seminel   _____

5. prostatitis   _____

6. vasektomy   _____

7. epididmis   _____

8. testes   _____

9. ejaculatory   _____

10. scrotum   _____

11. epididimitis   _____

12. balanitis   _____

VI.   Word Analysis: Word Roots, Combining Forms, Suffixes, and Prefixes Associated with the Male Reproductive System

Table 21-8 lists a number of terms with their pronunciations and definitions.

TABLE 21-8   WORD ANALYSIS: WORD ROOTS, COMBINING FORMS, SUFFIXES, AND PREFIXES ASSOCIATED WITH THE MALE REPRODUCTIVE SYSTEM

Term and Pronunciation	Brief Explanation
android (AN-droyd)	resembling a male
balanitis (bal-a-NĪ-tis)	inflammation of glans penis
epididymography (ep-i-did'-i-MOG-ra-fē)	an x-ray examination of the epididymis
orchiectomy (or-kē-EK-tō-mē)	removal of testes
prostatitis (pros-ta-TĪ-tis)	inflammation of the prostate gland
spermatogenesis (sper-mat-ō-JEN-e-sis)	formation of spermatozoa
testitis (tes-TĪ-tis)	inflammation of a testis
vasectomy (vas-EK-tō-mē)	removal of the vas deferens in part or completely
vesiculogram (ve-SIK-ū-lō-gram)	an x-ray of the seminal vesicles

1. Analyze each term.
2. Circle all prefixes, combining forms, word roots, and suffixes, and label them **p, cf, wr**, and **s**, respectively.
3. Check your answers (shown in Table 21-9).

B. Disorders, Pathological Conditions, and Surgical Procedures Associated with the Male Reproductive System

I.   Fill in the Blank

Fill in the blank with the appropriate term.

1. Failure of the testes to descend into the scrotum: _____
2. Narrowing of foreskin opening over the glans: _____
3. Enlargement of spermatic cord veins: _____

II.   Matching 1: Disorders and Pathological Conditions of the Male Reproductive System

Match the term to its meaning. (The same meaning may be used more than once.) Insert the appropriate letter in the space next to the question number.

Choices:

_____ 1. cryptorchidism
_____ 2. hypospadias
_____ 3. orchitis
_____ 4. benign prostatic hyperplasia
_____ 5. varicocele

a. nonmalignant overgrowth of prostate cells
b. failure of testes to descend
c. abnormal opening of urethra on underside of penis
d. inflammation of the testes
e. enlarged veins of spermatic cord

III.   Matching 2: Surgical and Related Procedures Involving the Male Reproductive System

Match the term to its meaning. (The same meaning may be used more than once.) Insert the appropriate letter in the space next to the question number.

		Choices:
_____ **1.** circumcision		**a.** surgical removal of the vas deferens
_____ **2.** castration		**b.** destruction of tissue with chemicals, an electric current, a hot iron, or by freezing
_____ **3.** cauterization		**c.** surgical removal of the testes
_____ **4.** vasectomy		**d.** surgical removal of the prepuce

IV.   Spell Check

Circle each incorrectly spelled term and write it correctly in the space provided.

1. seminoma   _____

2. epespadias   _____

3. prostatic   _____

4. caterization   _____

5. vazsectomy   _____

6. castration   _____

C. Medical Vocabulary Building

I.   Fill in the Blank

Fill in the blank with the appropriate term.

1. What is the term for prostate enlargement? _____

2. Give the term for excessive mammary gland development in a male. _____

3. A condition in which there is a small amount of sperm in semen is called _____.

4. An inflammation of the penis is known as _____.

5. The presence of sperm in semen is called _____.

II.   Spell Check

Circle each incorrectly spelled term and write it correctly in the space provided.

1. unuch   _____

2. jinecomastia   _____

3. oligospiremia   _____

4. penetis   _____

5. prostatomegaly   _____

6. spermatogenesis   _____

D. Sexually Transmitted Diseases (STDs) and Nonspecific Genital Infections

I.   Fill in the Blank

Fill in the blank with the appropriate term.

1. List three specific examples of bacteria-caused STDs.

a. _____

b. _____

c. _____

2. List four specific examples of virus-caused STDs.

a. _____

b. _____

c. _____

d. _____

3. Give two common nonspecific diseases found among men.

a. _____

b. _____

4. What does AIDS mean? _____

II.   Spell Check

Circle each incorrectly spelled term and write it correctly in the space provided.

1. gonorhea   _____

2. urethritis   _____

3. condilomata   _____

4. sifilis   _____

5. prostatitis   _____

6. candidiasis   _____

7. trichomoniasis   _____

8. vagenosis   _____

E. Abbreviations: Diseases and Disorders

I.   Matching

Match the abbreviation to its meaning. (The same meaning may be used more than once.) Insert the appropriate letter in the space next to the question number.

Choices:

_____ **1.** AZT   **a.** Kaposi's sarcoma

_____ **2.** Gc   **b.** pediatric AIDS

_____ **3.** HBV   **c.** gonorrhea

_____ **4.** CS   **d.** nongonococcal urethritis

_____ **5.** DGI   **e.** azidothymidine

_____ **6.** HSV   **f.** hepatitis B virus

_____ **7.** NGU   **g.** disseminated gonococcal infection

_____ **8.** KS   **h.** human papilloma virus

_____ **9.** PAIDS   **i.** herpes simplex virus

_____ **10.** HPV   **j.** congenital syphilis

II.   Spell Check

Circle each incorrectly spelled term and write it correctly in the space provided.

1. congitel   _____
2. papilloma   _____
3. sifilis   _____
4. gonorhea   _____
5. uretritis   _____
6. lymphogranuloma   _____

F. Increasing Your Medical Terminology Word Power 1

1. Read the following report.
2. Prepare to answer the questions at the end of the section.
3. Circle all unfamiliar terms with a red pencil.
4. Underline familiar terms with a blue pencil.
5. Use your knowledge of word elements, a medical dictionary, and the key terms to find the meaning of unfamiliar terms.

A Case of Early Syphilis

Key Terms

CAT   computerized axial tomography (CAT scan)

CSF   cerebrospinal (ser-e-bro-SPĪ-nal) fluid

EEG   electroencephalogram (e-lek-trō-en-SEF-a-lō-gram)

insomnia (in-SOM-nē-a)   inability to sleep or interrupted sleep

purulent (PŪR-ū-lent)   forming or containing pus

VDRL   Venereal Disease Research Laboratory test for syphilis

vertigo (VER-ti-gō)   a sensation of moving around in a space or of having objects spin around the person

B ACKGROUND

Central-nervous-system involvement in syphilis can occur as a later stage of this STD. Symptoms associated with the condition include continuous headache, vertigo, insomnia, and changes in personality.

C ASE HISTORY

A forty-year-old man who was referred to the Neurological Unit presented with a three-month history of a throbbing headache not relieved by aspirin or other pain relievers, constant and persistent throughout the day and occasionally aggravated at night, producing insomnia. No other symptoms were present.

General and neurologic examination was normal. Routine hematologic, biochemical, and urine analyses showed no abnormality. Skull x-rays, EEG, and CSF examinations were also normal. A CAT scan of the head was performed, which showed a small mass in the right cerebellar hemisphere of the brain. Three weeks later the patient developed a rash on his palms and thighs. No lesions were seen in the mouth.

The patient revealed that five months previously he had had sexual intercourse with a prostitute. A few days later he noticed a purulent urethral discharge, and he treated himself inadequately with oral penicillin.

A new examination that included a VDRL test of the CSF was performed, which was again normal. The patient was then treated with penicillin for twenty days. His headaches disappeared at the end of treatment. All skin lesions disappeared within two months.

Questions

I.   Fill in the Blank

Fill in the blank with the appropriate term.

1. A small mass was detected by a CAT head scan in the patient. Where was this mass located? _____
2. Explain the meaning of CSF. _____
3. What was the treatment used in this case? _____
4. On what body parts was a rash detected? _____
5. Did all signs and symptoms of the disease disappear after treatment? _____

II.   Spell Check

Circle each correctly spelled term in each of the following cases.

1. computerized, compooterized, computeurized
2. cerbrospinel, cerebrospinel, cerebrospinal
3. electroencephalogram, elektroencephalogram, electroencefalogram
4. insomnia, insomia, insommia
5. purrulent, purulent, purulint
6. venerreal, venereal, venireal
7. vertego, vertigo, virtigo

G. Increasing Your Medical Terminology Word Power 2

1. Read the following report.
2. Prepare to answer the questions at the end of the section.
3. Circle all unfamiliar terms with a red pencil.
4. Underline familiar terms with a blue pencil.
5. Use your knowledge of word elements, a medical dictionary, and the key terms to find the meaning of unfamiliar terms.

Erectile Dysfunction

Key Terms

cavernosal (kav'-er-NŌ-sal)   pertaining to hollow spaces; pertaining to erectile tissue

corpus (KŌR-pus) cavernosum (kav-er-NŌ-sum)   any erectile tissue; refers especially to the erectile structures such as the penis, clitoris of the female, and male and female urethra

detumescence (dē'-tū-MES-ens)   disappearance of swelling or enlargement

erectile (e-REK-tĭl)   ability to become erect

flaccid (FLAK-sid)   relaxed; flabby

hyperlipemia (hī'-per-lip-Ē-mē-a)   excessive quantity of fat in the blood

libido (li-BĒ-dō)   the sex drive, conscious or unconscious

prosthesis (PROS-thē-sis)   an artificial part or organ

psychogenic (sī-kō-JEN-ik)   of mental origin

revascularization (rē-vas'-kū-lar-i-ZĀ-shun)   restoration of blood flow to a body part

schizophrenia (skiz'-ō-FREN-ē-a)   a group of related mental disorders of unknown cause in which a special type of disordered thinking, affect, and behavior is present

transurethral (trans-ū-RĒ-thral)   pertains to an operation performed through the urethra

I NTRODUCTION

The inability to achieve and maintain an erection sufficient for satisfactory sexual intercourse is referred to as erectile dysfunction. Estimates indicate that this condition affects approximately 20 to 30 million men in the United States. This condition may be a result of neurologic, psychological, hormonal, arterial, or cavernosal impairment or from a combination of these factors.

P HYSIOLOGICAL ASPECTS OF PENILE ERECTION

Penile erection is a neuromuscular event regulated by psychological factors and hormone levels. On sexual stimulation, nerve impulses cause the release of neurotransmitters from cavernous nerves and of relaxing substances from penile endothelial cells. These actions not only cause a relaxation of smooth muscles in the arteries and arterioles supplying erectile tissue, but also a major increase in the blood flow to the penis. At the same time, additional events cause a rapid filling and expansion of the penile sinusoidal system, trapping blood within the corpora cavernosum and resulting in the raising of the penis to an erect position.

During sexual activities, certain penile muscles forcefully compress the base of the blood-filled corpora cavernosum and the penis becomes even harder. During this phase, blood inflow and outflow temporarily stops.

Detumescence or disappearance of the muscular erection can disappear due to various factors, including the cessation of neurotransmitter release. Contraction of the involved smooth muscles reopens the venous channels of the penis resulting in the trapped blood being expelled and the penis returning to a flaccid state.

P ATHOPHYSIOLOGY

Causes

Erectile dysfunction can be classified as psychogenic, organic (which includes arterial, cavernosal, hormonal, neurogenic, or drug-induced), or a combination of organic and psychogenic. The combined form is the most commonly found with patients. Features of only some of these causes will be described.

Common causes of psychogenic erectile dysfunction generally include lack of sexual arousability, obvious psychiatric disorders such as depression and schizophrenia, strained relationships, and performance anxiety.

Neurologic disorders such as Alzheimer's disease, stroke, and cerebral trauma often are the causes of erectile dysfunction. Usually the conditions cause a decreasing libido or prevent the initiation of an erection. In men with spinal cord injuries, the extent of erectile function depends mainly on the location and extent of the injury.

𝒟 YSFUNCTION AND AGING

Sexual function progressively decreases in healthy aging males. This situation can be recognized by several events including an increase of the length of inactive or resting periods between sexual stimulation and erection, less swollen erections, less forceful ejaculations, and a decrease in the ejaculatory volume. Individuals also experience a decrease in sensitivity to tactile stimulation. Serum testosterone concentrations also decrease.

𝒟 IAGNOSIS

Diagnosis of erectile dysfunction requires a thorough medical, sexual, and psychosocial history. This is especially important because the presenting signs or symptoms of a variety of diseases and/or disorders can cloud the actual condition and contribute to the wrong diagnosis. Such diseases and/or conditions include diabetes mellitus, coronary heart disease, hyperlipemia, hypertension, and pituitary tumors. A complete physical examination and appropriate laboratory tests, specifically to eliminate the possibility of the presence of these conditions, also should be performed.

𝒯 REATMENT

Since the early 1970s dramatic changes have occurred in the treatment of erectile dysfunction. From this time period approaches have included psychotherapy, the use of penile prostheses, intracavernous injection therapy, vacuum constriction devices, and revascularization. Transurethral and oral drug therapy are examples of the more recent additions.

Questions

I.   Matching

Match the term to its meaning. (The same meaning may be used more than once.) Insert the appropriate letter in the space next to the question number.

		Choices:
_____	**1.** cavernosal	**a.** pertaining to hollow spaces
_____	**2.** corpora	**b.** any erectile tissue
_____	**3.** detumescence	**c.** disappearance of swelling or enlargement
_____	**4.** flaccid	**d.** relaxed
_____	**5.** erectile	**e.** ability to become erect
_____	**6.** hyperlipemia	**f.** excessive quantity of fat in the blood
_____	**7.** revascularization	**g.** restoration of blood flow to a body part
_____	**8.** psychogenic	**h.** of mental origin
_____	**9.** prosthesis	**i.** an artificial part or organ
_____	**10.** libido	**j.** the sex drive, conscious or unconscious

II.   Spell Check

Circle each incorrectly spelled term and write it correctly in the space provided.

      1. cavirnosal   _____

      2. detumescence   _____

3. hyperlipidemia   _____
4. psychogenic   _____
5. schizofrenia   _____
6. corpora cavernossa   _____
7. flacid   _____
8. prostheses   _____
9. revaskularization   _____
10. transurethrel   _____

H. Increasing Your Medical Terminology Word Power 3

1. Read the following report.
2. Prepare to answer the questions at the end of the section.
3. Circle all unfamiliar terms with a red pencil.
4. Underline familiar terms with a blue pencil.
5. Use your knowledge of word elements, a medical dictionary, and the key terms to find the meaning of unfamiliar terms.

Chlamydial Infection of the Male Genital Tract

Key Terms

asymptomatic (a'-simp-tō-MAT-ik)   without symptoms

Chlamydia trachomatis (kla-MID-ē-a tra-KŌ-ma-tis)   a Gram-negative bacterial pathogen known for causing several sexually transmitted diseases and the eye disease *trachoma* (tra-KŌ-ma)

dysuria (dis-ū-RĒ-a)   painful or difficult urination

epididymitis (ep'-i-did'-i-MĪ-tis)   inflammation of the epididymis

leukocytosis (loo'-kō-sī-TŌ-sis)   increase in the number of leukocytes

mucoid (MŪ-koyd)   similar to mucus

mucopurulent (mū'-kō-PŪR-ū-lent)   consisting of mucus and pus

prostatitis (pros'-ta-TĪ-tis)   inflamed condition of the prostate gland

proximal (PROK-sim-al)   nearest the point of attachment; opposite of distal

tetracyclines (tet'-ra-SĪ-klēnz)   a group of broad-spectrum antibiotics

urethral (ū-RĒ-thral) congestion   a blockage of the canal used for urine discharge

urethral stricture (STRIK-chūr)   a narrowing of the urethra

urethritis (ū'-rē-THRĪ-tis)   inflammation of the urethra

1 NTRODUCTION

Chlamydial infection of the male genital tract was recognized in the early 1920s. It is one of the most common forms of chlamydial disease in the industrialized world.

H ISTOLOGY OF THE MALE GENITAL TRACT

The distal urethra (spongy urethra) is lined with stratified or pseudostratified columnar epithelium, with the exception of the wider end portion, which is lined by stratified squamous epithelium. The proximal urethra (membranous and prostatic urethra) is lined by transitional epithelia that are in contact with those of the urinary bladder.

Ducts from the prostate gland open into the proximal urethra and are largely lined by simple or pseudostratified columnar cells. The vas deferens and the vasa efferentia of the epididymis are also lined by columnar epithelium and open into the prostate urethra. The epithelium of the male genital tract is therefore a histological continuum and is largely composed of columnar cells that are particularly susceptible to infection by the bacterium *Chlamydia trachomatis*.

*P*ATHOGENESIS OF INFECTION

The columnar epithelium of the distal urethra is believed to become infected by chlamydiae during intercourse. The infection then spreads proximally, probably in continuity, until the entire urethra is involved. In some patients infection extends down the columnar epithelium of the vas deferens into the coiled tubes of the epididymis.

After entry into columnar cells by a mechanism that is not clearly understood, the infecting bacteria multiply, and subsequently infect many of the epithelial cells, which causes an inflammatory response, resulting in urethral congestion and leukocytosis.

*N*ON-GONOCOCCAL URETHRITIS

For the first four decades of the 20th century, non-gonococcal urethritis (NGU) was overshadowed by the bacterial STD gonorrhea, and was not thought to be very important. Today it is recognized as not only an important, but also a very common infection. More than 70,000 cases are reported each year from clinics for sexually transmitted diseases in Western industrialized countries.

Usually, but not invariably, NGU follows a change of sex partner. After an incubation period of between one and three weeks, the patient notices urethral irritation, dysuria, and a mucoid or mucopurulent urethral discharge. This is the typical presentation. But asymptomatic infections are not uncommon.

*C*OMPLICATIONS

Complications associated with NGU include urethral stricture, epididymitis, and prostatitis.

*L*ABORATORY DIAGNOSIS

Laboratory diagnosis depends on obtaining appropriate clinical specimens from infected individuals. Specimens are usually taken from the glans penis and the prostate gland. Once specimens are taken, special staining techniques are performed and attempts at culture are made.

*T*REATMENT

Tetracyclines generally are the antibiotics of choice for NGU cases. The duration of therapy is important. Effective regimens are usually a minimum of seven days' duration. Longer courses of treatment, lasting for three weeks or longer, are sometimes recommended.

Questions

I.   Matching

Match the term to its meaning. (The same meaning may be used more than once.)
Insert the appropriate letter in the space next to the question number.

Choices:

_____ 1. Chlamydia trachomatis
_____ 2. epididymitis
_____ 3. dysuria
_____ 4. mucoid
_____ 5. prostatitis
_____ 6. leucocytosis
_____ 7. mucopurulent
_____ 8. tetracyclines
_____ 9. stricture
_____ 10. urethritis

a. inflammation of the epididymis
b. a Gram-negative bacterial pathogen causing several sexually transmitted diseases
c. painful or difficult urination
d. inflamed condition of the prostate gland
e. similar to mucus
f. increase in the number of leukocytes
g. a group of broad-spectrum antibiotics
h. consisting of mucus and pus
i. a narrowing
j. inflammation of the urethra

II.   Spell Check

Circle each incorrectly spelled term and write it correctly in the space provided.

1. Chlamydia _____
2. gonococal _____
3. seudostratified _____
4. columnar _____
5. epididimis _____
6. leukocytosis _____
7. tetracyclines _____
8. disuria _____
9. mucopurulent _____
10. strictur _____

Term Search Challenge

Locate 16 terms in the puzzle.

1. Write the specific term next to its definition. Then find that term in the puzzle diagram and circle it.
2. Terms may be read from left to right, backward, up, down, or diagonally.
3. If a term appears more than once, circle it only once. (A term may be found inside others.)
4. Check your answers.

Clues:

1. Another term for sex cells _____
2. Structure used for sperm maturition _____
3. A testicular tumor _____
4. Male sex cells are produced in the _____ tubules

5. The surgical procedure that renders a male sterile

    _____

6. The pouch enclosing the primary male sex organ

    _____

7. The common tube of the male that serves for the passage of both urine and semen _____

8. Another term for foreskin _____

9. Two word roots for *testis* _____ and

    _____

10. Word root for *duct* or *vessel* _____

11. The typical primary lesion of syphilis _____

12. The term for an inflammation of the prostate gland

    _____

13. Term for the failure of the testis to descend _____

14. A castrated male _____

15. Terms for enlarged veins of spermatic cord associated with the testes

    _____

Term Search Puzzle

```
G  U  R  E  P  I  D  I  D  Y  M  I  S  C  A
A  T  E  S  T  O  S  E  U  N  U  C  H  R  V
M  V  C  L  I  T  O  R  I  S  I  N  D  Y  S
E  A  P  R  O  S  T  A  T  I  T  I  S  P  C
T  G  M  U  I  R  T  E  M  O  D  N  V  T  R
E  I  O  R  C  H  I  V  I  D  V  C  A  O  O
S  N  I  Z  I  C  H  A  N  C  R  E  R  R  T
E  A  G  H  M  E  N  S  T  R  U  A  I  C  U
S  E  M  I  N  I  F  E  R  O  U  S  C  H  M
U  V  A  S  T  E  R  C  G  R  T  S  O  I  T
A  A  V  L  U  V  U  T  E  R  U  S  C  D  E
P  R  E  P  U  C  E  O  C  O  L  P  E  I  S
O  N  E  M  O  V  A  M  A  R  E  O  L  S  T
S  E  M  E  N  T  T  Y  A  Z  Y  G  E  M  E
S  E  M  I  N  O  M  A  Z  O  A  C  N  T  S
```

The Female Reproductive System

"Age, I do abhor thee, youth, I do abhor thee . . . ."

—Shakespeare, *The Passionate Pilgrim*

INFORMATIONAL CHALLENGE

A. The Female Reproductive System

I.   Fill in the Blank

Fill in the blank with the appropriate term.

1. List six primary and accessory sex organs or structures of the female reproductive system.

   a. _____
   b. _____
   c. _____
   d. _____
   e. _____
   f. _____

2. List the three regions of the uterus.

   a. _____
   b. _____
   c. _____

3. What is the development period during which reproductive organs become functional? _____

4. Name the three layers of the uterus.

   a. _____
   b. _____
   c. _____

5. The oviducts are also known as the _____.

6. List two functions of the ovary.

   a. _____
   b. _____

7. List the structures that form the external female genitalia.

   a. _____
   b. _____

c. _____
d. _____
e. _____

II.   Matching: Structures and Functions of the Female Reproductive System

Match the term to its meaning. (The same meaning may be used more than once.)
Insert the appropriate letter in the space next to the question number.

Choices:

_____ **1.** ligaments
_____ **2.** fimbriae
_____ **3.** adnexa
_____ **4.** vulva
_____ **5.** cervix
_____ **6.** oviducts
_____ **7.** Bartholin's glands
_____ **8.** areola
_____ **9.** clitoris

a. ends of oviducts
b. ovaries and oviducts together
c. cordlike structures holding ovaries in place
d. tube-like structures through which ova pass to the uterus
e. area enclosing the female genitalia
f. lower part of uterus
g. structure that provides secretion that lubricates vaginal opening during sexual activity
h. a circular area of different pigmentation around the breast nipple
i. female equivalent of the penis

III.   Vision Quiz 1: The Female Reproductive System

Figure 22-7 shows the parts of the female reproductive system. Identify and write the name of the numbered body parts in the spaces provided.

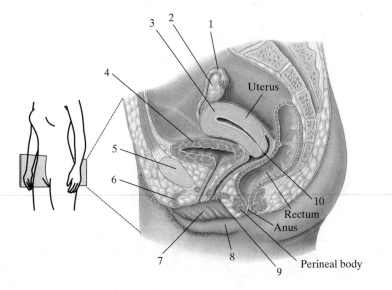

FIGURE 22-7   Vision Quiz 1. The female reproductive system.

Choices:

1. _____
2. _____
3. _____

a. oviduct
b. ovary
c. uterus

4. _____ **d.** urinary bladder
5. _____ **e.** clitoris
6. _____ **f.** vagina
7. _____ **g.** cervix
8. _____ **h.** labia majora
9. _____ **i.** labia minora
10. _____ **j.** urethra

IV.   Vision Quiz 2: Female External Genitalia

Figure 22-8 shows the female external genitalia. Identify and write the name of the numbered body parts in the spaces provided.

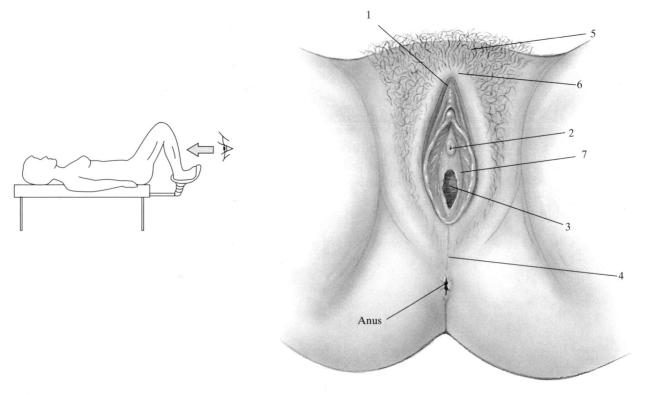

FIGURE 22-8   Vision Quiz 2. The female external genitalia.

Choices:

1. _____ **a.** clitoris
2. _____ **b.** mons pubis
3. _____ **c.** perineal body
4. _____ **d.** labia majora
5. _____ **e.** vaginal opening
6. _____ **f.** labia minora
7. _____ **g.** urethral opening

V.   Spell Check

Circle each incorrectly spelled term and write it correctly in the space provided.

1. genitalia   _____
2. pubis   _____

   3. klitoris   _____

   4. vajina   _____

   5. Falopian   _____

   6. endometrium _____

   7. cervix   _____

   8. vestibul   _____

   9. areola   _____

 10. ampulla   _____

B. *Menstruation, Pregnancy, and Menopause*

I.   Fill in the Blank

Fill in the blank with the appropriate term.

   1. List the four phases of menstruation.

       a. _____

       b. _____

       c. _____

       d. _____

   2. Give the term for painful menstruation. _____

   3. Give the specialties for the following:

       a. the study and treatment of the newborn _____

       b. pregnancy and the delivery of the fetus _____

       c. the female reproductive system in health and disease

        _____

       d. clinical conditions requiring the diagnosis, treatment, and management of a fetus _____

   4. What is the fertilized ovum called? _____

   5. The later stages of a developing individual is referred to as a(n)

     _____.

II.   Matching 1: General Terminology

Match the term to its meaning. (The same meaning may be used more than once.)
Insert the appropriate letter in the space next to the question number.

                                Choices:

_____ **1.** menses   **a.** menstrual cycle stop

_____ **2.** menopause   **b.** first menstrual cycle

_____ **3.** PMS   **c.** discharge of blood, other secretions,

_____ **4.** menarche   and destroyed cells of endometrium

                                d. depressed state of some women prior to menses

III.   Matching 2: Menstrual Cycle Phases

Match the term to its meaning. (The same meaning may be used more than once.)
Insert the appropriate letter in the space next to the question number.

                                Choices:

_____ **1.** postovulatory phase   **a.** release of an ovum

_____ **2.** ovulation   **b.** time between menses and ovulation

_____ 3. preovulatory phase
_____ 4. menses

c. time between ovulation and beginning of next menses
d. formation of corpus albicans
e. discharge of blood, other tissue fluid, and destroyed cells of the endometrium

IV.   Matching 3: Abnormal Uterine Bleeding

Match the term to its meaning. (The same meaning may be used more than once.) Insert the appropriate letter in the space next to the question number.

Choices:

_____ 1. absence of menstruation
_____ 2. large quantities of menstrual blood
_____ 3. spotting
_____ 4. excessive bleeding at time of menstrual period
_____ 5. heavy uterine bleeding with no regularity

a. hypomenorrhea
b. menometrorrhagia
c. amenorrhea
d. hypermenorrhea
e. menorrhagia

V.   Spell Check

Circle each incorrectly spelled term and write it correctly in the space provided.

1. menopase   _____
2. menarche   _____
3. fetis   _____
4. dismenorrhea   _____
5. gynecology   _____
6. premenstrual   _____
7. endometrium   _____
8. menses   _____
9. obstetriks   _____
10. hymin   _____
11. Grafean   _____
12. corpis hemmorrhagicum _____

C. Word Roots and/or Combining Forms for the Female Reproductive System

I.   Fill in the Blank

Fill in the blank with the appropriate term.

1. Give the combining form used for oviducts. _____
2. List 3 combining forms used for the uterus.

   a. _____
   b. _____
   c. _____

3. What is the combining form for the cervix? _____

II.   Matching: Combining Forms for the Female Reproductive System

Match the term to its meaning. (The same meaning may be used more than once.)
Insert the appropriate letter in the space next to the question number.

Choices:

_____	**1.** gynec/o	**a.** menses
_____	**2.** oophor/o	**b.** egg
_____	**3.** men/o	**c.** Bartholin's gland
_____	**4.** bartholin/o	**d.** perineum
_____	**5.** colp/o	**e.** uterus
_____	**6.** ov/o	**f.** woman
_____	**7.** vagin/o	**g.** ovary
_____	**8.** perine/o	**h.** vagina
_____	**9.** hyster/o	**i.** vulva
_____	**10.** vulv/o	

III.   Spell Check

Circle each incorrectly spelled term and write it correctly in the space provided.

1. colposcope   _____
2. episostenosis   _____
3. ovum   _____
4. vulvovaginites   _____
5. hysterodynia   _____
6. ocyte   _____
7. menorrhagia   _____
8. salpinkotomy   _____

IV.   Word Analysis: Word Roots, Combining Forms, Suffixes, and Prefixes
Associated with the Female Reproductive System

Table 22-11 lists a number of terms with their pronunciations and definitions.

**TABLE 22-11   WORD ANALYSIS: WORD ROOTS, COMBINING FORMS, SUFFIXES, AND
PREFIXES ASSOCIATED WITH THE FEMALE REPRODUCTIVE SYSTEM**

Term and Pronunciation	Brief Explanation
bartholinitis (bar-tō-lin-Ī-tis)	inflammation of the Bartholin's gland
cervical (SER-vi-kal)	pertaining to the cervix
colposcope (KOL-pō-skōp)	instrument used for the examination of the vagina (and cervix)
culdocentesis (kul-dō-sen-TĒ-sis)	surgical procedure to remove fluid from the vaginal cul-de-sac
episiostenosis (e-pi-sē-ō-ste-NŌ-sis)	narrowing of the vulvar opening
gynecology (gī-nē-KOL-ō-jē)	study of the female reproductive organs

(*Continued*)

TABLE 22-11   (CONTINUED)

Term and Pronunciation	Brief Explanation
hysterodynia (hist-ter-ō-DIN-ē-a)	uterine pain
menopause (MEN-ō-pawz)	end of menstruation
menorrhagia (men-ō-RĀ-jē-a)	excessive bleeding during a menstrual period
metrorrhea (me-trō-RĒ-a)	abnormal uterine discharge
oocyte (Ō-ō-sīt)	egg cell
ovariogenic (ō-vā'-rē-ō-JEN-ik)	produced by (originating in) the ovary
ovum (Ō-vum)	female reproductive cell
salpingotomy (sal-ping-OT-ō-mē)	incision of oviduct
uterogenic (ū-ter-ō-JEN-ik)	formed in the uterus
vaginal (VAJ-in-al)	pertaining to the vagina
vulvovaginitis (vul-vō-vaj-i-NĪ-tis)	inflammation of both the vulva and vagina

1. Analyze each term.
2. Circle all prefixes, combining forms, word roots, and suffixes, and label them **p**, **cf**, **wr**, and **s**, respectively.
3. Check your answers (shown in Table 22-12).

D. Disorders and Pathological Conditions of the Female Reproductive System

I.   Matching: Gynecologic Disorders and Pathological Conditions

Match the term to its meaning. (The same meaning may be used more than once.)

Choices:

_____ 1. cervical erosion
_____ 2. cystadenocarcinoma
_____ 3. endocervicitis
_____ 4. breast carcinoma
_____ 5. fibrocystic disease
_____ 6. endometriosis
_____ 7. benign tumor in the uterus
_____ 8. inflammation of the oviduct

a. a malignancy in which sacs occur during its development
b. inflammation of the lining of the cervix
c. presence of endometrial tissue in the pelvis
d. ulcers on cervical surface
e. small sacs of fluid in the breast
f. malignant tumor of the breast
g. fibroid
h. salpingitis

II.   Spell Check

Circle each incorrectly spelled term and write it correctly in the space provided.

1. cystadenoma   _____
2. fibroyd   _____
3. septik   _____
4. endometreosis   _____
5. salpingitis   _____

E. Operative and/or Clinical Procedures

I.   Matching: Gynecological Diagnostic and/or Surgical Procedures

Match the term to its meaning. (The same meaning may be used more than once.)
Insert the appropriate letter in the space next to the question number.

Choices:

_____ **1.** colpotomy
_____ **2.** amniocentesis
_____ **3.** cesarean (C) section
_____ **4.** dilation and curettage
_____ **5.** salpingotomy
_____ **6.** conization
_____ **7.** hysterectomy
_____ **8.** tubal ligation

a. analysis of fetal fluid
b. surgical removal of the uterus through the vagina or abdominal wall
c. incision into the vaginal wall
d. removal of cone-shaped tissue specimen
e. includes scraping and removing uteral lining
f. removal of a fetus by abdominal incision into the uterus
g. incision of an oviduct
h. sterilization procedure involving the tying of the oviducts

F. Medical Vocabulary Building

I.   Fill in the Blank

Fill in the blank with the appropriate term.

1. Pertaining to or resulting from sexual intercourse is called _____.

2. Give the term pertaining to the external female genitalia.

_____

II.   Matching

Match the term to its meaning. (The same meaning may be used more than once.)
Insert the appropriate letter in the space next to the question number.

Choices:

_____ **1.** anovular
_____ **2.** catamenia
_____ **3.** dyspareunia
_____ **4.** mammoplasty
_____ **5.** menometrorrhagia
_____ **6.** myometritis

a. the condition of a monthly uterine discharge of blood
b. pertaining to a lack of production and discharge of an ovum
c. difficult or painful sexual intercourse

_____ **7.** oligomenorrhea	**d.** inflammation of the muscular uterine wall
_____ **8.** panhysterectomy	
_____ **9.** postcoital	**e.** surgical repair of the breast
_____ **10.** pudendal	**f.** scanty monthly flow
_____ **11.** pyometritis	**g.** surgical excision of the entire uterus
_____ **12.** pyosalpinx	**h.** pertaining to after sexual intercourse
	i. pus accumulation in the oviduct (Fallopian tube)
	j. pus (purulent) inflammation of the uterus
	k. excessive uterine bleeding during and between the normal menstrual period
	l. pertains to the external female genitalia

G. Abbreviations

I.   Fill in the Blank: Disorders, Disease, and Procedures Used in Diagnosis and Treatment

Fill in the blank with the appropriate meaning.

1. DUB _____

2. Pap smear _____

3. PID _____

4. OB _____

5. MH _____

6. CS _____

7. D&C _____

8. STD _____

II.   Matching: Anatomy and Functions of the Female Reproductive System

Match the term to its meaning. (The same meaning may be used more than once.) Insert the appropriate letter in the space next to the question number.

Choices:

_____ **1.** luteninizing hormone	**a.** HCG
_____ **2.** follicle-stimulating hormone	**b.** LH
	c. GU
_____ **3.** human chorionic gonadotropin	**d.** FSH
	e. LMP
_____ **4.** genitourinary	**f.** PU
_____ **5.** last menstrual period	
_____ **6.** pregnancy urine	

H. Increasing Your Medical Terminology Word Power 1

1. Read the following report.

2. Prepare to answer the questions at the end of the section.

3. Circle all unfamiliar terms with a red pencil.

4. Underline familiar terms with a blue pencil.

5. Use your knowledge of word elements, a medical dictionary, and the key terms to find the meaning of unfamiliar terms.

Fallopian-Tube Carcinoma

Key Terms

cc cubic centimeter

diverticulitis (dī-ver-tik-ū-LĪ-tis) inflammation of the little inflated sacs (diverticula) of the colon

laparotomy (lap-ar-OT-ō-mē) surgical opening of the abdomen

leukorrhea (loo-kō-RĒ-a) white- or yellow-mucous vaginal or cervical discharge

nulligravida a woman who never became pregnant

palliation (pal-ē-Ā-shun) an easing or reducing of the effect

papillary (PAP-i-lar-ē) concerning or pertaining to a nipple or papilla

primipara (pri-MIP-a-ra) refers to a woman who has produced one infant weighing 500 grams

staging refers to a process of classifying tumors, especially malignancies

triad (TRĪ-ad) refers to any three items having something in common

unresectable (un-rē-SEK-ta-bl) not removable by surgical means

urinary incontinence inability to control urination

SUMMARY

Twenty-one patients with Fallopian-tube carcinoma from Haven Medical Center were reviewed. Most patients who died of this disease did so in the first two years after diagnosis, even following complete resection, clearly indicating the need for additional therapy such as whole abdomino-pelvic radiation. Chemotherapy for unresectable disease or recurrent disease was related in palliation with occasional prolonged survival.

INTRODUCTION

Carcinoma of the Fallopian tube is a rare cancer for which various surgical procedures, tumor grading systems, and different methods of postoperative management have been tried. The experience with Fallopian-tube carcinoma at Haven Medical Center from 1952 to 1982 was reviewed. These patients accounted for 0.4% of all gynecologic malignancies. Particular attention was directed to patient presentation, staging procedures, and the postoperative use of radiation and chemotherapy.

RESULTS

Patient Characteristics

The average age of the patients at initial presentation was fifty-five years with a range in age from thirty-four to eighty-two years. Six patients were either nulligravidas or primiparas (28.6%). The average parity was one with a range from zero to four.

The majority of patients presented with abnormal bleeding (52%), a pelvic mass (43%), or pain (38%), alone or in combination. One patient presented with abnormal cytology. Leukorrhea was found in three patients. One tumor was discovered incidentally during a hysterectomy. Two tumors were found at laparotomy, one for presumed diverticulitis and the other for presumed appendicitis. Another patient presented with a right pelvic mass. The classic diagnostic triad for Fallopian tube carcinoma of pain, bleeding, and leukorrhea was not found in any of the patients. However, the combination of a mass, bleeding, and leukorrhea was present in two patients.

In eight of the twenty-one patients, the tumor was on the right side (38.1%) and in twelve on the left side (57.1%). One patient had bilateral tumors at surgery.

Methods and Management

The primary therapy for Fallopian-tube carcinoma was surgical. Patients were categorized into three therapy regimens—surgery alone, surgery with postoperative radiation, and surgery with postoperative chemotherapy. The median follow-up time from diagnosis was four years with a range of seven months to twenty-three years.

Fourteen patients received postoperative radiation, and chemotherapy was used with four other patients. All therapy was individualized as determined by the treating gynecologist.

Questions

I.   Matching

Match the term to its meaning. (The same meaning may be used more than once.) Insert the appropriate letter in the space next to the question number

Choices:

_____ **1.** a woman who never became pregnant

a. triad

_____ **2.** returning or occurring at intervals

b. incontinence

_____ **3.** not removable by surgical means

c. unresectable

_____ **4.** white discharge or flow

d. cubic centimeter

_____ **5.** surgical opening of the abdomen

e. recurrent

_____ **6.** surgical removal of the uterus

f. nulligravida

_____ **7.** cc

g. leukorrhea

_____ **8.** an easing or reducing of the effect

h. laparotomy

_____ **9.** three items having something in common

i. hysterectomy

_____ **10.** inability to control urination

j. palliation

II.   Spell Check

Circle the correct form of the following items.

1. cubic, cubik, cubek
2. centimeter, sentimeter, centameter

   3. diverticulitis, divertikulitis, divirticulytis
   4. laparotomy, laperatomy, laperetomy
   5. abdoman, abdomen, adbomen
   6. leukorhea, leukorrhea, leukorrhae
   7. nullligravida, nullgraveda, nullgrevida
   8. palliation, pallietion, pallieashun
   9. primipara, primepeara, primepera
  10. incontinence, incontinance, inkontinence

I. *Increasing Your Medical Terminology Word Power 2*

   1. Read the following report.
   2. Prepare to answer the questions at the end of the section.
   3. Circle all unfamiliar terms with a red pencil.
   4. Underline familiar terms with a blue pencil.
   5. Use your knowledge of word elements, a medical dictionary, and the key terms to find the meaning of unfamiliar terms.

Condylomata Acuminata

Key Terms

benign (be-NĪN)   opposite of malignant

condyloma (kon-di-LŌ-ma)   a wartlike growth of the skin, usually seen on the external genitalia or near the anus

condylomata acuminata (kon-di-LŌ-ma-ta a-kyoo-min-NA-ta)   also known as genital warts; caused by certain papillomaviruses

cytotoxic (sī-tō-TOKS-ik)   destructive to cells

hyperplasia (hī-per-PLĀ-zē-a)   excessive production of normal cells

neoplasm (NĒ-ō-plazm)   a new and abnormal formation of tissue

papillomavirus (pap-i-LŌ-ma-VĪ-rus)   refers to a group of viruses known to cause tumors such as warts; certain ones are associated with causing sexually transmitted disease, genital warts, and some forms of genital cancers

papillary (PAP-i-lar-ē)   concerning a nipple or papilla

placenta (pla-SEN-ta)   the spongy connection between a mother and the developing fetus and through which the fetus receives its nourishment

I NTRODUCTION

The results of recent studies using highly specialized techniques indicate that a high percentage of precancers and invasive squamous neoplasms of the female genital tract contain the DNA sequences typical of certain human papillomaviruses. Other results suggest a close link between such viruses and the neoplastic process.

    Genital lesions of condylomata acuminata, or genital warts, are of significant public health importance because of the aforementioned carcinogenic potential, and the transmissibility both to sex partners and to the fetuses of infected pregnant women.

E PIDEMIOLOGY

Warts, both genital and skin, are caused by different papillomaviruses. Such viruses also have distinct clinical effects. Human papillomavirus infection produces obvious condylomas and macroscopically invisible forms of epithelial hyperplasia. The incubation period for warts lesions to appear ranges from six weeks to eight months, with an average of three months. These lesions are primarily seen in sexually mature persons.

Genital warts are sexually transmitted tumors affecting the genitalia, anorectal region and, less frequently, the urethral mucosa, bladder, and ureters. An infected mother may transmit the viral infection to her newborn, even when clinical evidence of maternal infection is absent. The route of transmission is via the blood that crosses the placenta.

The infecting virus is presumably acquired by infants at birth, and laryngeal papillomas develop most frequently during the first seven years of life. In childhood, recurrence does occur after excision. Unfortunately, the virus will persist if regression does not occur in puberty.

CLINICAL FEATURES

Typically, genital warts are discrete, well-differentiated single or multiple papillary growths. They may appear on or about the genitalia, perineum, or anal area. The lesions are white to gray in color, and exhibit a so-called "cauliflower-like" appearance. Penile warts usually occur on surfaces subject to injury, such as the frenulum, corona, or inner surface of the prepuce. Intraurethral warts can occur, with the meatus being the most commonly affected. Vaginal warts are most common on the labia, and less common on other parts of the vulva and the perineum. Cervical warts are not uncommon.

COMPLICATIONS

During pregnancy, genital warts tend to grow rapidly. If massive warts block the birth canal, cesarean section may be required for delivery. Following delivery the warts may decrease in size.

DIAGNOSIS

The diagnosis of genital warts is made on clinical grounds, and should be a consideration whenever large, multiple, cauliflower masses are observed in the anogenital region of patients. Furthermore, genital warts should be differentiated from other conditions causing general types of growths. These include carcinomas and benign neoplasms.

TREATMENT

Cytotoxic, destructive, or surgical methods can be used to treat genital warts. The method selected varies from case to case. Treatment should be sought at the earliest possible opportunity.

Questions

I.   Matching

Match the term to its meaning. (The same meaning may be used more than once.) Insert the appropriate letter in the space next to the question number.

Choices:

_____ **1.** benign
_____ **2.** condyloma
_____ **3.** condylomata acuminata
_____ **4.** cytotoxic
_____ **5.** hyperplasia
_____ **6.** neoplasm
_____ **7.** papillomavirus
_____ **8.** papillary
_____ **9.** placenta

a. genital warts
b. opposite of malignant
c. a wartlike growth on the skin, usually seen on the external genitalia or near the anus
d. destructive to cells
e. a new and abnormal formation of tissue
f. excessive production of normal cells
g. a group of viruses known to cause tumors such as warts
h. concerning a nipple or papilla
i. the spongy connection between a mother and the developing fetus and through which the fetus receives its nourishment

II.   Spell Check

Circle the correct form of the following terms.

1. benine, benign, benin
2. condylomas, condelomas, condylowmas
3. condyloma accuminata, condyloma acumineta, condylomata acuminata
4. cytotoxic, sitotoxic, cytotxik
5. hyperplazia, hyperplazea, hyperplasia
6. neoplasm, neoplazam, neoplsim
7. papilovirus, papillomavirus, pappillovirus
8. papilley, papillary, papillery
9. palsenta, placenta, pleacenta

J. Increasing Your Medical Terminology Word Power 3

1. Read the following report.
2. Prepare to answer the questions at the end of the section.
3. Circle all unfamiliar terms with a red pencil.
4. Underline familiar terms with a blue pencil.
5. Use your knowledge of word elements, a medical dictionary, and the key terms to find the meaning of unfamiliar terms.

A Randomized Trial Comparison of Total Mastectomy and Radical Mastectomy with Radiation Therapy

Key Terms

axilla (ak-SIL-a)   the armpit

en bloc **(en blok)**   in surgery, the entire removal, or as a lump

mastectomy (mas-TEK-tō-mē)   removal of a breast

metastasis (mē-TAS-ta-sis)   movement of cells from one part of the body to another

node (nōd)   a swelling; constricted region

postoperative   following a surgical operation

radical (RAD-i-kal) mastectomy   removal of an entire breast

*I*NTRODUCTION

The role of radical mastectomy in cases of breast cancer, as compared with extensive surgery, has been a matter of significant debate. The Halsted radical mastectomy approach, an *en bloc* removal of the breast, muscles of the chest wall, and contents of the axilla, was the "traditionally established and standardized operation" for patients with breast cancer no matter the stage for most of the 20th century. By the mid-1960s, however, dissatisfaction with the results obtained following radical mastectomy, and information from a variety of sources regarding other approaches, led a number of surgeons to support more extensive surgery and still others to advocate more limited types of operations. The availability of new findings concerning tumor metastases also provided a basis for the suggestion that less radical surgery might be just as effective as the more extensive operations that were being used to treat patients with breast cancer.

In 1971, a well-designed study was initiated to resolve this controversy. The principal aims of the study were to determine whether patients with either clinically negative or clinically positive axillary nodes who received local or regional treatments other than mastectomy would have outcomes similar to those obtained with radical mastectomy.

*M*ETHODS

Between June 1972 and October 1975, after obtaining written informed consent, 1,755 women with primary operable breast cancer were randomly assigned to treatment. The study involved the examination and the statistical comparison of the medical records of a total of 1,097 women with clinically negative axillary nodes who underwent radical mastectomy, total mastectomy without dissection but with postoperative irradiation, or total mastectomy and axillary dissection only in the event their nodes became positive. A total of 658 patients with clinically positive axillary nodes either underwent radical mastectomy or underwent total mastectomy without axillary dissection, but with postoperative irradiation.

*R*ESULTS

The findings of the statistical analysis of this study showed no significant differences among the three groups of women with negative nodes, or between the two groups of women with positive nodes in relation to disease-free survival, relapse-free survival, distant disease-free survival, or overall survival.

*C*ONCLUSIONS

The results of this study confirm the findings of earlier studies showing no advantage from radical mastectomy.

Questions

I.   Matching

Match the term to its meaning. (The same meaning may be used more than once.) Insert the appropriate letter in the space next to the question number.

Choices:

_____ **1.** axilla
_____ **2.** *en bloc*
_____ **3.** mastectomy
_____ **4.** metastasis
_____ **5.** node
_____ **6.** postoperative
_____ **7.** radical mastectomy

a. in surgery, the entire removal, or as a lump
b. removal of a breast
c. the armpit
d. a swelling; constricted region
e. movement of cells from one part of the body to another
f. following a surgical operation
g. removal of an entire breast

II. Spell Check

Circle each correct form of the following terms.

  1. axillery, axilary, axillary
  2. nods, nodes, noodes
  3. en blok, enblok, en bloc
  4. mastectomy, masectomy, matectomie
  5. metestases, metastases, metasteses
  6. postoperetive, postoperative, postoparative
  7. radicle, radicale, radical

Term Search Challenge

Locate 16 terms in the puzzle.

  1. Write the specific term next to its definition. Then find that term in the puzzle diagram and circle it.
  2. Terms may be read from left to right, backward, up, down, or diagonally.
  3. If a term appears more than once, circle it only once. (A term may be found inside others.)
  4. Check your answers.

Clues:

  1. Removal of the vagina _____
  2. Condition in which there is an abnormal cervical or vaginal white to yellowish mucus discharge _____
  3. Pear-shaped, thick-walled, muscular organ situated in the pelvis between the urinary bladder and the rectum _____
  4. Lower part of the uterus extending from the isthmus to the vagina

  _____
  5. Inflammation of the cervix _____
  6. Absence of menstruation _____
  7. Painful menses _____
  8. Abbreviation for premenstrual syndrome _____
  9. Female reproductive (sex) cells (plural form) _____
  10. The two female reproductive glands that produce ova after puberty

  _____
  11. Abbreviation for pelvic inflammation caused by a number of infectious disease agents _____
  12. Uterine tube inflammation _____

13. The first menstrual cycle _____
14. Cessation of menses and the reproductive period of life

    _____

15. Lack of breast development _____
16. Abbreviation for gynecology _____

Term Search Puzzle

```
E   S   G   E   P   R   C   L   O   S   C   O   P   A   O
R   D   Y   S   M   E   N   O   R   R   H   E   A   L   L
V   A   N   O   S   M   N   V   N   N   Y   Y   M   P   P
I   N   P   Q   M   E   N   A   R   C   H   E   A   I   E
C   A   R   S   U   T   E   R   U   S   L   U   S   N   C
I   L   S   T   L   L   F   I   U   T   V   X   T   G   T
T   Y   U   T   V   L   M   E   O   P   Q   R   I   I   O
I   S   R   O   L   X   P   S   T   F   T   S   A   T   M
S   C   E   R   V   I   X   Y   S   E   A   E   A   I   Y
W   O   T   A   M   E   N   O   R   R   H   E   A   S   R
L   E   U   K   O   R   R   H   E   A   O   C   S   H   R
R   P   I   L   M   E   N   O   P   A   U   S   E   N   O
D   I   T   S   Y   P   H   V   P   P   Y   O   G   D   I
P   D   E   L   V   I   S   A   C   H   A   N   C   R   O
```

Obstetrics, Fetology, and Neonatology

"Each organic being is striving for life ... each has to struggle for life ... the vigorous survive and multiply."

—Charles Darwin

INFORMATIONAL CHALLENGE

A. Fertilization and Prenatal Development

I.   Fill in the Blank

Fill in the blank with the appropriate term.

1. The ovarian structure that releases a mature ovum is called a(n) _____ follicle.
2. A fertilized egg is also known as a(n) _____.
3. Fertilization normally takes place in the _____.
4. Three processes in the development of a new individual are _____, _____, and _____.
5. List the primary germ-cell layers.
   a. _____
   b. _____
   c. _____
6. List the four embryonic membranes.
   a. _____
   b. _____
   c. _____
   d. _____

II.   Matching 1: Fertilization and Early Development

Match the term to its meaning. (The same meaning may be used more than once.) Insert the appropriate letter in the space next to the question number.

_____ 1. hollow ball of cells developing from a zygote
_____ 2. outer rim of cells of a blastocyst that will develop into fetal membranes
_____ 3. inner lining of the uterus
_____ 4. embryonic layer

_____ **5.** sac containing amnion, yolk sac, and embryo

_____ **6.** term for the developing individual until the end of the eighth week of pregnancy

_____ **7.** developing individual from the end of the eighth week of fetal development until birth

_____ **8.** structure that supports the embryonic and fetal development during the remaining months of pregnancy

_____ **9.** another term for pregnancy

_____ **10.** hormone used in tests to indicate pregnancy

Choices:

a. trophoblast	**g.** fetus
b. blastocyst	**h.** embryo
c. endoderm	**i.** gestation period
d. endometrium	**j.** human chorionic gonadotropin
e. gestation	**k.** placenta
f. chorionic vesicle	

III.   Matching 2: Fetal Development, Embryonic Membranes, and Hormonal Changes

Match the term to its meaning. (The same meaning may be used more than once.) Insert the appropriate letter in the space next to the question number.

_____ **1.** germ-cell layer that gives rise to the reproductive organs and most of the urinary system

_____ **2.** germ-cell layer that gives rise to the lining of the body cavities and the skin

_____ **3.** germ-cell layer that gives rise to the lungs and structures of the gastrointestinal system

_____ **4.** hormone that stimulates breast development and milk production

_____ **5.** lower levels of this hormone in women may lead to osteoporosis

_____ **6.** another term for birth

_____ **7.** most common form of fetal presentation in labor

_____ **8.** the fetal presentation in which the fetal buttocks occurs first

Choices:

a. ectoderm	**e.** parturition
b. mesoderm	**f.** human placental lactogen
c. cephalic presentation	**g.** estrogen
d. endoderm	**h.** breech presentation

IV.   Spell Check

Circle each incorrectly spelled term and write it correctly in the space provided.

1. coitis   _____

2. trofoblast   _____

3. anmion   _____

4. embreo

   5. plascental   _____
   6. parturition   _____
   7. amniosentesis   _____
   8. chorion   _____
   9. gestation   _____
   10. gonadotropin   _____

V.   Vision Quiz: Fetal Development, Fetology

Figure 23-9 shows a fetus. Identify and write the letters of the numbered body regions in the spaces provided.

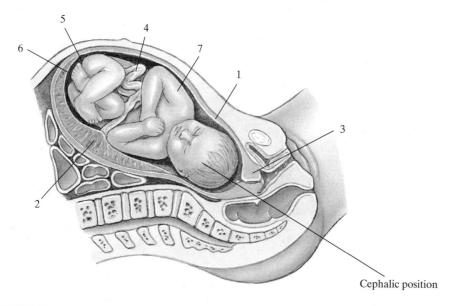

FIGURE 23-9   Vision Quiz. The Fetus.

Choices:

_____ **1.**		**a.** cervix
_____ **2.**		**b.** placenta
_____ **3.**		**c.** uterine wall
_____ **4.**		**d.** umbilical cord
_____ **5.**		**e.** amniotic fluid or amnion
_____ **6.**		**f.** fetus
_____ **7.**		**g.** amniotic membrane

B. Word Elements Associated with Obstetrics, Fetology, and Neonatology

I.   Matching 1: Word Roots and/or Combining Forms

Match the term to its meaning. (The same meaning may be used more than once.) Insert the appropriate letter in the space next to the question number.

Choices:

_____ **1.** cervic		**a.** vagina
_____ **2.** colp/o		**b.** cervix
_____ **3.** cept		**c.** receive

_____ **4.** perineum	**d.** birth
_____ **5.** toc	**e.** month
_____ **6.** epis/o	**f.** vulva
_____ **7.** ovul	**g.** ovary
_____ **8.** hyster/o	**h.** pregnancy
_____ **9.** uter	**i.** uterus
_____ **10.** gravid/o	**j.** perineo
_____ **11.** nat	**k.** ovum
_____ **12.** oo	**l.** partum
_____ **13.** pelvi	**m.** pelvis
_____ **14.** partum	

II. Matching 2: Prefixes and Suffixes

Match the term to its meaning. (The same meaning may be used more than once.)
Insert the appropriate letter in the space next to the question number.

Choices:

_____ **1.** pertaining to	**a.** ante-
_____ **2.** before	**b.** -al
_____ **3.** inflammation	**c.** -itis
_____ **4.** process	**d.** -osis
_____ **5.** condition of	**e.** -ion
_____ **6.** many	**f.** multi-
_____ **7.** excision	**g.** -ectomy
_____ **8.** new	**h.** neo-
_____ **9.** none	**i.** nulli-
_____ **10.** after	**j.** post-

III. Spell Check

Circle each incorrectly spelled term and write it correctly in the space provided.

1. antinatal   _____

2. epiziotomy   _____

3. intrauterine   _____

4. nullipara   _____

5. primipara   _____

6. endometreosis   _____

7. hematosalpink   _____

8. multipara   _____

9. ogenesis   _____

10. salpingectomy   _____

IV. Word Analysis: Word Roots, Combining Forms, Suffixes, and Prefixes
Associated with Obstetrics, Fetology, and Neonatology

Table 23-11 lists a number of terms with their pronunciations and definitions.

TABLE 23-11   WORD ANALYSIS: WORD ROOTS, COMBINING FORMS, SUFFIXES, AND PREFIXES ASSOCIATED WITH OBSTETRICS, FETOLOGY, AND NEONATOLOGY

Term and Pronunciation	Definition
abortion (a-BŌR-shun)	premature termination of pregnancy
amniocentesis (am'-ni-ō-sen-TĒ-sis)	surgical puncture of the amniotic sac to obtain a fluid sample
anovular (an-ŌV-ū-lar)	lack of ovum production and discharge
antenatal (an'-tē-NĀ-tal)	before birth or labor
antepartum (an'-tē-PAR-tum)	before the beginning of labor
cervicitis (ser-vi-SĪ-tis)	inflammation of the cervix
colpoperineoplasty (kol'-pō-per'-in-Ē-ō-plas'-tē)	surgical repair of the vagina and the perineum
colposcope (KOL-pō-skōp)	instrument used for the examination of the vagina and cervix
conception (kon-SEP-shun)	union of sperm and ovum; fertilization
contraception (kon'-tra-SEP-shun)	prevention of conception
dystocia (dis-TŌ-sē-a)	difficult and painful childbirth
embryologist (em'-brē-ol-Ō-jist)	specialist in the study of embryos
episiotomy (e-pis'-i-OT-ō-mē)	incision of the perineum to prevent tearing and to aid in delivery
eutocia (ū-TŌ-sē-a)	normal birth
fibroma (fī-BRŌ-ma)	fibrous tissue tumor
hematosalpinx (hē'-ma-tō-SAL-pinks)	collection of blood in oviducts
hysterectomy (his'-ter-EK-tō-mē)	surgical excision of the uterus
hysterotomy (his'-ter-OT-ō-mē)	incision of the uterus, cesarean section
intrauterine (in'-tra-Ū-ter-in)	within the uterus
mastitis (mas-TĪ-tis)	inflammation of the breast
multigravida (mul'-ti-GRAV-i-da)	woman who has been pregnant two or more times
multipara (mul'-TIP-a-ra)	woman who has borne two or more children
myometritis (mī'-ō-mē-TRĪ-tis)	inflammation of the muscular wall of the uterus

(Continued)

TABLE 23-11   (CONTINUED)

Term and Pronunciation	Definition
neonatal (nē'-ō-NĀ-tal)	newborn (first 4 weeks after birth)
nullipara (nul-IP-a-ra)	woman who has borne no children
oogenesis (ō'-ō-JEN-ē-sis)	ovum formation
oophoritis (ō'-of-ō-RĪ-tis)	inflammation of an ovary
pelvimetry (pel-VIM-et-rē)	pelvis measurement to determine its capacity and diameter
postpartum (pōst-PAR-tum)	after labor
prenatal (prē-NĀ-tal)	before birth
primipara (prī-MIP-a-ra)	woman who is bearing her first child
pseudocyesis (sū'-dō-sī-Ē-sis)	false pregnancy
pyosalpinx (pī'-ō-SAL-pinks)	accumulation of pus in the oviduct
retroversion (ret'-rō-VER-zhun)	being turned backward
salpingectomy (sal'-pin-JEK-tō-mē)	surgical excision of oviduct
trimester (trī-MES-ter)	three months
vaginitis (vaj'-in-Ī-tis)	inflammation of the vagina

1. Analyze each term.
2. Circle all prefixes, combining forms, word roots, and suffixes and label them **p**, **cf**, **wr**, and **s**, respectively.
3. Check your answers (shown in Table 23-12).

C. Obstetrical Complications, Disorders, Diseases, and Pathological Conditions

I.   Matching

Match the term to its meaning. (The same meaning may be used more than once.) Insert the appropriate letter in the space next to the question number.

Choices:

_____ 1. abruptio placentae
_____ 2. amnionitis
_____ 3. chorioamnionitis
_____ 4. choriocarcinoma
_____ 5. dystocia
_____ 6. eclampsia
_____ 7. ectopic pregnancy

a. inflammation of the chorion and amnion
b. premature detachment of the placenta after the twentieth week of pregnancy
c. inflammation of the amnion
d. cancerous chorion tumor

_____ **8.** embryotocia
_____ **9.** hysterorrhexis
_____ **10.** hydatidiform mole
_____ **11.** tubal pregnancy

e. seizures and coma between the twentieth week of pregnancy and the first week following birth; caused by high blood pressure and kidney disorders

f. difficult labor

g. pregnancy occurring outside of the uterus

h. rupture of the uterus

i. a cystic mass that develops in place of a normal placenta and fetus

j. abortion

k. pregnancy occurring in the oviduct

II. Spell Check

Circle each incorrectly spelled term and write it correctly in the space provided.

1. abruptea _____

2. placentae _____

3. chorriocarcinoma _____

4. eclampsea _____

5. hysterorrheksis _____

6. chorioamnyonitis _____

7. amnionitis _____

8. dystocia _____

9. embriotocia _____

10. salpingocyesis _____

D. Neonatal Disorders and Defects

I.   Matching 1: Neonatal Disorders and Defects

Match the term to its meaning. (The same meaning may be used more than once.)
Insert the appropriate letter in the space next to the question number.

Choices:

_____ **1.** congenital anomaly
_____ **2.** erythroblastosis fetalis
_____ **3.** esophageal atresia
_____ **4.** hyaline membrane disease
_____ **5.** microcephalus
_____ **6.** omphalitis
_____ **7.** omphalocele
_____ **8.** pyloric stenosis
_____ **9.** spina bifida

a. newborn condition resulting in erythrocyte destruction resulting from an incompatibility between the mother's and fetus' blood

b. abnormality present at birth

c. respiratory distress syndrome of the newborn

d. congenital absence of a part of the esophagus

e. inflammation of the umbilicus

f. fetus with a very small head

g. congenital herniation of a portion of the intestine through the abdominal wall at the umbilicus (navel)

h. narrowing of the pyloric sphincter

i. congenital defect in the vertebral column caused by the failure of the vertebral arch to fuse

II.   Matching 2: Genetically Related Conditions

Match the term to its meaning. (The same meaning may be used more than once.)
Insert the appropriate letter in the space next to the question number.

_____   **1.** Down's syndrome
_____   **2.** Klinefelter's syndrome
_____   **3.** Turner's syndrome
_____   **4.** XXX female

Choices:

     a. occurs in males; resulting from an extra X chromosome producing a XXY condition

     b. chromosome abnormality caused by an additional chromosome associated with the twenty-first pair; results in characteristic facial changes, increased susceptibility to infections, mental capabilities lower than normal, and stunted growth

     c. condition resulting from extra X chromosome; affected individuals generally appear normal; however, have decreased mental capabilities

     d. results from a loss of one sex chromosome; found in females; affected individuals have underdeveloped ovaries and secondary sex characteristics are lacking; menstruation does not occur

III.   Spell Check

Circle each incorrectly spelled term and write it correctly in the space provided.

     1. hydrocephallus   _____
     2. tracheoesofageal   _____
     3. Klinefelter's   _____
     4. karyotype   _____
     5. omphalocele   _____
     6. spina bifida   _____
     7. fiztula   _____
     8. erythroblastosus   _____
     9. atrezhia   _____
   10. pyloric   _____

E. Obstetrical Diagnostic Tests and Procedures

I.   Matching

Match the term to its meaning. (The same meaning may be used more than once.)
Insert the appropriate letter in the space next to the question number.

_____   **1.** amniocentesis   _____   **7.** fetometry
_____   **2.** amniography   _____   **8.** laparoscopy
_____   **3.** amnioscopy   _____   **9.** obstetrical sonogram
_____   **4.** endovaginal sonogram   _____ **10.** pelvimetry
_____   **5.** fetal monitoring   _____ **11.** pregnanediol test
_____   **6.** fetograph   _____ **12.** pregnancy test

Choices:

   a. x-ray filming of the amniotic cavity; introduction of contrast material into amniotic fluid results in outlining of the amniotic cavity and fetus

   b. surgical procedure to aspirate amniotic fluid for diagnostic purposes associated with the fetus

   c. ultrasound image of the uterus, uterine tubes, and ovaries

   d. visual examination of the amniotic cavity and the fetus

   e. visual examination of the abdominal cavity with the aid of a laparoscope; procedure used to examine the ovaries and uterine tubes

   f. use of an electronic device for the simultaneous recording of fetal heart rate and uterine contractions

   g. measurement to determine fetal size

   h. x-ray filming of the fetus

   i. ultrasound image of pregnant uterus to determine state of fetal development

   j. measurement of mother's pelvis to determine ability of fetus to pass through it

   k. a urine test to detect menstrual disorders or possibility of abortion

   l. test performed on urine or blood to detect human chorionic gonadotropin hormone

II.   Spell Check

Circle each incorrectly spelled term and write it correctly in the space provided.

   1. amnieocentesis _____
   2. amnioscopy _____
   3. fetograph _____
   4. pelvimetry _____
   5. amniografy _____
   6. endovaginel _____
   7. laparoskopy _____
   8. pregnanidiol _____

F. Obstetric Surgical Procedures and Treatment

I.   Matching

Match the term to its meaning. (The same meaning may be used more than once.) Insert the appropriate letter in the space next to the question number.

_____ **1.** amniofusion   _____ **6.** meconium aspiration
_____ **2.** amniotomy   _____ **7.** perineotomy
_____ **3.** cesarean section   _____ **8.** therapeutic abortion
_____ **4.** episiotomy   _____ **9.** tocolytic agent use
_____ **5.** hormone replacement therapy

Choices:

    a. surgical delivery of a baby; incision is made through the abdomen and uterus

    b. incision of the perineum during delivery to prevent perineum tearing and to aid in delivery

    c. introduction of an isotonic or similar solution into the amniotic sac to relieve fetal distress

    d. incision into the amnion; ruptures fetal membrane to induce labor

    e. use of specific hormones to boost deficiency or to regulate hormone production

    f. fetal aspiration of amniotic fluid containing newborn feces

    g. incision of the perineum

    h. abortion induced by mechanical means or the use of drugs for medical consideration

    i. the use of drugs to stop labor contractions

II.   Spell Check

Circle each incorrectly spelled term and write it correctly in the space provided.

    1. amniofussion   _____

    2. cesarean   _____

    3. meconium   _____

    4. amneiotomy   _____

    5. epiziotomy   _____

    6. pereneotomy   _____

G. Medical Vocabulary Building

I.   Matching

Match the term to its meaning. (The same meaning may be used more than once.) Insert the appropriate letter in the space next to the question number.

_____	**1.** Braxton-Hicks contraction		_____	**6.** macrosomia
			_____	**7.** meconium
_____	**2.** cephalopelvic disproportion		_____	**8.** morula
			_____	**9.** ovum transfer
_____	**3.** effacement		_____	**10.** polyhydramnios
_____	**4.** hyperemesis gravidarum		_____	**11.** spermicidals
_____	**5.** lochia		_____	**12.** surrogate mother

Choices:

    a. excessive and severe vomiting that results in maternal dehydration and weight loss

    b. conditions preventing normal delivery through birth canal, includes baby's head either too large or too small

    c. irregular and nonproductive uterine contractions that occur throughout pregnancy

    d. uterine discharge of blood, mucus, and tissue during first two weeks following childbirth

    e. cervix dilation during normal delivery, permitting passage of fetus

f. large-bodied baby, commonly seen in diabetic pregnancies

g. a solid mass of cells resulting from cell division after fertilization

h. first feces of newborn

i. a fertilization method for women who cannot conceive; a donor ovum is impregnated within the donor's body by artificial insemination and later transferred to the recipient female

j. various creams, jellies, foams, etc. containing agents that kill spermatozoa

k. excessive amniotic fluid

l. a female who contracts and serves to bear a child for another

II.   Spell Check

Circle each incorrectly spelled term and write it correctly in the space provided.

1. cephelopelvic   _____

2. hyperimesis   _____

3. macrosomia   _____

4. morula   _____

5. effasement   _____

6. lokchia   _____

7. mekonium   _____

8. polyhydramneos   _____

H. Pregnancy- and Obstetric-Related Abbreviations

I.   Definitions

Write the meanings of the following abbreviations in the spaces provided.

1. AB _____

2. AH _____

3. CDC _____

4. CS _____

5. CIS _____

6. CST _____

7. Cx _____

8. DUB _____

9. ECC _____

10. EDB _____

II.   Matching 1: Pregnancy- and Obstetric-Related Abbreviations, Part 1

Match the term to its meaning. (The same meaning may be used more than once.) Insert the appropriate letter in the space next to the question number.

Choices:

_____ **1.** EDC   **a.** endometrial biopsy

_____ **2.** EDD   **b.** estimated date of confinement

_____ **3.** EMB   **c.** expected date of delivery

_____ **4.** FHR   **d.** gamete intrafallopian transfer

_____ **5.** GIFT   **e.** fetal heart rate

_____ **6.** grav I   **f.** hormone replacement therapy

_____ **7.** HRT   **g.** hysterosalpingography
_____ **8.** HSG   **h.** pregnancy one
_____ **9.** IUD   **i.** intrauterine growth retardation
_____ **10.** IUGR   **j.** intrauterine device
_____ **11.** IUP   **k.** intrauterine pregnancy
_____ **12.** L&D   **l.** labor and delivery

III.   Matching 2: Pregnancy- and Obstetric-Related Abbreviations, Part 2

Match the term to its meaning. (The same meaning may be used more than once.) Insert the appropriate letter in the space next to the question number.

Choices:

_____ **1.** LMP   **a.** last menstrual period
_____ **2.** multip.   **b.** normal spontaneous delivery
_____ **3.** NSD   **c.** multipara
_____ **4.** OB   **d.** pelvic inflammatory disease
_____ **5.** PID   **e.** premenstrual syndrome
_____ **6.** PMS   **f.** obstetrics
_____ **7.** SVD   **g.** spontaneous delivery
_____ **8.** TAH   **h.** total abdominal hysterectomy
_____ **9.** TSS   **i.** toxic shock syndrome
_____ **10.** UC   **j.** uterine contraction

IV.   Spell Check

Circle each incorrectly spelled term and write it correctly in the space provided.

1. alfa-fetoprotein   _____
2. cesarrean   _____
3. diethylstillbesterol   _____
4. curetage   _____
5. intrafallopian   _____
6. hysterosalpingography   _____
7. luteinizing   _____
8. spontaneous   _____
9. histerektomy   _____
10. chorionic   _____
11. dysfunctional   _____
12. graveda   _____
13. gonadotropin   _____
14. intrauterine   _____
15. multiparus   _____
16. syndrome   _____

I. *Abbreviations Associated with Neonatology and Related Topics*

I.   Definitions

Write the meanings of the following abbreviations in the spaces provided.

1. AFP _____
2. AGA _____

   3. DNA _____

   4. ECMO _____

   5. FECG _____

   6. FHR _____

   7. FHT _____

   8. FTND _____

   9. HDN _____

 10. IgG _____

II.   Matching 1: Abbreviations Associated with Neonatology and Related Topics

Match the term to its meaning. (The same meaning may be used more than once.) Insert the appropriate letter in the space next to the question number.

Choices:

_____	**1.** IVF-ET	**a.** low birth weight
_____	**2.** LBW	**b.** newborn
_____	**3.** LGA	**c.** in vitro fertilization and embryo transfer
_____	**4.** NB	**d.** large for gestational age
_____	**5.** Para 2-0-1-2	**e.** pediatrics
_____	**6.** peds	**f.** 2 full-term infants, 0 premature, 1 abortion, and 2 live births
_____	**7.** Rh neg	**g.** rhesus positive
_____	**8.** Rh pos	**h.** Rhesus negative
_____	**9.** SGA	**i.** small for gestational age

III.   Matching 2: Abbreviations Used for Fetal Presentations

Match the term to its meaning. (The same meaning may be used more than once.) Insert the appropriate letter in the space next to the question number.

Choices:

_____	**1.** LSA	**a.** breech
_____	**2.** LMA	**b.** face
_____	**3.** LScA	**c.** transverse
_____	**4.** LScP	**d.** vertex
_____	**5.** LMP	
_____	**6.** RSA	
_____	**7.** LSP	
_____	**8.** LMT	
_____	**9.** RMT	
_____	**10.** RSP	
_____	**11.** RMA	
_____	**12.** RMP	
_____	**13.** RScA	
_____	**14.** RScP	
_____	**15.** LOA	
_____	**16.** ROA	
_____	**17.** ROT	

J. Increasing Your Medical Terminology Word Power 1

1. Read the following report.
2. Prepare to answer the questions at the end of the section.
3. Circle all unfamiliar terms with a red pencil.
4. Underline familiar terms with a blue pencil.
5. Use your knowledge of word elements, a medical dictionary, and the key terms to find the meaning of unfamiliar terms.

Neonatal Brain Tumors

Key Terms

astrocytoma (as-trō-sī-TŌ-ma)   tumor composed of astrocytes (star-shaped supportive nerve cells)

calcification (kal-si-fi-KĀ-shun)   depositing of calcium in tissue

ependymoma (ep-en-di-MŌ-ma)   tumor of the membrane lining the central canal of the spinal cord

germinoma (jer-mi-NŌ-ma)   tumor developing from the germ cells in the testis or ovary

hydrocephalus (hī-drō-SEF-a-lus)   accumulation of cerebrospinal fluid in the ventricles of the brain

meningioma (men-in-jē-Ō-ma)   slow-growing tumor that originates in one of the meninges

supratentorial (soo-pra-ten-TŌ-rē-al)   supporting structure found between the cerebrum and cerebellum

teratoma (ter-a-TŌ-ma)   congenital tumor containing one or more of the primary embryonic germ layers

I NTRODUCTION

Neonatal brain tumors are those that present clinically within the first two months of life. They are rare and present in only 0.5%–1.9% of all pediatric brain tumors (those in individuals under the age of fifteen).

There have been many reported cases and numerous review articles on neonatal brain tumors, including more than 2,000 pathologic cases, but most lack radiologic correlation.

C ASE STUDY

Forty-five pathologically proven cases of neonatal brain tumors (diagnosed in neonates within 60 days of birth) were reviewed from neuroradiology records dating back to 1964. Computerized tomography (CT) was performed in twenty-four cases, MR in five, sonography in six, and angiography in seven. Two-thirds of the lesions were supratentorial. The most common histology was a tumor composed of poorly differentiated tissues; twelve were teratomas. In addition, there were nine astrocytomas and twelve cases each of ependymoma and germinoma. The dominant CT appearance, regardless of histology, was a large lesion with associated hydrocephalus.

Coarse calcification was a constant feature in the teratomas. Prognosis was poor overall, with the longest survival seen in astrocytoma cases.

Questions

I.   Fill in the Blank

Fill in the blank with the appropriate term.

1. A tumor consisting of star-shaped supportive nerve cells is called a(n) _____.

2. When are neonatal brain tumors usually present clinically? _____

3. How many of the lesions were found between the cerebrum and cerebellum? _____

4. What was the major CT finding regardless of histology? _____

5. The term used for a slow-growing tumor originating in one of the meninges is _____.

6. The depositing of calcium in tissues is called _____.

7. A congenital tumor containing one or more primary embryonic germ layers is known as a(n) _____.

II.   Matching

Match the term to its meaning. (The same meaning may be used more than once.) Insert the appropriate letter in the space next to the question number.

Choices:

_____ **1.** astrocytoma
_____ **2.** calcification
_____ **3.** ependymoma
_____ **4.** germinoma
_____ **5.** hydrocephalus
_____ **6.** meningioma
_____ **7.** supratentorial
_____ **8.** teratoma

a. tumor of the membrane lining the central canal of the spinal cord
b. tumor composed of astrocytes
c. depositing of calcium in tissue
d. slow-growing tumor that originates in one of the meninges
e. tumor developing from the germ cells in the testis or ovary
f. accumulation of cerebrospinal fluid in the ventricles of the brain
g. congenital tumor containing one or more of the primary embryonic germ layers
h. supporting structure found between the cerebrum and cerebellum

K. Increasing Your Medical Terminology Word Power 2

1. Read the following report.
2. Prepare to answer the questions at the end of the section.
3. Circle all unfamiliar terms with a red pencil.
4. Underline familiar terms with a blue pencil.
5. Use your knowledge of word elements, a medical dictionary, and the key terms to find the meaning of unfamiliar terms.

Neural Tube Defects

Key Terms

anencephaly (an'-en-SEF-a-lē)   congenital condition in which there is an absence of a brain and spinal cord

anomaly (a-NOM-a-lē)   irregularity; deviation from normal

congenital (kon-JEN-i-tal)   present at birth

craniorachischisis (krā'-nē-ō-ra-KIS-ki-sis)   congenital fissure of the skull and spine

dysraphism (dis-RA-fizm)   failure of fusion of parts that normally fuse; failure of raphe (a ridge) formation

encephalocele (en-SEF-a-lō-sēl)   protrusion of the brain through a cranial fissure

folic (FŌ-lik) acid   member of the vitamin B complex; used in treatment of folic-acid-deficiency disease and sprue

iniencephaly (IN-ē-en-SEF-a-lē)   congenitally and deformed fetus resulting in the brain and spinal cord occupying a single cavity

in utero **(in Ū-ter-ō)**   within the uterus

mutation (mū-TĀ-shun)   permanent genetic change

occult spina bifida (ū-KULT SPĪ-na BI-fid-a)   failure of vertebrae to close without a hernial protrusion

spina bifida (SPĪ-na BI-fid-a)   congenital defect in the walls of the spinal canal caused by a lack of connection between the vertebral laminae

teratogenetic (ter'-a-tō-je-NET-ik)   development of abnormal structures in an embryo resulting in a severely deformed fetus

I NTRODUCTION

The two most common forms of neural tube defects in the United States, namely, spinal bifida and anencephaly, occur in 1 in 1,000 pregnancies. Worldwide it is believed that there are 300,000 or more per year with these defects. Although these severe conditions have been recognized for centuries, never before has progress been so rapid and significant as in the last decade, especially in the area of prevention. The results of several studies indicate that at least one-half of neural-tube-defect cases could be prevented if women consumed sufficient quantities of the B vitamin folic acid before conception and during early pregnancy.

Increasingly, new research findings are uncovering the biochemistry, developmental biology, and molecular genetics associated with neural tube defects. Such studies also are providing bases for new prevention strategies. The current recommendations of the Institute of Medicine and the United States Public Health Service propose that women who could become pregnant consume 400 micrograms of folic acid daily.

C LINICAL FEATURES

Although most studies of neural tube defects have considered only spina bifida or anencephaly, the clinical range also includes craniorachischisis, encephalocele, and iniencephaly. The latter two conditions are relatively rare but tend to appear in geographic areas that have a high rate of neural tube defects, such as northern China.

Another neural tube defect, spina bifida occulta, which is the mildest form of spinal dysraphism, is frequently not included in neural-tube-defect studies. This is because the condition often remains undetected and because of uncertainty concerning its relationship to overt spina bifida.

Neural tubes can be categorized as open (if neural tissue is exposed or covered by a membrane) or as closed (if the defect is covered by normal skin). About 20 percent of affected infants have other congenital anomalies. Genetic abnormalities that include chromosomal defects, single gene mutations, and teratogenic causes have been found in fewer than 10 percent of affected infants.

DEVELOPMENTAL FEATURES

Development and closure of the neural tube are normally completed within 28 days of conception. This is usually before most women are aware that they are pregnant. It is generally accepted that neural tube defects result from the failure of the neural tube to close, although it has also been suggested that a closed tube may reopen in certain cases.

CONSEQUENCES

Anencephaly and spina bifida are significant factors in fetal and infant mortality. About 4,000 fetuses are affected per year in the United States. One-third of the affected fetuses are lost as a result of spontaneous or elective abortion. All infants with anencephaly are stillborn or die shortly after birth, whereas many infants with spina bifida now survive. The survival of such infants usually is the result of extensive medical and surgical care. The risk of early death among infants with open spina bifida varies significantly worldwide.

In addition to the emotional drain of spina bifida, the estimated monetary cost is overwhelming. In the United States, for example, the total cost of care and treatment during the 1990s was estimated to be approximately $294,000 per infant.

TREATMENT

Damage to open neural tissues during development is progressive and appears to result from toxic substances in the amniotic fluid as well as injury to the neural tissue through contact with the uterine wall and birth canal. The current approaches being used to possibly decrease the severity of the condition include cesarean section, surgical treatment *in utero*, and attempts to prevent secondary disabilities by means of hormone treatments. There is no question that medical care for people who are born with neural tube defects is complicated and challenging.

PRIMARY PREVENTION

The primary approach to reducing neural tube defects is through better nutrition. The link between nutrition and the occurrence of neural tube defects provides a powerful tool for primary prevention. The urgent challenge facing medical and public health officials is how to translate this knowledge into practice. This will require increasing the consumption of foods now fortified with folic acid, taking vitamin supplements containing folic acid, and improving the knowledge of women and medical professionals as to the benefits of folic acid in preventing neural tube defects.

Questions

I.   Matching

Match the term to its meaning. (The same meaning may be used more than once.) Insert the appropriate letter in the space next to the question number.

Choices:

_____ **1.** anencephaly
_____ **2.** anomaly
_____ **3.** congenital
_____ **4.** craniorachischisis
_____ **5.** encephalocele
_____ **6.** dysraphism
_____ **7.** folic acid
_____ **8.** iniencephaly
_____ **9.** *in utero*
_____ **10.** mutation
_____ **11.** spina bifida
_____ **12.** teratogenic

a. abnormality, irregularity
b. congenital condition in which there is an absence of a brain and spinal cord
c. congenital fissure of the skull and spine
d. present at birth
e. failure of fusion of parts that normally fuse; failure of raphe (a ridge) formation
f. congenitally deformed fetus resulting in the brain and spinal cord occupying a single cavity
g. a member of the vitamin B complex; used in treatment of folic-acid-deficiency disease and sprue
h. within the uterus
i. congenital defect in the walls of the spinal canal caused by a lack of a connection between the vertebrae laminae
j. permanent genetic change
k. development of abnormal structures in an embryo resulting in a severely deformed fetus
l. protrusion of the brain through a cranial fissure

II.   Spell Check

Circle each incorrectly spelled term and write it correctly in the space provided.

1. anensephaly   _____
2. congenital   _____
3. disraphism   _____
4. ineincephaly   _____
5. teratogenic   _____
6. anomalies   _____
7. craniorakhischisis _____
8. encefhlocele   _____
9. spina bifida   _____
10. folic   _____

L. Increasing Your Medical Terminology Word Power 3

1. Read the following report.
2. Prepare to answer the questions at the end of the section.
3. Circle all unfamiliar terms with a red pencil.
4. Underline familiar terms with a blue pencil.
5. Use your knowledge of word elements, a medical dictionary, and the key terms to find the meaning of unfamiliar terms.

Neonatal Hyperbilirubinemia

Key Terms

basal ganglia (BĀ-sal GANG-lē-a)   four masses of gray matter located deep in the cerebral hemispheres

bilirubin (bil-i-ROO-bin)   orange-colored or yellowish pigment in bile

biliverdin (bil-i-VER-din)   greenish pigment in bile formed by the oxidation of bilirubin

conjugated (KON-jū-gā-ted)   linked, joined

deciliter (DES-i-lē-ter)   metric measurement, equal to 0.1 liter

enterohepatic (en'-ter-ō-hē-PAT-ik)   pertaining to the intestines and liver

heme (hēm)   iron-containing non-protein portion of the hemoglobin molecule

hemolysis (hē-MOL-i-sis)   destruction of red blood cells

hyperbilirubinemia (hi'-per-bil'-i-roo-bin-Ē-mē-a)   excessive amount of bilirubin in the blood

jaundice (JAWN-dis)   condition characterized by yellowness of the skin, whites of the eyes, and body fluids due to excess bilirubin in the blood

kernicterus (ker-NIK-ter-us)   hemolytic jaundice of the newborn (icterus neonatorum)

milligram (MIL-i-gram)   one-hundredth of a gram

neurotoxic (nū'-rō-TOKS-ik)   poisonous to nerve cells

senescent (se-NES-ent)   old

unconjugated (un-KON-jū-gāt-ed)   not joined or connected

I NTRODUCTION

Icterus neonatorum, or neonatal jaundice, has been known as a clinical entity for over one century. The term "kernicterus" was introduced to clinical medicine in the early 1900s to specify the yellow staining of the basal ganglia found in infants who died of severe jaundice. Treatment of infants with jaundice from the 1950s through the 1970s was exceptionally aggressive because of the high incidence of kernicterus and hemolytic disease of the newborn. During the 1980s and 1990s the management of jaundice in infants changed. It appeared that too many infants were being treated for the condition unnecessarily. The picture of the disease became blurred because newborns were being discharged from hospitals sooner after their birth, thus limiting the ability of physicians to detect jaundice during the period when the serum levels of bilirubin were likely to rise. Because of these and other factors, physicians became less likely to treat jaundice in neonates, which unfortunately led to reports of fatal kernicterus.

P ATHOPHYSIOLOGY

Neonatal hyperbilirubinemia develops from a predisposition to the production of bilirubin in newborns and their limited ability to excrete it. Infants, especially preterm infants, have higher rates of bilirubin production than adults because their red blood cells have a shorter life span. In newborns, unconjugated bilirubin is not readily excreted and the ability to conjugate bilirubin is limited. Together these factors led to a high concentration of serum bilirubin in the first day of life in full-term infants, and up to the first week in pre-term infants, and some full-term Asian infants. Bilirubin concentrations decline during the next several weeks and eventually reach values similar to those found in adults. Exaggerated levels occur when the bilirubin concentrations reach 7 to 17 milligrams per deciliter. Concentrations above 17 mg/dl cause pathologic jaundice and can usually be diagnosed. Of primary concern with exaggerated hyperbilirubinemia is the potential for neurotoxic effects and general cellular injury. Bilirubin can impair nerve conduction, particularly in the auditory nerve, and interfere with DNA synthesis.

*C*AUSES

The main source of bilirubin is the breakdown of hemoglobin in senescent or hemolyzed red blood cells. Heme is broken down enzymatically by heme oxygenase, resulting in the release of iron and the formation of carbon monoxide and biliverdin. Biliverdin is further degraded to bilirubin by the enzyme biliverdin reductase. Bilirubin then passes through the liver and is changed into an excretable conjugated form that enters the lumen of the small intestine. This form of bilirubin can be degraded by bacteria so that it can be reabsorbed into the circulation.

Increased production of bilirubin, deficiency of hepatic uptake, impaired conjugation of bilirubin, and increased enterohepatic circulation of bilirubin are responsible for most cases of pathologic jaundice in newborns. It should be noted that increased bilirubin production occurs in infants with blood-group incompatibilities, red blood cell-enzyme deficiencies, defects in red blood cell construction, or deficiencies in the enzyme responsible for bilirubin conjugation.

Questions

I.   Matching

Match the term to its meaning. (The same meaning may be used more than once.) Insert the appropriate letter in the space provided next to the question number.

_____ **1.** bilirubin	Choices:
_____ **2.** biliverdin	**a.** greenish pigment in bile formed by the oxidation of bilirubin
_____ **3.** conjugated	**b.** linked, joined
_____ **4.** enterohepatic	**c.** orange-colored or yellowish pigment in bile
_____ **5.** heme	**d.** iron-containing non-protein portion of the hemoglobin molecule
_____ **6.** hemolysis	**e.** destruction of red blood cells
_____ **7.** hyperbilirubinemia	**f.** pertaining to the intestines and liver
_____ **8.** jaundice	**g.** excessive amount of bilirubin in the blood
_____ **9.** kernicterus	**h.** poisonous to nerve cells
_____ **10.** neurotoxic	**i.** condition characterized by yellowness of the skin, whites of the eyes, and body fluids due to excess bilirubin in the blood
_____ **11.** senescent	**j.** hemolytic jaundice of the newborn (icterus neonatorum)
_____ **12.** unconjugated	**k.** not joined or connected
	l. old

II.   Spell Check

Circle each incorrectly spelled term and write it correctly in the space provided.

1. billirubin   _____
2. deciliter   _____
3. hyperbilirubenimia _____
4. kernikterus   _____
5. senesent   _____
6. biliverdin   _____
7. enterohepathic   _____
8. jaundice   _____
9. miligram   _____
10. unconjugated   _____

Term Search Challenge

Locate 14 terms in the puzzle.

1. Write the specific term next to its definition. Then find that term in the puzzle diagram and circle it.
2. Terms may be read from left to right, backward, up, down, or diagonally.
3. If a term appears more than once, circle it only once. (A term or abbreviation may be found inside others.)
4. Check your answers.

Clues:

1. Voluntary prevention of pregnancy _____
2. Uterine development of an individual _____
3. Vascular structure that provides nutrition for the fetus _____
4. Removal of a fetus by means of an incision into the uterus _____
5. Yellowish fluid secreted by the breast during pregnancy and up to 3 days after delivery _____
6. Term meaning "before birth" _____
7. Normal uterine contractions that result in the delivery of the fetus _____
8. Inability to conceive _____
9. Innermost fetal membrane, which forms the bag of waters and encloses the fetus _____
10. Unborn offspring in the post-embryonic period after the major body structures have been formed _____
11. Abnormal fluid collection in ventricles of the brain, resulting in an enlargement of the head _____
12. Term meaning "before the proper time" _____
13. Another term for the viral disease German measles _____
14. Abbreviation for *in vitro* fertilization and embryo transfer _____

Term Search Puzzle

```
P  R  E  G  N  A  N  C  Y  A  B  X  T  R  O
L  P  I  E  S  M  U  T  R  A  P  E  T  N  A
A  R  N  S  E  C  C  O  N  M  J  R  A  C  C
C  E  C  T  C  O  J  I  O  N  S  U  T  E  O
E  G  I  A  T  C  R  R  O  I  M  O  N  A  N
N  N  S  T  I  S  R  N  E  O  S  J  E  R  T
T  A  I  I  O  T  O  T  O  N  I  J  Y  D  R
A  N  O  O  N  R  B  R  R  U  B  E  L  L  A
Y  C  N  N  T  I  A  U  M  M  O  N  O  T  C
X  V  T  N  C  O  L  O  S  T  R  U  M  O  E
O  S  T  E  R  I  L  I  T  Y  I  N  M  A  P
N  T  I  V  F  E  T  V  E  L  V  E  T  U  T
O  H  Y  D  R  O  C  E  P  H  A  L  U  S  I
G  L  M  P  R  E  M  A  T  U  R  E  O  T  O
C  E  S  A  R  E  A  N  N  S  U  T  E  F  N
```

CHAPTER 24

The Nervous System

"Health is a state of complete physical, mental, and social well-being and not merely the absence of disease or infirmity . . . ."

—Preamble of the World Health Organization Center

INFORMATIONAL CHALLENGE

A. The Neuron

I.   Fill in the Blank

Fill in the blank with the appropriate term.

   1. The basic unit of the nervous system is the _____.
   2. Messages are transmitted to other cells in the nervous system by electrical signals known as _____or _____.

II.   Matching: Cells and Functions of the Nervous System

Match the term to its meaning. (The same meaning may be used more than once.) Insert the appropriate letter in the space next to the question number.

Choices:

_____ **1.** astrocyte	**a.** covering for axons
_____ **2.** myelin	**b.** produces myelin
_____ **3.** synapse	**c.** help to remove dead neurons from CNS
_____ **4.** oligodendrite	**d.** star-shaped support cell
_____ **5.** satellite cells	**e.** myelinated neurons of the PNS
_____ **6.** Schwann cells	**f.** site where one neuron contacts a target cell
_____ **7.** microglia	**g.** associated with ganglia
_____ **8.** dendrite	**h.** contains nucleus and most other cell organelles
_____ **9.** axon	**i.** serves as the cable for impulse transmission to other cells
_____ **10.** cell body	**j.** receives impulses and transmits them to cell body

III.   Spell Check

Circle each incorrectly spelled term and write it correctly in the space provided.

1. neuroglia   _____

2. Schwan's   _____

3. myelin   _____

4. neurotransmitten   _____

5. nuron   _____

6. synapse   _____

IV.   Vision Quiz: The Motor Neuron and Its Parts

Figure 24-10 shows the parts of neurons. Using the choices given, identify and write the letter of the numbered structures in the spaces provided next to the question number.

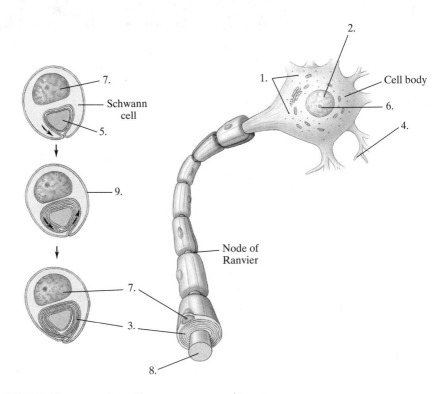

Schwann cell

Node of Ranvier

Cell body

FIGURE 24-10   Vision Quiz. The motor neuron and its parts.

Choices:

_____ **1.**   **a.** cell body

_____ **2.**   **b.** axon

_____ **3.**   **c.** dendrites

_____ **4.**   **d.** nucleus of cell body

_____ **5.**   **e.** neurolemma of Schwann cell

_____ **6.**   **f.** nucleolus

_____ **7.**   **g.** myelin sheath of Schwann cell

_____ **8.**   **h.** Schwann cell nucleus

_____ **9.**

B. The Human Brain and Its Organization and Structure

I.   Fill in the Blank

Fill in the blank with the appropriate term.

   1. The two main parts of the central nervous system are the
         _____ and the _____.
   2. Two types of nerves found with the peripheral nervous system are
         _____ and _____.
   3. The nerve portions of the autonomic nervous system are subdivided
         into the _____ and _____ divisions.
   4. The liquid circulating within the ventricles of the brain is called
         _____ fluid.
   5. The depressions of the cerebral cortex are called
         _____.
   6. The convolutions of the cerebral cortex are called
         _____.
   7. The two parts of the diencephalon are the _____
         and the _____.

II.   Matching: CNS Parts and Functions

Match the term to its meaning. (The same meaning may be used more than once.)
Insert the appropriate letter in the space next to the question number.

                                              Choices:

_____ **1.** cranial nerves   **a.** part of the nervous system regulat-
_____ **2.** pia mater   ing involuntary vital functions
_____ **3.** dura mater   **b.** membranes covering the brain and
_____ **4.** autonomic nervous system   spinal cord
_____ **5.** meninges   **c.** fluid within the ventricles of the brain
_____ **6.** brain stem   **d.** 12 pairs of nerves emerging from
_____ **7.** cerebrospinal fluid   the cranial cavity through various
_____ **8.** spinal cord   openings in the skull
_____ **9.** pons   **e.** outermost meninx of the brain and
                                             the spinal cord
                                         f. stem-like portion of the brain con-
                                             necting the cerebrospinal hemi-
                                             spheres with the spinal cord
                                         g. part of the central nervous system
                                             within the spinal canal
                                         h. innermost meninx covering the
                                             brain and spinal cord
                                         i. connects parts of the diencephalon

III.   Spell Check

Circle each incorrectly spelled term and write it correctly in the space provided.

   1. sulki   _____
   2. parietal   _____
   3. ocipital   _____
   4. thalmus   _____
   5. cerbellum   _____

   6. subarachnoid _____
   7. gyri _____
   8. meninx _____
   9. hypothlamus _____
   10. oblongata _____

IV.   Vision Quiz 1: The Human Brain

Figure 24-11 shows a sagittal view of the CNS. Using the choices given, identify and write the letter of the numbered structures in the spaces provided next to the question number.

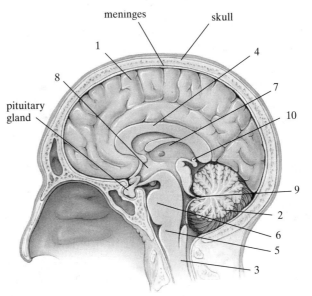

FIGURE 24-11   Vision Quiz. The human brain.

Choices:

_____ 1.   **a.** spinal cord
_____ 2.   **b.** cerebrum
_____ 3.   **c.** medulla oblongata
_____ 4.   **d.** hypothalamus
_____ 5.   **e.** fornix
_____ 6.   **f.** cerebellum
_____ 7.   **g.** corpus callosum
_____ 8.   **h.** midbrain
_____ 9.   **i.** thalamus
_____ 10.   **j.** pons
                       k. fourth ventricle
                       l. pituitary

V.   Vision Quiz 2: The Lobes and Sulci of the Brain

Figure 24-12 shows the lobes of the brain and its main sulci. Using the choices given, identify and write the letter of the numbered structures in the spaces provided next to the question number.

                       Choices:

_____ 1.   **a.** parietal lobe
_____ 2.   **b.** temporal lobe

_____ **3.**
_____ **4.**
_____ **5.**
_____ **6.**
_____ **7.**
_____ **8.**

c. frontal lobe
d. occipital lobe
e. lateral sulcus
f. precentral sulcus
g. postcentral sulcus
h. central sulcus

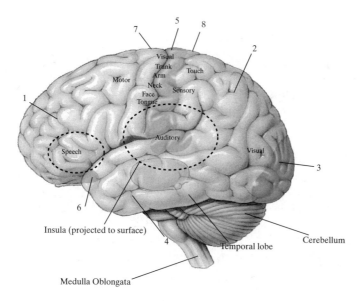

FIGURE 24-12   Vision Quiz. The lobes and sulci of the brain.

C. *Cranial Nerves*

I.   Matching: Cranial Nerves, Functions, and Associations

Match the term to its meaning. (The same meaning may be used more than once.)
Insert the appropriate letter in the space next to the question number.

Choices:

_____ **1.** olfactory
_____ **2.** auditory
_____ **3.** glossopharyngeal
_____ **4.** optic
_____ **5.** oculomotor
_____ **6.** trigeminal
_____ **7.** abducens
_____ **8.** facial
_____ **9.** vagus
_____ **10.** spinal
_____ **11.** hypoglossal
_____ **12.** trochlear

a. tongue and pharynx
b. vision
c. hearing
d. eye movements
e. muscles turning eye outward
f. sense of smell
g. voice and swallowing
h. muscles of the face, ears, and scalp
i. neck muscles
j. beneath the tongue
k. facial movements
l. eye muscles

II.   Spell Check

Circle each incorrectly spelled term and write it correctly in the space provided.

     1. olefactory   _____

     2. oculomotor   _____

    3. trochler   _____

    4. trigerminal   _____

    5. abducens   _____

    6. fasial   _____

    7. glossopharyngeal   _____

    8. vegas   _____

    9. hypoglosal   _____

    10. auditory   _____

D. Components of the Peripheral Nervous System (PNS)

I.   Fill in the Blank

Fill in the blank with the appropriate term.

    1. All nervous tissue outside the CNS belongs to the _____ nervous system.

    2. The PNS consists of two subdivisions known as the _____ nervous system and the _____ nervous system.

    3. The _____ nervous system constantly controls the body's vital functions.

    4. _____ nerves carry signals to the CNS.

    5. _____ nerves carry signals away from the CNS.

II.   Matching

Match the term to its meaning. (The same meaning may be used more than once.) Insert the appropriate letter in the space next to the question number.

Choices:

_____ **1.** afferent division of the PNS

_____ **2.** postganglionic fiber

_____ **3.** mixed nerves

_____ **4.** efferent division of the PNS

_____ **5.** alpha receptor

_____ **6.** beta receptor

_____ **7.** reflex action

_____ **8.** nicotinic receptor

_____ **9.** patellar reflex

_____ **10.** Babinski's sign

_____ **11.** Achilles reflex

a. belongs to sympathetic system

b. regulates responses such as pupil dilation

c. carry signals from and away from CNS

d. carries signals to the CNS from sensory organs

e. inhibits uterine contraction and heart stimulation

f. carries signals from the CNS to effector organs

g. belongs to parasympathetic system

h. extend to effector organs, where they control organ function

i. automatic uncontrolled response to stimuli

j. extension of big toe when side of the foot is stimulated

k. ankle-jerk response

l. knee-jerk response

III.   Spell Check

Circle each incorrectly spelled term and write it correctly in the space provided.

1. anesthesiologist   _____
2. pateller   _____
3. Achiles   _____
4. automic   _____
5. muscarinic   _____
6. nicotinic   _____
7. beta   _____
8. parasympathetic   _____
9. abdominal   _____
10. Babinski's   _____

E. Word Roots and/or Combining Forms for the Nervous System

I.   Fill in the Blank

Fill in the blank with the appropriate term.

1. Two word roots used for the brain are _____ and
_____.
2. The combining form used for spinal cord is _____.
3. What is the combining form for nerve? _____
4. Two combining forms for ganglion are _____ and
_____.

II.   Matching 1: Word Roots and/or Combining Forms Associated with
the Anatomy and/or Functions of the Nervous System, Part 1

Match the term to its meaning. (The same meaning may be used more than once.)
Insert the appropriate letter in the space next to the question number.

                                    Choices:

_____ **1.** plex   **a.** cerebellum
_____ **2.** cerebr/o   **b.** network, nerve
_____ **3.** neuro   **c.** pons
_____ **4.** thalam   **d.** dura mater
_____ **5.** cerebell   **e.** cerebrum
_____ **6.** dur   **f.** nerve
_____ **7.** pont   **g.** thalamus
_____ **8.** radicul/o   **h.** (nerve) root

III.   Matching 2: Word Roots and/or Combining Forms Associated with
the Anatomy and/or Functions of the Nervous System, Part 2

                                    Choices:

_____ **1.** gli/o   **a.** sheath
_____ **2.** poli/o   **b.** "glue" (supportive and connecting
_____ **3.** ventricul/o   parts of the nervous system)
_____ **4.** thec   **c.** thin, slender

_____ **5.** lept/o
_____ **6.** mening/o
_____ **7.** esthesi
_____ **8.** my/o

d. ventricles of the brain
e. gray matter of the brain and spinal cord
f. membrane
g. muscle
h. feeling

IV.   Spell Check

Circle each incorrectly spelled term and write it correctly in the space provided.

1. algesick   _____
2. cerabeller   _____
3. encephlitis   _____
4. gangliitis   _____
5. kineesiology   _____
6. meningococus   _____
7. disphagia   _____
8. pontobulbar   _____
9. radiculopathy   _____
10. theecal   _____

V.   Word Analysis: Word Roots and/or Combining Forms for the Nervous System

Table 24-12 lists a number of terms with their pronunciations and definitions.

TABLE 24-12   WORD ANALYSIS: WORD ROOTS AND COMBINING FORMS FOR THE NERVOUS SYSTEM

Term and Pronunciation	Definition
algesic (al-JĒ-sik)	painful
cerebellar (ser-e-BEL-ar)	pertaining to the cerebellum
cerebrovascular (ser-ē-brō-VAS-kū-lar)	blood vessels of the brain
subdural (sub-DŪ-ral)	beneath the dura mater
encephalitis (en-sef-a-LĪ-tis)	inflammation of the brain
dysesthesia (dis-es-THĒ-zē-a)	abnormal or painful sensation on the skin
gangliitis (gang-lē-Ī-tis)	inflammation of a ganglion
ganglionectomy (gang-lē-ō-NEK-tō-mē)	excision of a ganglion
glial (GLĪ-al)	neurological supportive-tissue glia, or neuroglia
kinesiology (ki-nē-sē-OL-ō-jē)	study of muscles and body movements

(Continued)

TABLE 24-12   (CONTINUED)

Term and Pronunciation	Definition
leptomeningitis (lep-tō-men-in-JĪ-tis)	inflammation of the (thin) pia and arachnoid membranes
meningioma (men-in-jē-Ō-ma)	tumor of the meninges (arachnoid)
meningococcus (men-in-gō-KOK-us)	bacterium that attacks the meninges
neurorrhaphy (nū-ROR-a-fē)	suturing nerve (endings)
dysphasia (dis-FĀ-zē-a)	difficulty speaking; due to brain lesion
plexitis (plek-SĪ-tis)	inflammation of a nerve network (plexus)
poliomyelopathy (pōl-ē-ō-mī-el-OP-a-thē)	any disease of the gray matter of the spinal cord
pontobulbar (pon-tō-BUL-bar)	pertaining to the pons and the medulla oblongata
radiculopathy (rā-dik-ū-LOP-a-thē)	any disease condition of spinal nerve roots
thalamic (thal-AM-ik)	pertaining to the thalamus
thecal (THĒ-kal)	pertaining to a sheath (covering)
ventriculitis (ven-trik-ū-LĪ-tis)	inflammation of brain ventricles

1. Analyze each term.
2. Circle all combining forms and word roots and label them **cf** and **wr**, respectively.
3. Check your answers (shown in Table 24-13).

F. Nervous System Diseases and Disorders

I.   Fill in the Blank

Fill in the blank with the appropriate term.

1. The general term used to indicate an inflammation of the meninges is _____.
2. The term for an inflammation of nerves is _____.
3. Two viral diseases of the nervous system are _____ and _____.

II.   Matching

Match the term to its meaning. (The same meaning may be used more than once.) Insert the appropriate letter in the space next to the question number.

Choices:

_____ 1. cerebrovascular accident
_____ 2. epilepsy
_____ 3. hydrocephalus
_____ 4. encephalitis
_____ 5. zoster
_____ 6. Huntington's chorea
_____ 7. multiple sclerosis
_____ 8. Parkinson's disease
_____ 9. sciatica
_____ 10. organic brain syndrome

a. inflammation of the brain
b. interruption of blood supply to the brain
c. continual occurrence of rapid, jerky, involuntary movements
d. swelling of brain ventricles caused by local blockage
e. seizure disorder
f. shingles; acute viral infection of cerebral or spinal nerves
g. any acute or chronic mental disorder caused by impairment of brain tissue function
h. severe pain in the leg along the course of the sciatic nerve
i. progressive, degenerative neurologic disorder characterized by resting tremor
j. sclerotic patches scattered along the brain and spinal cord

III.   Spell Check

Circle each incorrectly spelled term and write it correctly in the space provided.

1. ensephalitis   _____
2. epilepsy   _____
3. siezure   _____
4. sklerosis   _____
5. Alzheimer's   _____
6. sciatica   _____
7. khorea   _____
8. Parkenson's   _____
9. cerebrovascular   _____
10. apoplexy   _____

G. CNS Associated Diagnostic and Clinical Procedures

I.   Matching 1: CNS Associated Diagnostic and Clinical Procedures

Match the term to its meaning. (The same meaning may be used more than once.) Insert the appropriate letter in the space next to the question number.

Choices:

_____ 1. pneumoencephalography
_____ 2. myelography
_____ 3. echoencephalography
_____ 4. cerebral angiography
_____ 5. PET
_____ 6. brain scan

a. injection of contrast material to obtain x-rays of brain vessels
b. recording brain structure with sound
c. injection of dye into spinal fluid to obtain x-rays of the spinal cord

_____ **7.** electroencephalography
_____ **8.** ventriculogram
_____ **9.** lumbar puncture

d. injection of air by spinal puncture to obtain x-rays of the brain

e. recording electrical brain impulses

f. injection of radioactive chemicals through the brain

g. procedure used to follow the brain's metabolism of glucose

h. procedure to obtain x-rays after the direct injection of air into cerebral ventricles

i. procedure used to obtain cerebrospinal fluid

II.   Matching 2: Surgical Procedures

Match the term to its meaning. (The same meaning may be used more than once.) Insert the appropriate letter in the space next to the question number.

Choices:

_____ **1.** radicotomy
_____ **2.** neurectomy
_____ **3.** neurorrhaphy
_____ **4.** ganglionectomy
_____ **5.** neurotomy
_____ **6.** neurolysis
_____ **7.** neuroplasty
_____ **8.** stereotaxis
_____ **9.** trephination

a. incision of a nerve

b. incision into a nerve root

c. ganglion excision

d. suture of a nerve

e. nerve excision

f. separating a nerve from an adhesion

g. cutting out a circular piece of bone from the skull

h. method of precisely locating brain areas for surgery

i. surgical repair of a nerve

III.   Spell Check

Circle each incorrectly spelled term and write it correctly in the space provided.

1. mylography   _____
2. pneumoencephalography _____
3. emision   _____
4. ventriculography   _____
5. ganglionectomy   _____
6. neurorhaphy   _____
7. radicotomy   _____
8. trephination   _____

H. Medical Vocabulary Building

I.   Matching

Match the term to its meaning. (The same meaning may be used more than once.) Insert the appropriate letter in the space next to the question number.

_____ **1.** atelomyelia
_____ **2.** cephalalgia
_____ **3.** cordotomy

_____ **4.** diplegia
_____ **5.** diskectomy
_____ **6.** epidural

	7. hemianopsis		14. phagomania
	8. hypermnesia		15. achiomyelitis
	9. hypnology		16. sympathectomy
	10. logomania		17. vagotomy
	11. meningopathy		18. agoraphobia
	12. myelophthisis		19. akathisia
	13. oligodendroglioma		20. endorphins

Choices:

    a. imperfect development of the spinal cord

    b. head pain

    c. surgical incision into the spinal cord; usually done for pain relief

    d. surgical incision of an intervertebral disk

    e. paralysis of identical parts on both sides of the body

    f. situated on the dura mater

    g. blindness of half the field of vision in one or both eyes

    h. excellent memory of date, names, and details

    i. the study of sleep

    j. excessive, continuous, and repetitive flow of speech

    k. any disease involving the meninges

    l. wasting away of the spinal cord

    m. malignant tumor originating from and consisting of oligodendroglia

    n. spinal cord inflammation

    o. abnormal craving (madness) for food

    p. surgical incision of the vagus nerve

    q. surgical excision of a portion of the sympathetic nervous system

    r. inability to remain still

    s. abnormal fear of being in public places

    t. brain-produced chemical substances that act as natural analgesics

II.   Spell Check

Circle each incorrectly spelled term and write it correctly in the space provided.

    1. endorfins   _____

    2. rachomyelitis   _____

    3. myelofthisis   _____

    4. diskectomy   _____

    5. cordotomy   _____

    6. akathisia   _____

    7. oligodendroglioma   _____

    8. hypermnesia   _____

    9. atelomyelia   _____

    10. epidurel   _____

I. *Abbreviations Associated with the Nervous System*

I.   Definitions

Write the meanings of the following abbreviations.

    1. CVA _____

    2. DT _____

3. OBS _____

4. EEG _____

II.   Matching

Match the term to its meaning. (The same meaning may be used more than once.)
Insert the appropriate letter in the space next to the question number.

Choices:

_____ **1.** central nervous system	**a.**	CSF
_____ **2.** electroencephalogram	**b.**	CNS
_____ **3.** cerebrospinal fluid	**c.**	PEG
_____ **4.** pneumoencephalography	**d.**	EEG
_____ **5.** acetylcholine	**e.**	CVA
_____ **6.** cerebrovascular accident	**f.**	Ach
_____ **7.** multiple sclerosis	**g.**	MS

J. Increasing Your Medical Terminology Word Power 1

1. Read the following report.
2. Prepare to answer the questions at the end of the section.
3. Circle all unfamiliar terms with a red pencil.
4. Underline familiar terms with a blue pencil.
5. Use your knowledge of word elements, a medical dictionary, and the
   key terms to find the meaning of unfamiliar terms.

Brain Tumors

Key Terms

astrocytoma (as-trō-sī-TŌ-ma)   tumor consisting of astrocytes

ataxia (ā-TAK-sē-a)   defective muscular coordination and movement

hemiparesis (hem-ē-PAR-ē-sis)   paralysis of one side of the body

medulloblastoma (me-dūl-ō-blas-TŌ-ma)   malignant tumor that often invades
the meninges and is found in the roof of the fourth ventricle and cerebellum

meningioma (men-in-jē-Ō-ma)   slow-growing tumor that starts in the arachnoidal tissue

neoplasm (NĒ-ō-plazm)   a new and abnormal growth

pneumoencephalography (nū'-mō-en-sef-a-LOG-ra-fē)   procedure used to obtain x-rays of the brain following injection of air by means of a lumbar puncture

1 NTRODUCTION

Brain tumors develop in approximately 35,000 adult Americans each year. These can
be divided into primary tumors (those arising from the brain and its coverings) and
metastatic tumors (those arising elsewhere in the body).

In children, astrocytomas and medulloblastomas are the most common tumors;
in adults, the most common are metastatic tumors, astroglial neoplasms, and meningiomas. Recent evidence indicates that the incidence of primary tumors among the
elderly is increasing.

More adults die each year of primary brain tumors than of Hodgkin's disease or multiple sclerosis. Malignant gliomas alone account for 2.5% of deaths due to cancer and are the third leading cause of death from cancer in persons 15 to 34 years of age.

There is little information about the relation of environmental factors to primary brain tumors. Cranial irradiation and exposure to some chemicals may lead to an increased incidence of both astrocytomas and meningiomas. Head injury may increase the development of meningiomas but does not appear to cause astrocytomas.

*D*IAGNOSIS

Brain tumors present a variety of clinical patterns, depending on the type of tumor and its location. Possible signs include seizures, visual or hearing loss, hemiparesis, numbness or ataxia, double vision, and headache.

CT and MRI techniques have caused a major revolution in providing direct views of tumors and in diagnosis. The two imaging techniques used a decade ago, conventional brain scanning and pneumoencephalography, are not helpful today.

*T*REATMENT

Surgery is part of initial management of virtually all brain tumors; it established the diagnosis and relieves pressure quickly. Radiation therapy plays a central role in the management of malignant tumors. Chemotherapy has had limited effectiveness. However, there is an increasing tendency to use combination chemotherapy as the primary therapy instead of radiation for malignant tumors in children under the age of two years.

Questions

I.   Matching

Match the term to its meaning. (The same meaning may be used more than once.) Insert the appropriate letter in the space next to the question number.

Choices:

_____ **1.** hemiparesis
_____ **2.** ataxia
_____ **3.** metastatic
_____ **4.** pneumoencephalography
_____ **5.** astrocytoma
_____ **6.** meningioma
_____ **7.** medulloblastoma
_____ **8.** Hodgkin's disease
_____ **9.** neoplasm

a. slow-growing tumor that starts in arachnoidal tissue
b. defective muscular coordination
c. paralysis of one side of the body
d. tumor consisting of astrocytes
e. malignant tumor that invades the meninges and found in the roof of the cerebellum
f. new and abnormal growth
g. disease of unknown cause producing enlargement of lymphoid tissue and invasion of other tissues
h. x-ray procedure involving the injection of air by lumbar puncture
i. change in the location of a cancer

II.   Spell Check

Circle each incorrectly spelled term and write it correctly in the space provided.

1. sclerosis _____
2. metastik _____
3. ataxea _____
4. astrocytoma _____
5. Hogkin's _____
6. hemeparesis _____
7. pneumoensephalography _____
8. medulablastoma _____

K. *Increasing Your Medical Terminology Word Power 2*

1. Read the following report.
2. Prepare to answer the questions at the end of the section.
3. Circle all unfamiliar terms with a red pencil.
4. Underline familiar terms with a blue pencil.
5. Use your knowledge of word elements, a medical dictionary, and the key terms to find the meaning of unfamiliar terms.

Multiple Brain Abscesses

Key Terms

abscess (AB-ses)   localized collection of pus

brucellosis (broo-sel-Ō-sis)   bacterial disease acquired by ingesting contaminated milk or dairy products; the bacteria belong to the genus of *Brucella* (broo-SEL-a)

CAT   computerized axial tomography

CSF   cerebrospinal fluid

hepatosplenomegaly (hep-a-tō-sple-nō-MEG-a-lē)   enlargement of both the liver and spleen

lethargy (LETH-ar-jē)   sluggishness

lymphadenopathy (limf-ad-ē-NOP-a-thē)   disease of the lymph nodes

papilledema (pap-il-ē-DĒ-ma)   swelling and inflammation of the optic nerve at the point of its entrance into the eyeball

quadriplegia (kwad-ri-PLĒ-jē-a)   paralysis of both arms and legs, usually the trunk

WBC   white blood cell count

*C*ASE REPORT

A four-year-old male, who had been in good health until one month before admission, was admitted to the hospital in January 2000 with a history of weakness, fever, nausea and vomiting, headache, and lethargy of four weeks' duration. Physical examination revealed a marked hepatosplenomegaly and cervical lymphadenopathy. The neurologic status was normal. The pupils were equally round and reactive. However, ophthalmological examination revealed a mild papilledema. WBC and differential counts were within normal limits. Analysis of cerebrospinal fluid (CSF) was normal.

Serologic investigation revealed antibodies against brucellosis. The first blood culture for bacterial disease agents was negative. Treatment consisted of a combination of oral tetracycline for 21 days and intramuscular streptomycin for 14 days in adequate pediatric doses.

After completing the course of therapy, a brain CAT was taken in February 2000 because of persistent headaches and a mild papilledema. Six multiple abscesses in the brain, approximately 2 × 2 to 4 × 4 cm in diameter, were found. The patient was transferred to the department of neurosurgery. After a surgical drainage of the abscesses, the patient developed temporary quadriplegia. However, within six weeks he recovered without residual signs and symptoms after repeated drainages. Repeat cultures from blood and abscess material were positive for the causative bacterial pathogen.

On the last CAT scan, obtained in September 2000, the multiple abscesses had disappeared completely.

Questions

I.   Fill in the Blank: Multiple Brain Abscesses

Fill in the blank with the appropriate term.

1. The term for the enlargement of both the liver and spleen is

   _____.

2. What did the initial physical examination of the patient reveal?

   _____

3. What were the findings on initial ophthalmological examination?

   _____

4. Was the first blood culture positive or negative for brucellosis?

   _____

5. What were the two antibiotics used in the treatment for the patient?

   _____

6. What were the routes of administration for the two antibiotics used in treatment? _____

   _____

7. Why was a brain CAT taken in February? _____

8. What were the dimensions of the brain abscesses shown in the CAT?

   _____

9. Was the treatment given to the patient successful in eliminating the multiple abscesses? _____

II.   Spell Check

Circle each incorrectly spelled term and write it correctly in the space provided.

1. absces   _____
2. brucellosis   _____
3. cerebrospinal   _____
4. nurosurgery   _____
5. differential   _____
6. hepatosplenomegaly   _____

7. papiledema   _____

8. quadriplegea   _____

L. *Increasing Your Medical Terminology Word Power 3*

1. Read the following report.
2. Prepare to answer the questions at the end of the section.
3. Circle all unfamiliar terms with a red pencil.
4. Underline familiar terms with a blue pencil.
5. Use your knowledge of word elements, a medical dictionary, and the key terms to find the meaning of unfamiliar terms.

Pontine Hydatid Cyst: An Unusual Case

Key Terms

ataxic (a-TAK-sik) gait   uncoordinated walking

cerebropontine (ser'-ē-brō-PON-tēn)   refers to the connection between the medulla and cerebrum

hydatid (HĪ-da-tid) cyst   cyst produced by young stages of the sheep tapeworm

hypoesthesia (hī'-pō-es-THĒ-zē-a)   dulled sensitivity to touch

inhomogenous (in-hō'-mō-jē-NĒ-us)   lacking uniformity

multicystic   having many cysts

neurinoma (nū-ri-NŌ-ma)   tumor of a peripheral nerve arising from a Schwann cell sheath

otitis (ō-TĪ-tis) media   middle ear infection

paresthesia (par'-es-THĒ-zē-a)   sensation of numbness or tingling

pontine (PON-tēn)   rounded projection on the ventral surface of the brain stem

scolex (SKŌ-lex)   head of a tapeworm

spasm (SPAZ-em)   involuntary sudden movement or convulsive muscular contraction

supratentorial (soo'-pra-ten-TŌ-rē-al)   above the tentorium; the process of the dura mater between the cerebrum and cerebellum supporting the occipital lobes

tactile (TAK-til)   sensation of touch

I NTRODUCTION

Cerebral localization of young forms of the sheep tapeworm, *Echinococcus granulosus* (ē-kī'-nō-KOK-us gran'-ū-LŌ-sus), is a rare occurrence and usually produces single large cysts located in the supratentorial compartment. This report concerns the finding of a pontine hydatid cyst next to a multicystic neurinoma in a cerebropontine site.

C ASE REPORT

A 62-year-old male presented with recurrent right facial pain, right facial spasms, dizziness, nausea, and vomiting. He also complained of progressive numbness of the left leg. The patient's medical history included complete hearing loss in his right ear dating from a childhood episode of otitis media.

Neurologic examination revealed an ataxic gait, hyperreflexic weakness, and tactile and vibratory hypoesthesia of the left leg. Paresthesia was also found associated with the right trigeminal nerve. A cranial magnetic resonance image (MRI) showed an inhomogenous mass in the right cerebellopontine (CP) site and the internal auditory canal that was separated by a thin layer from a round cyst in the mid-pons. The pontine lesion had a considerable mass. No abnormalities of the supratentorial compartment were observed except for a moderate enlargement of the third ventricle.

D IAGNOSIS AND TREATMENT

Three weeks after the MRI, the patient underwent surgery for the removal of the CP mass and the pontine-associated cyst. Histologic examination of the materials removed showed the CP mass to be an acoustic neurinoma and the cyst to be a hydatid cyst containing numerous tapeworm scoleces. Subsequent hepatic sonographic examination revealed two clinically inactive hydatid cysts in the patient. After specific inquiry, the patient indicated that 35 years earlier he had worked as a mason for one year near a sheep slaughter in Argentina.

Questions

I.   Matching

Match the term to its meaning. (The same meaning may be used more than once.) Insert the appropriate letter in the space next to the question number.

Choices:

_____ **1.** ataxic gait
_____ **2.** hypoesthesia
_____ **3.** hydatid cyst
_____ **4.** multicystic
_____ **5.** inhomogenous
_____ **6.** neurinoma
_____ **7.** paresthesia
_____ **8.** otitis media
_____ **9.** scolex
_____ **10.** tactile
_____ **11.** spasm
_____ **12.** supratentorial

a. cyst produced by young sheep tapeworms
b. uncoordinated walking
c. lack of uniformity
d. many cysts
e. middle ear infection
f. tumor of a peripheral nerve arising from a Schwann cell sheath
g. sensation of numbness or tingling
h. convulsive muscular contraction
i. head of a tapeworm
j. above the tentorium
k. sensations of touch
l. dulled sensitivity to touch

II.   Spell Check

Circle each incorrectly spelled term and write it correctly in the space provided.

1. hipoesthesia   _____

2. inhomojenous   _____

3. neurinoma   _____

4. ponteen   _____

5. supratentorial   _____

6. skolex   _____

7. atacksic   _____

8. tacteel   _____

Term Search Challenge

Locate 18 terms in the puzzle.

1. Write the specific term next to its definition. Then find that prefix in the puzzle diagram and circle it.

2. Terms may be read from left to right, backward, up, down, or diagonally.

3. If a term appears more than once, circle it only once. (A term may be found inside others.) Check your answers.

Clues:

1. Central nervous system consists of the _____ and the _____ cord.

2. Peripheral nerves that function involuntarily or automatically without conscious control belong to the _____ nervous system.

3. Collections of nerve tissue outside of the brain and spinal cord (*plural*) _____

4. Individual nerve cell _____

5. The largest part of the brain _____

6. The outer nervous tissue of the cerebrum _____

7. Outermost meninx is the dura _____

8. Branching fiber of nerve cell that is the first part to receive the nervous impulse _____

9. Combining form for the brain _____

10. The space between neurons, through which nerve impulse jumps from one nerve cell to another _____

11. Spaces or canals within the middle part of the cerebrum _____

12. The coverings of the brain and spinal cord _____

13. Nerves that carry impulses toward the brain _____

14. Microscopic fiber that carries the nervous impulse along a nerve _____

15. Abbreviation for cerebrospinal fluid _____

16. Nerves that carry impulses away from the brain and spinal cord to the muscles and _____

17. Combining form for nerve _____

Term Search Puzzle

```
B  S  F  S  C  A  C  O  M  A  P  E  V  C  A
O  R  P  T  O  O  H  O  R  U  E  N  E  E  U
D  S  A  I  F  O  R  S  M  A  P  C  N  R  T
Y  L  T  I  N  R  T  T  A  S  O  E  T  E  O
P  A  L  O  N  A  L  L  E  A  C  P  R  B  N
X  Y  A  I  G  E  L  P  T  X  N  H  I  R  O
C  S  M  G  A  N  G  L  I  A  Y  A  C  U  M
M  R  P  Y  P  P  A  L  S  Y  S  L  L  M  I
A  P  A  I  E  P  A  L  S  S  E  O  E  T  C
T  A  X  N  N  L  P  A  R  E  S  I  S  F  F
E  L  O  H  I  A  O  D  E  N  D  R  I  T  E
R  S  N  I  L  A  L  A  F  F  E  R  E  N  T
V  E  A  C  E  T  L  C  H  O  L  I  N  E  G
E  F  F  E  R  E  N  T  S  Y  N  A  P  S  E
N  E  U  R  O  N  M  E  N  I  N  G  E  S  E
```

Selected Aspects of Psychiatry and Mental Illness

"The key to the understanding of the essence of conscious mental processes lies in the region of the unconscious. . . ."

—Karl Gustav Carus (1789–1869)

INFORMATIONAL CHALLENGE

A. An Introduction to Psychiatry and Psychological Tests

I.   Fill in the Blank

Fill in the blank with the appropriate term.

1. A(n) _____ is the medical specialist who deals with the diagnosis, treatment, and prevention of mental illness.
2. A(n) _____ is a nonmedically educated individual who is trained in methods of psychotherapy, analysis, and research techniques.
3. A medical specialist trained in the use of psychoanalysis is a _____.
4. The specialist dealing with the legal aspects of psychiatry is called a _____.

II.   Matching: Psychological Tests

Match the term to its meaning. (The same meaning may be used more than once.) Insert the appropriate letter in the space next to the question number.

_____ 1. Thematic Apperception Test
_____ 2. Wechsler Adult Intelligence Test
_____ 3. Bender-Gestalt Test

Choices:
a. intelligence test
b. pictures are used to make or to form a story
c. inkblots are used to bring out associations

_____ **4.** Rorschach Test or technique

_____ **5.** Goodenough-Harris Drawing Test

_____ **6.** Minnesota Multiphasic Personality Inventory

_____ **7.** Draw-a-Person Test

_____ **8.** Adaptive Behavior Scales

_____ **9.** Bayley Scales of Infant Development

d. individual is asked to draw geometric designs

e. used to reveal personality characteristics such as an ability to relate to others

f. individual is asked to draw a body

g. evaluates abilities and habits in behavioral areas

h. evaluates mental and psychomotor development in children under two years of age

III.   Spell Check

Circle each incorrectly spelled term and write it correctly in the space provided.

1. pychiatry   _____

2. psychologist   _____

3. psychology   _____

4. forensic   _____

5. Rorshach   _____

6. Apperception   _____

7. Gestalt   _____

8. multiphasic   _____

B. Mental or Psychiatric Disorders and Illnesses

I.   Fill in the Blank

Fill in the blank with the appropriate term.

1. The fear of high places is called _____.

2. Alternating moods of mania and depression are known as _____ illness.

3. Illnesses triggered by emotional factors are known as being _____.

4. A personality disorder in which the individual is continually suspicious and mistrustful of others is referred to as a(n) _____ state.

5. Sexual disorders are divided into two types: _____ and _____.

6. The presence of a persistent delusion (false belief) not caused by any other mental disorder is typical of the psychiatric disorder known as a(n) _____ disorder.

7. The psychiatric condition in which an individual's mental conflicts are expressed as physical signs and symptoms is called a(n) _____ disorder.

II.   Matching 1: Psychiatric Signs and Symptoms

Match the term to its meaning. (The same meaning may be used more than once.) Insert the appropriate letter in the space next to the question number.

Choices:

_____ **1.** amnesia

_____ **2.** autism

a. false personal belief

b. loss of memory

_____ **3.** delusion
_____ **4.** dysphoria
_____ **5.** apathy
_____ **6.** hypochondria
_____ **7.** aggression
_____ **8.** paranoia
_____ **9.** hallucination

c. complete withdrawal
d. lack of interest
e. hostile attitude
f. an exaggerated feeling of sadness
g. imagining illnesses
h. overly suspicious and feeling persecuted
i. hearing or seeing things not present

III.   Matching 2: Psychiatric or Mental Disorders

_____ **1.** affective disorders
_____ **2.** psychoses
_____ **3.** neurosis
_____ **4.** personality disorder
_____ **5.** organic mental disorders
_____ **6.** disorders suggesting organic disease

_____ **7.** sexual disorder
_____ **8.** anxiety disorder
_____ **9.** psychoactive-substance use disorder
_____ **10.** delusional disorder
_____ **11.** sexual disorders
_____ **12.** somatoform disorders

Choices:

a. all mental disorders that have no obvious demonstrable organic basis
b. a major disturbance of thinking and behavior in which contact with reality is lost
c. mental disturbances caused by brain lesions
d. a long-lasting, poor adaptation of behavior suggesting a distortion of personality development
e. condition in which there is an alteration of moods
f. conditions involving distress and inappropriate tension
g. voluntary or involuntary production of symptoms to obtain medical attention
h. psychological sexual identity differs from a physical one
i. condition in which the presence of a persistent delusion (false belief) is not caused by any other mental disorder
j. disorders associated with the regular use of psychoactive substances that affect the CNS
k. disorders in which sexual arousal requires unusual fantasies
l. a disorder in which an individual's mental problems are expressed as physical signs

IV.   Spell Check

Circle each incorrectly spelled term and write it correctly in the space provided.

1. amesia   _____
2. autism   _____
3. hallucination   _____
4. hypocondria   _____
5. narcissism   _____
6. uphoria   _____
7. schizofrenia   _____

8. transsexualism _____

9. anorexia _____

10. bulimia _____

C. Word Elements Associated with Psychiatry

I. Fill in the Blank

Fill in the blank with the appropriate term.

1. List three combining forms to indicate the mind.

_____, _____, and

_____

2. Give the suffix for fear. _____

II. Matching

Match the term to its meaning. (The same meaning may be used more than once.) Insert the appropriate letter in the space next to the question number.

Choices:

_____ 1. phas/o   **a.** self

_____ 2. psych/o   **b.** mind

_____ 3. -thymia   **c.** feeling

_____ 4. auto-   **d.** speech

_____ 5. -phoria   **e.** sleep

_____ 6. -somnia   **f.** obsessive occupation

_____ 7. -mania   **g.** movement

_____ 8. -kinesia   **h.** body

_____ 9. somat/o   **i.** down

_____ 10. cata-   **j.** split

_____ 11. schiz/o

III. Spell Check 1

Circle each incorrectly spelled term and write it correctly in the space provided.

1. phonofobia _____

2. psychiatrist _____

3. shizophrenia _____

4. psychosomatic _____

5. pyromania _____

6. euphoria _____

7. catatonic _____

8. dysthymia _____

IV. Spell Check 2

Circle each incorrectly spelled term and write it correctly in the space provided.

1. delirum _____

2. pychiaty _____

3. Wechsler _____

4. Minnesota _____

5. pneumoencephalogram _____

6. electroshock   _____

7. Apperception   _____

V.   Word Analysis: Word Elements Associated with Psychiatry

Table 25-8 lists a number of terms with their pronunciations and definitions.

TABLE 25-8   WORD ANALYSIS: WORD ELEMENTS ASSOCIATED WITH PSYCHIATRY

Term and Pronunciation	Brief Explanation
aphasia (a-FĀ-zē-a)	absence or impairment of the ability to speak
dysphoria (dis-FŌ-rē-a)	exaggerated feeling of depression; discomfort
autism (AW-tizm)	a form of thinking in which the attention is fixed on the individual's own ego (self-centered), and with a complete disregard for reality
catatonia (kat-a-TŌ-nē-a)	a phase of schizophrenia in which the individual is not able to move or talk
cyclothymic (sī-klō-THĪ-mik)	pertaining to cyclic variation in moods of a manic-depressive individual; mood swings
hyperkinesis (hī-per-ki-NĒ-sis)	abnormally increased muscular movement and activity
kleptomania (klep-tō-MĀ-nē-a)	impulsive stealing
mental (MEN-tal)	pertaining to the mind
psychiatrist (sī-KĪ-a-trist)	a physician who specializes in the study, prevention, and treatment of mental disorders
psychosomatic (sī-kō-sō-MAT-ik)	pertaining to the relationship between the mind and body
pyrophobia (pī-rō-FO-bē-a)	abnormal fear of fire
schizophrenia (skiz-ō-FREN-ē-a)	group of severe mental disorders marked by disturbances in behavior, ability to think logically, and hallucinations (ha-loo-si-NĀ-shuns)

1. Analyze each term.
2. Circle all prefixes, word roots, combining forms, and suffixes and label them **p, wr, cf**, and **s**, respectively.
3. Check your answers (shown in Table 25-9).

D. *Medical Vocabulary Building*

I.   Matching

Match the term to its meaning. (The same meaning may be used more than once.)
Insert the appropriate letter in the space next to the question number.

_____ 1. atelomyelia	_____ 11. meningopathy
_____ 2. cephalalgia	_____ 12. myelophthisis
_____ 3. cordotomy	_____ 13. oligodendroglioma
_____ 4. diplegia	_____ 14. phagomania
_____ 5. diskectomy	_____ 15. rachiomyelitis
_____ 6. epidural	_____ 16. sympathectomy
_____ 7. hemianopsis	_____ 17. vagotomy
_____ 8. hypermnesia	_____ 18. agoraphobia
_____ 9. hypnology	_____ 19. akathisia
_____ 10. logomania	_____ 20. endorphins

Choices:

a. a condition of imperfect spinal cord development
b. head pain
c. surgical incision into the spinal cord; usually done for pain relief
d. surgical incision of an intervertebral disk
e. paralysis of identical parts of both sides of the body
f. pertaining to a position situated on the dura mater
g. blindness of half the field of vision in one or both eyes
h. a condition in which there is an excellent recall (memory) of dates, names, and details of events
i. the study of sleep
j. an excessive, continuous, and repetitious flow of speech; seen in certain forms of mental illness such as monomania
k. any disease involving the meninges
l. a wasting away of the spinal cord
m. a malignant tumor originating from and consisting of oligodendroglia
n. spinal cord inflammation
o. an abnormal craving (madness) for food
p. surgical incision of the vagus nerve
q. surgical excision of a portion of the sympathetic nervous system
r. an inability to remain still
s. abnormal fear of being alone in public places
t. brain-produced chemical substances that act as natural analgesics

II. Spell Check

Circle each incorrectly spelled term and write it correctly in the space provided.

1. endofins _____
2. rachomyelitis _____
3. myelofthisis _____
4. diskectomy _____
5. cordotomy _____
6. akathisia _____
7. oligodendroglioma _____
8. hypermnesia _____
9. atelomyelia _____
10. epidurel _____

E. *Abbreviations Associated with Mental Disorders, Psychiatric Tests, and Professional Organizations*

I.   Matching 1: Mental Disorders and Therapy

Match the term to its meaning. (The same meaning may be used more than once.)
Insert the appropriate letter in the space next to the question number.

Choices:

_____	**1.** EST	**a.** organic brain syndrome
_____	**2.** OBS	**b.** delirium tremens
_____	**3.** CR	**c.** electroshock therapy
_____	**4.** CA	**d.** *Diagnostic and Statistical Manual of Mental Disorders*
_____	**5.** DT	
_____	**6.** DSM	**e.** electroconvulsive therapy
_____	**7.** CVA	**f.** cerebrovascular accident
_____	**8.** ECT	**g.** conditioned reflex
_____	**9.** SR	**h.** chronologic age
		i. stimulus response

II.   Matching 2: Psychiatric Tests and Associated Organizations

Choices:

_____	**1.** ADA-MHA	**a.** American Board of Psychiatry and Neurology
_____	**2.** ABPN	
_____	**3.** MMPI	**b.** Alcohol, Drug Abuse, and Mental Health Administration
_____	**4.** MHA	
_____	**5.** NIMH	**c.** Child's Apperception Test
_____	**6.** TAT	**d.** Mental Health Association
_____	**7.** WISC	**e.** National Institute for Mental Health (U.S.)
_____	**8.** CAI	
		f. Thematic Apperception Test
		g. Minnesota Multiphasic Personality Inventory
		h. Wechsler Intelligence Scale for Children

F. *Increasing Your Medical Terminology Word Power 1*

1. Read the following report.
2. Prepare to answer the questions at the end of the section.
3. Circle all unfamiliar terms with a red pencil.
4. Underline familiar terms with a blue pencil.
5. Use your knowledge of word elements, a medical dictionary, and the key terms to find the meaning of unfamiliar terms.

Insomnia

Key Terms

anxiety (ang-ZĪ-e-tē)   feelings of worry, uneasiness, or fear, especially of the future

apnea (AP-nē-a)   temporary stopping of breathing

hypnotic medications   drugs capable of inducing sleep

insomnia (in-SOM-nē-a)   inability to sleep, difficulty staying asleep, or awakening early

myoclonus (mī-OK-lō-nus)   muscle twitching

psychotherapy (sī-kō-THER-a-pē)   treating diseases such as nervous disorders by mental approaches rather than by physical means such as surgery, and so on

I NTRODUCTION

Insomnia is considered to be the most common sleep complaint. Surveys of large percentages of the general population indicate that about one-third of those asked complain of sleeping difficulty. Among the various medical specialists, psychiatrists report the highest percentage of patients who complain of insomnia.

Although it is rare before the age of twenty, more than 40% of the general population report insomnia after the age of sixty. The complaint is most frequent among women and persons in lower economic groups. Several characteristic behaviors are related to insomnia. During the day and at bedtime, individuals report difficulty relaxing and frequently describe themselves as tense, anxious, worried, and depressed.

C AUSES

The most common complaint of insomniacs (in-SOM-nē-aks) is simply difficulty falling asleep, difficulty in staying asleep, or awakening early. Sleeping difficulties often begin before the age of forty and may continue for many years.

Medical conditions, particularly those involving pain, discomfort, anxiety, or depression, commonly cause sleep difficulty. Such conditions also may include cardiovascular (kar-dē-ō-VAS-kū-lar), pulmonary, gastrointestinal, renal, endocrine, and neurological disorders. Several stimulant drugs and the large quantities of caffeine (kaf-EEN) contained in coffee, tea, or cola drinks, if taken close to bedtime, may cause difficulty falling asleep. Sleep apnea and myoclonus at night are infrequent causes.

S OME APPROACHES TO MANAGEMENT

The key to dealing successfully with insomnia may require evaluating the entire person and not focusing only on the symptom of insomnia. Approaches used to promote better sleep include general measures such as daily activity and exercise before bedtime, reducing or eliminating factors that interrupt sleep, relaxation training, and other activities that can reduce stress. More specific approaches can involve psychotherapy and hypnotic medications.

Questions

I.   Fill in the Blank

Fill in the blank with the appropriate term.

  1. What percentage of the general population reports insomnia after the age of sixty? _____

  2. What are the most common complaints of insomniacs?

  _____

3. What stimulant drug may cause difficulty falling asleep?

_____

4. What is the term for a temporary cessation of breathing?

_____

5. What is the term for muscle twitching? _____

II.   Spell Check

Circle each incorrectly spelled term and write it correctly in the space provided.

1. anziety   _____
2. apnea   _____
3. myoclonus   _____
4. sikotherapy   _____
5. insonmiac   _____
6. psychatrist   _____

G. Increasing Your Medical Terminology Word Power 2

1. Read the following report.
2. Prepare to answer the questions at the end of the section.
3. Circle all unfamiliar terms with a red pencil.
4. Underline familiar terms with a blue pencil.
5. Use your knowledge of word elements, a medical dictionary, and the key terms to find the meaning of unfamiliar terms.

Depression Among Women in Their Reproductive Years

Key Terms

antidepressant (an'-ti-dē-PRES-sant)   usually a medication that acts to prevent, cure, or relieve depression

bloating (BLŌ-ting)   refers to causing swelling or being swollen

comorbid (kō-MOR-bid)   pertains to acting together to cause a condition

dysphoric (dis-FŌ-rik)   pertaining to being depressed

exacerbate (eks-AS-er-bāte)   to increase or aggravate severity of a condition

insomnia (in-SOM-nē-a)   inability to sleep at times when one is expected to do so

labile (LĀ-bīl)   unsteady; rapidly changing

migraine (MĪ-grān)   severe sudden headaches, frequently on one side of the head; usually accompanied by blurred and disordered vision and nausea

psychosis (sī-KŌ-sis)   mental disorder causing personality disintegration and loss of contact with reality

psychotic (sī-KOT-ik)   pertains to psychosis or to be affected by psychosis

psychotropic (sī-kō-TRŌ-pik)   medications that affect psychological function, behavior, or experience

sequela (sē-KWĒ-la)   a condition following and resulting from a disease; _plural,_ sequelae

serotonin (ser-ō-TŌN-in)   a chemical found in platelets, gastrointestinal mucosa, and other locations; causes constriction of blood vessels

symptomatic (simp-tō-MAT-ik)   concerning a symptom

toxicity (toks-IS-i-tē)   extent or degree of being poisonous

I NTRODUCTION

Major depression is recognized as a significant worldwide public health problem. Depressive disorders are the most common psychiatric problems encountered in primary-care settings, and in the United States the economic cost associated with them rivals that of cardiovascular disease.

Although depression is not considered a gender-specific disorder, clear differences exist in the occurrence of depressive syndromes in men and women. A number of studies indicate that women experience depression more often and in different ways than men. Indeed, women present major depression twice as often as men. The reasons for the differences are unclear, but both biological and psychological factors are believed to play a role. The above-mentioned findings have led to new research investigations concerning specific mood syndromes such as premenstrual dysphoric disorder (PMDD) and postpartum depression (PPD).

Certain comorbid conditions with sign-and-symptom profiles similar to depression, such as anxiety disorders and thyroid gland disorders, have a higher incidence in women than in men. Growing lines of evidence also indicate that normal fluctuations in certain reproductive hormone levels uncover depressive symptoms in women who are more valuable for this type of study of from a genetic and/or psychologic standpoint. From a psychosocial perspective, the continuing struggle to cope with ever-changing societal roles may offer insight into women's higher incidence of depression.

P REMENSTRUAL DYSPHORIC DISORDER

The cause, diagnosis, and treatment of premenstrual dysphoric disorder (PMDD) have been the subjects of a significant body of research. Although many women experience some degree of discomfort in the week before menses, only a small percentage of them, 5 to 7%, have the signs and symptoms typical of true PMDD. Patients with this disorder are usually symptomatic only during the 7 to 10 days before menses. Other conditions such as major depression and thyroid disorders persist throughout the menstrual cycle. The condition of possible PMDD patients should be differentiated from other medical or psychiatric disorders. Patients who present with PMDD should clearly undergo a complete physical examination that concentrates on any and all possible causes of their range of signs and symptoms such as bloating, food cravings, labile mood, and poor concentration. A key symptom that often causes an individual to seek treatment is severe irritability. In addition, some medical conditions such as migraine headaches may be exacerbated during the premenstrual period, which makes diagnosis of PMDD even more difficult.

T REATMENT

Once PMDD is diagnosed, a number of treatment options are available. These include psychotropic and hormonal therapies. However, the most promising appears to be the use of selective serotonin reuptake inhibitor antidepressants. Doses prescribed are generally the starting doses used to treat depression. The most problematic side effect noted is sexual dysfunction. This problem should be brought to the attention of the patient and discussed honestly before treatment is started.

$\mathcal{D}$ EPRESSION DURING AND FOLLOWING PREGNANCY

The lifetime risk of depression for women aged 25 to 44 years of age ranges from 10 to 25 percent. At one time pregnancy was regarded as being protective against the risk of a psychiatric disorder. However, numerous studies have shown that pregnant and nonpregnant women have an equivalent risk of depression. Patients who are coping with depression issues may be in one of the following categories:

1. Women planning a pregnancy, yet who require supportive maintenance therapy for their pregnancy;

2. Pregnant women who become depressed;

3. Women who have an unexpected pregnancy while taking an antidepressant.

Although initiating or continuing antidepressant medication during pregnancy always deserves concern, both physicians and patients need to recognize the risks of untreated depression, which include malnutrition, insomnia, possible use of illicit substances, refusal of prenatal care, and psychotic disorders. Psychosis is of particular concern because it may include delusions or hallucinations that result in behavior that could endanger the patient and/or the fetus.

The evaluation of the use of antidepressant medication for pregnant patients should take into consideration factors such as the risk of fetal malformation, neonatal toxicity, and behavioral sequelae caused by drug exposure. To date, no psychotropic medication has been approved by the United States Food and Drug Administration (FDA) for use by pregnant women. Most antidepressant drugs are classified as FDA category C, which includes drugs that have either demonstrated harmful effects on lower animals or for which studies with humans are lacking.

Questions

I.   Matching

Match the term to its meaning. (The same meaning may be used more than once.) Insert the appropriate letter in the space next to the question number.

_____	**1.** bloating		_____	**7.** migraine
_____	**2.** comorbid		_____	**8.** psychosis
_____	**3.** dysphoric		_____	**9.** psychotic
_____	**4.** exacerbate		_____	**10.** psychotropic
_____	**5.** insomnia		_____	**11.** sequela
_____	**6.** labile		_____	**12.** toxicity

Choices:

a. to increase or aggravate severity of condition
b. pertains to acting together to cause a condition
c. refers to causing swelling or being swollen
d. inability to sleep at times when one is expected to do so
e. pertaining to being depressed
f. unsteady
g. mental disorder causing personality disintegration and loss of contact with reality

    h. severe sudden headaches, frequently on one side of the head; usually accompanied by blurred and disordered vision together with nausea

    i. medications that affect psychic function, behavior, or experience

    j. pertains to or affected by psychosis

    k. a condition following and resulting from a disease

    l. extent or degree of being poisonous

II.   Spell Check

Circle each incorrectly spelled term and write it correctly in the space provided.

    1. antidepresant _____

    2. exaserbated _____

    3. labile _____

    4. postpartum _____

    5. secuelae _____

    6. disphoric _____

    7. insomnia _____

    8. migraine _____

    9. psykhotropic _____

    10. serotonen _____

H. Increasing Your Medical Terminology Word Power 3

    1. Read the following report.

    2. Prepare to answer the questions at the end of the section.

    3. Circle all unfamiliar terms with a red pencil.

    4. Underline familiar terms with a blue pencil.

    5. Use your knowledge of word elements, a medical dictionary, and the key terms to find the meaning of unfamiliar terms.

Selected Aspects of Alzheimer's Disease

Key Terms

acetylcholine (as-e'-til-KŌ-lēn)   a chemical known to play an important role in nerve impulse transmissions at synapses

amyloid (AM-i-loyd)   a protein-polysaccharide complex having starch-like properties produced and deposited in tissues during certain pathological situations.

apolipoprotein (ap'-ō-lip'-ō-PRŌ-tēn)   a nonlipid protein portion of a lipoprotein; functions include binding to specific enzymes

cognitive (KOG-ni-tiv) function   refers to the mental process by which knowledge is acquired

dementia (dē-MEN-shē-a)   a severe impairment of cognitive (intellectual) function that is usually progressive and that interferes with normal occupational and social activities

microglia (mī-KROG-lē-a)   nervous tissue that forms the supportive elements of the nervous system

neurofibril (nū-rō-FĪ-bril)   many extremely small fibrils (threads) that extend in every direction in the nerve cell body; *neurofibrilla* (nū-rō-FI-bril-a) extend into the axon and dendrites of the cell

neuropathological (nū'-rō-path'-ō-LOJ-i-kal)   pertaining to disease of nerves

preclinical (prē-KLIN-i-kal)   occurring before diagnosis of a definite disease is possible

I NTRODUCTION

The German neurologist Alois Alzheimer, in 1907, identified the disease that bears his name. The condition, *Alzheimer's* (ALTS-hī-merz) *disease*, is generally described as a chronic disorder with a gradual onset and slow progressive course that typically results in an inevitable deterioration of cognitive function. This general description can apply to several illnesses, called dementias, in which parts of the brain stop working, causing disruptions in emotional stability, memory, judgment, and reasoning ability. Most dementias occur more frequently as people age. About 15 percent of persons who reach the age of 65 will develop some type of dementia. Furthermore, by age 85 the proportion increases to at least 35 percent. Of all the dementias, Alzheimer's disease is the most common.

F EATURES OF THE DISEASE

Microscopic views of the brains of patients with Alzheimer's disease show extensive loss of nerve cells in certain regions, including the hippocampus, a center for memory, and the cerebral cortex, the part involved in language, memory, reasoning, and other important thought processes. Early research findings demonstrated that the dying neurons communicate by means of the neurotransmitter acetylcholine, which is ultimately broken down by the enzyme acetylcholinesterase.

Other observable findings in the brains of patients include the presence of clusters of proteins and accumulations of beta-amyloid proteins. The protein clusters occur in these two forms inside nerve cells that are called neurofibrillary tangles, spring-like threads that appear as pairs of strands wound around each other. In the 1980s the tangles were found to consist of a particular protein called *tau*. The amyloid protein deposits occur in the spaces between neurons, causing nearby nerve cells to appear swollen and deformed. The amyloid protein accumulations, sometimes referred to as senile or amyloid plaques, are generally accompanied by reactive inflammatory cells known as microglia. Such cells are part of the brain's immune system and, according to some viewpoints, might actually be trying to remove damaged neurons and the amyloid protein.

O CCURRENCE AND CONTRIBUTING FACTORS

Exactly when the neuropathological changes appear clinically is not known. One of the major areas of research is the identification of the signs and specific indicators, known as markers, of its preclinical phase. Prospective studies of patients without clinically evident dementia show that subtle signs and symptoms may develop several years, or even decades, before dementia can be diagnosed. Affected individuals experiencing the initial preclinical phase have a mild impairment of verbal memory, with later difficulty in their ability to pay attention and in their language capability, spatial orientation, and psychomotor speed.

Persons without dementia who are at increased risk for Alzheimer's disease include individuals who have a family history of Alzheimer's disease, Down's syndrome, and a particular genetic factor known as the apolipoprotein E gene.

Questions

I.   Matching

Match the term to its meaning. (The same meaning may be used more than once.) Insert the appropriate letter in the space next to the question number.

_____ **1.** acetylcholine   _____ **6.** microglia
_____ **2.** amyloid   _____ **7.** neurofibril
_____ **3.** apolipoprotein   _____ **8.** neuropathological
_____ **4.** cognitive function   _____ **9.** preclinical
_____ **5.** dementia

Choices:

a. a nonlipid protein portion of a lipoprotein; functions include binding to specific enzymes

b. a chemical known to play an important role in nerve impulse transmissions

c. a protein-polysaccharide complex having starch-like properties, produced and deposited in tissues during certain pathological situations

d. a severe impairment of cognitive (intellectual) function that is usually progressive and that interferes with normal occupational and social activities

e. nervous tissue that forms the supportive elements of the nervous system

f. refers to the mental process by which knowledge is acquired

g. pertaining to diseases of nerves

h. many extremely small fibrils (threads) that extend in every direction in the nerve cell

i. occurring before diagnosis of a definite disease is possible

II.   Spell Check

Circle each incorrectly spelled term and write it correctly in the space provided.

1. aceylcholinesterase _____
2. Alzehimer's   _____
3. dementias   _____
4. neurofibrilary   _____
5. neurotransmitter   _____
6. acetylcholin   _____
7. cognitive   _____
8. mikrogalia   _____
9. newropathological   _____
10. amyliod   _____

Term Search Challenge

Locate 14 terms in the puzzle.

1. Write the specific term next to its definition. Then find that term in the puzzle diagram and circle it.

2. Terms may be read from left to right, backward, up, down, or diagonally.

3. If a term appears more than once, circle it only once. (A term or abbreviation may be found inside others.)

4. Check your answers.

Clues:

1. any morbid fear _____

2. sleepwalking _____

3. false beliefs resulting from unconscious needs _____

4. false sensory perceptions without actual external stimulation

_____

5. clinical drugs producing hallucinations _____

6. abbreviation for intelligence quotient _____

7. term for loss of memory _____

8. term for condition in which the individual is completely withdrawn and is unable to communicate _____

9. term for an exaggerated feeling of well-being _____

10. term for a state of morbid sadness, dejection, or melancholy

_____

11. self-love or infatuation _____

12. a phase of schizophrenia in which the individual is not able to move or talk _____

13. term for increased muscular movement and activity

_____

14. a physician who specializes in the study, prevention, and treatment of mental disorders _____

Term Search Puzzle

```
D  Y  S  P  H  O  R  I  A  O  P  Q  N  R  D
T  S  I  R  T  A  I  H  C  Y  S  P  O  S  E
P  H  O  B  I  A  L  O  S  A  N  G  I  T  L
H  A  L  L  U  C  I  N  O  G  E  N  S  X  U
N  U  E  M  S  I  L  U  B  M  A  N  M  O  S
A  T  R  C  A  T  A  T  O  N  I  A  E  W  I
R  I  N  C  A  A  L  I  F  O  R  N  R  S  O
C  S  J  R  M  D  E  P  R  E  S  S  I  O  N
I  M  A  K  N  R  H  F  I  L  A  A  E  V  S
S  A  S  A  E  D  E  U  P  H  O  R  I  A  L
S  T  N  F  S  L  O  S  G  E  T  Z  O  O  A
I  I  Q  A  I  A  N  M  L  E  I  N  A  X  N
S  I  S  E  N  I  K  R  E  P  Y  H  A  T  E
M  H  A  L  L  U  C  I  N  A  T  I  O  N  S
```

CHAPTER 26

The Sense Organs: Eye and Ear

"It is characteristic of Science and Progress that they continually open new fields to our vision."

—Louis Pasteur

INFORMATIONAL CHALLENGE

A. Eye Structure and Function

I.   Fill in the Blank

Fill in the blank with the appropriate term.

1. The area of sharpest vision in the retina is known as the
   _____.
2. The two main cavities of the eye are the _____
   chamber and the _____ chamber.
3. The pigmented portion of the eye is called the
   _____.
4. The portion of the eye that bends (refracts) and focuses light on the
   fovea centralis is the _____.
5. The two types of light-sensitive or photosensitive cells found in the
   eye are the _____ and the
   _____.

II.   Matching

Match the term to its meaning. (The same meaning may be used more than once.)
Insert the appropriate letter in the space next to the question number.

_____ **1.** conjunctiva   _____ **6.** cornea
_____ **2.** lacrimal gland   _____ **7.** vitreous humor
_____ **3.** sclera   _____ **8.** optic disk
_____ **4.** pupil   _____ **9.** macula lutea
_____ **5.** retina

Choices:

a. gives shape to and protects the eye
b. opening in the center of the lens
c. lining of the eyelid
d. contains the photoreceptors of the eye
e. contains the vitreous humor

f. secretes tears
g. outer surface of the eye
h. the area where the optic nerve joins the retina
i. the yellow spot in the retina containing the fovea centralis

III.   Spell Check

Circle each incorrectly spelled term and write it correctly in the space provided.

1. vitreos _____
2. sclera _____
3. coroid _____
4. iri _____
5. acommodation _____
6. conjunctiva _____
7. lakrimal _____
8. pupil _____

IV.   Vision Quiz: Structures of the Eye

Figure 26-9 shows the structures of the eye. Identify and write the name of the numbered components in the spaces provided.

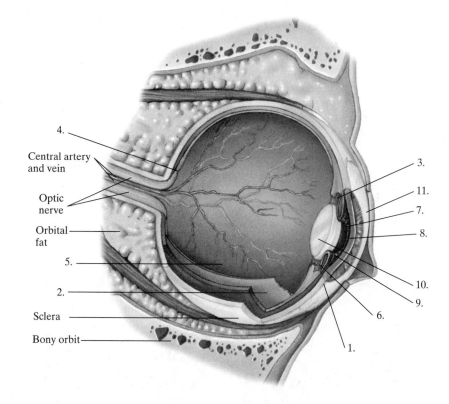

FIGURE 26-9   Vision Quiz. The internal anatomy of the eye.

Choices:

1. _____   **a.** conjunctiva
2. _____   **b.** anterior chamber
3. _____   **c.** optic nerve
4. _____   **d.** posterior chamber

5. _____	**e.** lens
6. _____	**f.** iris
7. _____	**g.** sclera
8. _____	**h.** posterior cavity
9. _____	**i.** retina
10. _____	**j.** fovea centralis
11. _____	**k.** cornea

B. Word Elements Associated with the Eye

I.   Fill in the Blank

Fill in the blank with the appropriate term.

1. Give two combining forms for eyelid. _____ and
   _____

2. List three word roots for eye. _____,
   _____, and _____

3. Give three word roots for pupil. _____,
   _____, and _____

II.   Matching 1: Combining Forms and/or Word Roots for the Eye, Part 1

Match the term to its meaning. (The same meaning may be used more than once.)
Insert the appropriate letter in the space next to the question number.

Choices:

_____ **1.** ambly	**a.** water
_____ **2.** choroid/o	**b.** pupil
_____ **3.** aque	**c.** iris
_____ **4.** kerat/o	**d.** eyelid
_____ **5.** cycl/o	**e.** dull
_____ **6.** palpebr	**f.** choroid layer
_____ **7.** blephar	**g.** cornea
_____ **8.** core/o	**h.** lacrimal duct
_____ **9.** dacry/o	**i.** ciliary body of the eye
_____ **10.** irid/o	

III.   Matching 2: Combining Forms and/or Word Roots for the Eye, Part 2

Match the term to its meaning. (The same meaning may be used more than once.)
Insert the appropriate letter in the space next to the question number.

Choices:

_____ **1.** lacrim/o	**a.** glassy
_____ **2.** sclera/o	**b.** uvea
_____ **3.** presb/o	**c.** retina
_____ **4.** vitra	**d.** old age
_____ **5.** uve	**e.** tear duct
_____ **6.** retin/o	**f.** sclera
_____ **7.** phot/o	**g.** crystalline lens of the eye
_____ **8.** phac/o	**h.** light
_____ **9.** phak/o	

IV.   Spell Check

Circle each incorrectly spelled term and write it correctly in the space provided.

1. dacryohea   _____
2. keretoconjunctivitis   _____
3. corneal   _____
4. blefaritis   _____
5. scleritis   _____
6. corectasis   _____
7. aqeous   _____
8. retinopathy   _____
9. uvel   _____
10. ophthalmalgia   _____

V.   Word Analysis: Word Roots, Combining Forms, and Suffixes Associated with the Eye

Table 26-14 lists a number of terms with their pronunciations and definitions.

TABLE 26-14   WORD ANALYSIS: WORD ROOTS, COMBINING FORMS, AND SUFFIXES ASSOCIATED WITH THE EYE

Term and Pronunciation	Brief Explanation
amblyopia (am-blē-Ō-pē-a)	dim or dull vision
aqueous (A-kwē-us)	pertaining to water
blepharitis (blef-ar-Ī-tis)	inflammation of eyelid edges
choroidoretinitis (kō-royd-ō-ret-in-Ī-tis)	inflammation of the choroids and retina
conjunctivoma (kon-junk-ti-VŌ-ma)	a tumor of the conjunctiva
corectasis (kor-EK-ta-sis)	dilation of the pupil
coreometer (kō-rē-OM-e-ter) corneal (KOR-nē-al)	instrument used to measure the pupil pertaining to the cornea
cyclectomy (sī-KLEK-tō-mē)	excision of a portion of the ciliary body of the eye
dacryorrhea (dak-rē-ō-RĒ-a)	excessive flow of tears
iridocystectomy (ir-i-dō-sis-TEK-tō-mē)	excision of a cyst from the iris
iritis (i-RĪT-is)	inflammation of the iris
keratoconjunctivitis (ker-a-tō-con-junk-ti-VĪ-tis)	inflammation of the cornea and conjunctiva

(Continued)

TABLE 26-14 (CONTINUED)

Term and Pronunciation	Brief Explanation
lacrimal (LAK-rim-al)	pertaining to tears
palpebritis (pal-pe-BRĪ-tis)	inflammation of the eyelid
oculopupillary (ok-ū-lō-PYŪ-pi-lar-ē)	pertaining to the pupil of the eye
ophthalmalgia (of-thal-MAL-jē-a)	eye pain
optical (OP-ti-kal)	pertaining to the eye, or vision
phacolysis (fa-KOL-i-sis)	destruction of the crystalline lens

1. Analyze each term.
2. Circle all combining forms, word roots, and suffixes, and label them **cf**, **wr**, and **s**, respectively.
3. Check your answers (shown in Table 26-16).

C. Eye Disorders and Diseases

I.   Matching 1: Focusing Defects and Problems

Match the term to its meaning. (The same meaning may be used more than once.) Insert the appropriate letter in the space provided next to the question number.

Choices:

_____ 1. normal vision
_____ 2. uneven focusing
_____ 3. farsightedness
_____ 4. near-sightedness
_____ 5. loss of eyeball elasticity
_____ 6. close objects are blurred
_____ 7. abnormal increase in intraocular pressure
_____ 8. abnormality in position of the eye
_____ 9. clouding of the lens
_____ 10. separation of visual layer from underlying pigment layer of the eye

a. hyperopia
b. myopia
c. emmetropia
d. astigmatism
e. presbyopia
f. retinal detachment
g. cataract
h. strabismus
i. glaucoma

II.   Matching 2: Eye Infections, Irritations, and Related Conditions

Match the term to its meaning. (The same meaning may be used more than once.) Insert the appropriate letter in the space provided next to the question number.

Choices:

_____ 1. infection of the eyelash
_____ 2. stye

a. conjunctivitis
b. chalazion

_____ **3.** inflammation of conjunctiva

_____ **4.** inflammation of the cornea

_____ **5.** blocked sebaceous gland ducts

_____ **6.** nvoluntary, rapid eye movement

c. keratitis

d. nystagmus

e. hordeolum

f. blepharitis

III.   Matching 3: Procedures for Diagnosis and Treatment

Match the term to its meaning. (The same meaning may be used more than once.)
Insert the appropriate letter in the space provided next to the question number.

_____ **1.** use of light beam to detect refraction problems

_____ **2.** visual examination of eye's interior

_____ **3.** measurement of intraocular pressure

_____ **4.** examination of anterior chamber angle

_____ **5.** a test for vision clarity

_____ **6.** measures range of vision (peripheral vision)

_____ **7.** use of fluorescein dye for examination of blood flow in the eye

_____ **8.** restoring normal eye coordination

_____ **9.** used for blood coagulation in the eye's interior

Choices:

a. gonioscopy

b. retinoscopy

c. ophthalmoscopy

d. visual acuity

e. tonometry

f. visual field testing

g. orthoptic training

h. fluorescein angiography

i. laser photocoagulation

IV.   Spell Check

Circle each incorrectly spelled term and write it correctly in the space provided.

1. strabissmus _____

2. amblyopia _____

3. ophthamology _____

4. optomitrist _____

5. hordeolum _____

6. glaucoma _____

7. tonommetry _____

8. goniscopy _____

D. *Medical Vocabulary Building*

I.   Matching

Match the term to its meaning. (The same meaning may be used more than once.)
Insert the appropriate letter in the space next to the question number.

Choices:

_____ **1.** anisocoria

_____ **2.** aphakia

_____ **3.** cycloplegia

_____ **4.** dacryoma

a. the absence of the crystalline lens

b. unequal pupils

c. a tumor-like swelling caused by tear duct blockage

_____ **5.** ectropion

_____ **6.** iridodesis

_____ **7.** iridotasis

_____ **8.** nyctalopia

_____ **9.** optomyometer

_____ **10.** phacolysis

_____ **11.** entropion

_____ **12.** miotic

_____ **13.** trichiasis

_____ **14.** pterygium

d. ciliary muscle paralysis

e. a process turning the edge of an eyelid outward

f. stretching of the iris

g. surgical binding of a part of the iris to form an artificial one

h. night blindness

i. instrument used to measure eye muscle strength

j. surgical destruction of crystalline lens

k. pertaining to an agent that causes contraction of the pupil

l. inward turning of the lower eyelid margin

m. abnormal triangular fold of membrane that extends from the conjunctiva to the cornea

n. ingrowing eyelashes that rub against the cornea resulting in eyeball irritation

II.   Spell Check

Circle each incorrectly spelled term and write it correctly in the space provided.

1. terygium _____

2. facolysis _____

3. iridasis _____

4. aphakia _____

5. entropion _____

6. nyctalopia _____

7. irdodesis _____

8. anisocoria _____

E. Abbreviations Used with the Eye

I.   Matching 1: Abbreviations Associated with the Eye, Part 1

Match the term to its meaning. (The same meaning may be used more than once.) Insert the appropriate letter in the space next to the question number.

Choices:

_____ **1.** accommodations   **a.** astigm

_____ **2.** myopia   **b.** VA

_____ **3.** astigmatism   **c.** cyl

_____ **4.** visual acuity   **d.** accom

_____ **5.** cylindrical lens   **e.** OU

_____ **6.** left eye   **f.** OD

_____ **7.** each eye   **g.** oph

_____ **8.** right eye   **h.** OS

_____ **9.** ophthalmology   **i.** myop

II.   Matching 2: Abbreviations Associated with the Eye, Part 2

Match the term to its meaning. (The same meaning may be used more than once.) Insert the appropriate letter in the space next to the question number.

Choices:

_____ **1.** c gl
_____ **2.** EM
_____ **3.** IOP
_____ **4.** s gl
_____ **5.** VF
_____ **6.** VE
_____ **7.** Tn
_____ **8.** PD
_____ **9.** PERRLA

a. emmetropia (normal vision)
b. visual efficiency
c. without correction (without glasses)
d. intraocular pressure
e. correction with glasses
f. intraocular tension
g. interpupillary distance
h. visual field
i. pupils equal, round, and reactive to light with accommodation

III.   Meanings of Abbreviations Used with the Eye

Give the meanings of the following abbreviations in the spaces provided.

1. accom _____
2. astigm _____
3. ARMD _____
4. EM _____

F. Structure and Function of the Ear

I.   Fill in the Blank

Fill in the blank with the appropriate term.

1. Another term for eardrum is _____.
2. List the three bones, or ossicles, of the ear. _____,
_____, _____
3. The inner ear, or _____, contains the functional
organs for hearing and equilibrium (balance).
4. The specific passages in the inner ear that are associated with maintaining balance are the _____.

II.   Matching: Structures and Functions Associated with the Ear

Match the term to its meaning. (The same meaning may be used more than once.)
Insert the appropriate letter in the space next to the question number.

Choices:

_____ **1.** cerumen
_____ **2.** Eustachian tube
_____ **3.** endolymph
_____ **4.** oval window
_____ **5.** saccules
_____ **6.** utricle
_____ **7.** spiral organ (organ of Corti)
_____ **8.** auricle
_____ **9.** auditory canal

a. a membrane between the middle and inner ears
b. contains sound receptors that change mechanical vibrations into nerve impulses
c. fluid in the inner ear
d. external part of the ear
e. equalizes pressure on both sides of the eardrum
f. auditory meatus
g. earwax
h. a small, saclike inner ear structure associated with balance

III.   Spell Check

Circle each incorrectly spelled term and write it correctly in the space provided.

1. labrinth   _____

2. cochlea   _____

3. osicles   _____

4. tympanic   _____

5. meatis   _____

6. eustachian   _____

7. utricle   _____

8. sacule   _____

IV.   Vision Quiz: Parts of the Ear

Figure 26-10 shows the structures of the ear. Identify and write the name of the numbered components in the spaces provided.

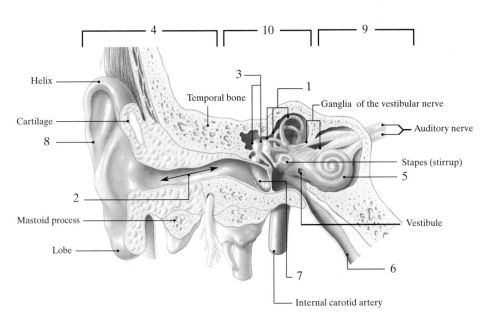

FIGURE 26-10   Vision Quiz. The anatomy of the ear.

Choices:

1. _____   **a.** outer ear

2. _____   **b.** semicircular canals

3. _____   **c.** auditory meatus

4. _____   **d.** ear ossicles

5. _____   **e.** middle ear

6. _____   **f.** auricle

7. _____   **g.** cochlea

8. _____   **h.** tympanic membrane

9. _____   **i.** eustachian tube

10. _____   **j.** inner ear

G. Word Elements Associated with the Ear

I.   Fill in the Blank

Fill in the blank with the appropriate term.

   1. Give two combining forms for hearing. _____,

   _____

   2. List two combining forms for the ear. _____,

   _____

II.   Matching: Word Roots and/or Combining Forms Associated with the Ear

Match the term to its meaning. (The same meaning may be used more than once.)
Insert the appropriate letter in the space next to the question number.

Choices:

_____ **1.** ear   **a.** ot
_____ **2.** eardrum   **b.** staped
_____ **3.** eustachian tube   **c.** salping/o
_____ **4.** stapes   **d.** auri
_____ **5.** hearing   **e.** audi/o
_____ **6.** mastoid process   **f.** tympan/o
_____ **7.** cerumen   **g.** mastoid
_____ **8.** eardrum   **h.** cerumin
                                               i. myring/o
                                               j. acous

III.   Spell Check

Circle each incorrectly spelled term and write it correctly in the space provided.

   1. tympanotomy   _____
   2. stapectomy   _____
   3. auriscope   _____
   4. ceruminosis   _____
   5. otites   _____
   6. myringomicosis _____
   7. audiometer   _____
   8. acoustic   _____

IV.   Word Analysis: Word Roots, Combining Forms, and Suffixes Associated with the Ear

Table 26-15 lists a number of terms with their pronunciations and definitions.

TABLE 26-15   WORD ANALYSIS: WORD ROOTS, COMBINING FORMS, AND SUFFIXES ASSOCIATED WITH THE EAR

Terms and Pronunciation	Brief Explanation
acoustic (a-KOOS-tik)	pertaining to hearing
audiometer (aw-dē-OM-e-ter)	an instrument used to test hearing

(Continued)

TABLE 26-15 (CONTINUED)

Terms and Pronunciation	Brief Explanation
auriscope[a] (AW-ri-skop)	instrument used to visually examine the ear
ceruminosis (se-roo-mi-NŌ-sis)	abnormal (excessive) secretion of cerumen
mastoiditis (mas-toyd-Ī-tis)	inflammation of the mastoid process
myringomycosis (mir-in-gō-mi-KŌ-sis) otitis (ō-TĪ-tis)	fungus infection of the eardrum inflammation of the ear
salpingopharyngeal (sal-ping-gō-fa-RIN-jē-al)	pertaining to the eustachian tube and throat
stapedectomy (stā-pe-DEK-tō-mē)	excision of the stapes
tympanotomy (tim-pan-OT-ō-mē)	incision into tympanic membrane

[a]Another term is otoscope.

1. Analyze each term.
2. Circle all combining forms, word roots, and suffixes, and label them **cf, wr,** and **s,** respectively.
3. Check your answers (shown in Table 26-16).

H. Hearing Disorders, Diseases, and Tests

I.   Matching 1: Infections and Other Abnormalities Involving the Ear

Match the term to its meaning. (The same meaning may be used more than once.) Insert the appropriate letter in the space next to the question number.

Choices:

_____ 1. inflammation of the middle ear with serum accumulation

_____ 2. inflammation of the air cells of the mastoid process

_____ 3. an infection of the external ear

_____ 4. condition involving recurring vertigo and tinnitus

_____ 5. progressive breakdown of normal bone around the oval window

_____ 6. hearing loss associated with aging

_____ 7. benign tumor of the acoustic cranial nerve

_____ 8. inflammation of the eardrum

a. external otitis
b. Meniere's disease
c. otosclerosis
d. mastoiditis
e. serous otitis media
f. presbycusis
g. acoustic neuroma
h. myringitis

II.   Matching 2: Procedures to Detect and Treat Ear Abnormalities

Choices:

_____ **1.** otoscopy
_____ **2.** audiometry
_____ **3.** myringotomy

a. evaluation of hearing levels
b. visual examination of the ear with an otoscope
c. surgical incision of the eardrum

III.   Spell Check

Circle each incorrectly spelled term and write it correctly in the space provided.

1. otoscopy   _____
2. Miniere's   _____
3. presbicusis   _____
4. virtigo   _____
5. tinitus   _____
6. otitis   _____

I. Medical Vocabulary Building

I.   Matching

Match the term to its meaning. (The same meaning may be used more than once.)
Insert the appropriate letter in the space next to the question number.

Choices:

_____ **1.** endaural
_____ **2.** labyrinthectomy
_____ **3.** myringectomy
_____ **4.** mastoidalgia
_____ **5.** otomycosis
_____ **6.** fenestration

a. pertaining to within the ear
b. surgical excision of the labyrinth
c. mastoid pain
d. surgical excision of the tympanic membrane
e. fungus infection of the ear
f. surgical operation in the inner ear labyrinth to restore hearing

II.   Spell Check

Circle each incorrectly spelled term and write it correctly in the space provided.

1. fenstration   _____
2. miringectomy   _____
3. endaural   _____
4. otomycosis   _____
5. mastoidalgia   _____
6. labrinthectomy   _____

J. Abbreviations Associated with the Ear and Hearing

I.   Matching

Match the term to its meaning. (The same meaning may be used more than once.)
Insert the appropriate letter in the space next to the question number.

Choices:

_____ **1.** ENT
_____ **2.** AS

a. otology
b. right ear

_____ **3.** Oto   **c.** left ear

_____ **4.** AD   **d.** ear, nose, and throat

_____ **5.** AC   **e.** eustachian tube function

_____ **6.** ETF   **f.** air conduction

_____ **7.** HD   **g.** bone conduction

_____ **8.** PE tube   **h.** hearing distance

_____ **9.** BC   **i.** polyethylene-ventilating-tube placement in the eardrum

K. Increasing Your Medical Terminology Word Power 1

1. Read the following report.
2. Prepare to answer the questions at the end of the section.
3. Circle all unfamiliar terms with a red pencil.
4. Underline familiar terms with a blue pencil.
5. Use your knowledge of word elements, a medical dictionary, and the key terms to find the meaning of unfamiliar terms.

Glaucoma

Key Terms

atrophy (AT-rō-fē) a wasting; decrease in the size of an organ or tissue

excavation (eks-ka-VĀ-shun) forming a cavity

gonioscopy (gō-nē-OS-kop-ē) procedure used to determine presence of blockage in the entrance to the anterior chamber of the eye

opthalmoscopy (of-thal-MOS-kō-pē) examination of the interior of the eye

tonometry (tōn-OM-e-trē) measurement of tension of part of the body such as the eye

visual field testing measuring or determining the ability to see objects in an area under varying levels of lighting

O VERVIEW

The term glaucoma includes a group of diseases sharing the pathologic features of intraocular pressure, excavation, and atrophy of the optic-nerve head and visual field loss. Although it may occur at any age, it is found mainly in the elderly.

C AUSES

Glaucoma results from an imbalance between the production of aqueous humor and its outflow from the anterior portion of the eye. In the normal eye, the fluid circulates within the anterior portion, filling the anterior and posterior chambers and maintaining the intraocular pressure without which the eye would collapse.

T YPES

There are several types of glaucoma, including *open-angle glaucoma, angle-closure glaucoma,* and *secondary glaucoma.* The open-angle form is by far the most common. On examination, the eye appears to be anatomically normal, but functionally the flow of the aqueous humor is blocked.

Angle-closure glaucoma occurs when a part of the anterior chamber narrows. In this type of glaucoma, the flow of aqueous humor from the posterior chamber through the pupil into the anterior chamber is partially blocked, thus increasing the pressure in the posterior chamber compared with that in the anterior chamber.

Secondary glaucoma is the term applied to all forms of glaucoma in which the elevated intraocular pressure is caused by another pathologic process within the eye. The disease changes the structures in portions of the anterior chamber, limiting the outflow of aqueous humor and causing the intraocular pressure to rise.

E ARLY DETECTION

To diagnose glaucoma early—before significant, irreversible ocular damage occurs—screening for the disease is done. It identifies an elevated intraocular pressure or an abnormal appearance of the optic disk, thus providing evidence supporting a suspicion of glaucoma. If either, or both, of these findings is present, referral to an ophthalmologist is indicated for a diagnostic evaluation and treatment.

Four specific tests are then performed to determine the presence or absence of glaucoma. These are *tonometry* (to determine intraocular pressure), *opthalmoscopy, gonioscopy*, and *visual field testing*.

Most forms of glaucoma can be treated successfully if the disorder is discovered early in its course.

Questions

I.   Fill in the Blank

Fill in the blank with the appropriate term.

1. List three types of glaucoma. _____,

_____,

_____.

2. Which type of glaucoma is the most common?

_____

3. List four specific tests used to detect the presence of glaucoma.

_____, _____,

_____, _____

II.   Matching

Match the term to its meaning. (The same meaning may be used more than once.) Insert the appropriate letter in the space next to the question number.

Choices:

_____ **1.** atrophy
_____ **2.** excavation
_____ **3.** tonometry
_____ **4.** ophthalmoscopy
_____ **5.** gonioscopy
_____ **6.** intraocular
_____ **7.** glaucoma
_____ **8.** angle-closure glaucoma

a. procedure to measure tension
b. forming a cavity
c. procedure to examine an eye's interior
d. a wasting
e. procedure to detect a blockage of the anterior chamber
f. imbalance between aqueous humor production and its outflow from the anterior part of the eye
g. within the eye
h. condition caused by a narrowing of a part of the anterior chamber of the eye

III.   Spell Check

Circle each incorrectly spelled term and write it correctly in the space provided.

1. gluacoma   _____
2. atrophy   _____
3. intocular   _____
4. opthalmoscopy _____
5. tonometry   _____
6. excavation   _____

L. Increasing Your Medical Terminology Word Power 2

1. Read the following report.
2. Prepare to answer the questions at the end of the section.
3. Circle all unfamiliar terms with a red pencil.
4. Underline familiar terms with a blue pencil.
5. Use your knowledge of word elements, a medical dictionary, and the key terms to find the meaning of unfamiliar terms.

Uveitis

Key Terms

biopsy (BĪ-op-sē)   surgical removal of a small piece of living tissue for microscopic examination, usually for diagnostic purposes

inflammation   tissue reaction to injury

intraocular   within the eyeball

uveitis (ū-vē-Ī-tis)   inflammation of the entire uvea or any part of this eye structure

vascular (VAS-kū-lar)   pertains to blood vessels

𝒰 VEITIS

Uveitis is the term used to describe many forms of intraocular inflammation involving parts of, or the entire, *uvea* (Ū-vē-a). Closely located ocular structures such as the retina, cornea, and optic nerve may also be affected.

Uveitis is derived from the Latin *uva*, or "grape": a peeled blue grape has a bluish vein structure that resembles the middle, vascular layer of the uvea. The uvea consists of the iris anteriorly and the ciliary body and choroid layer posteriorly. Inflammation of the anterior uvea is termed *anterior uveitis*, or *iridocyclitis* (ir-id-ō-sī-KLĪ-tis). If only the iris is involved, the condition is called *iritis* (i-RĪ-t-is). Inflammation of the ciliary body is *cyclitis* (sik-LĪ-tis), and *choroidal inflammation* is termed *choroiditis* (kō-royd-Ī-tis). In clinical usage, "uveitis" has come to describe most forms of intraocular inflammation.

Uveitis is associated with significant disease states including loss of the eye, loss of vision, or opposite-eye inflammation. In most cases of uveitis, diagnosis is established on the basis of a thorough review of the patient's history, a review of body systems that may be contributing to the disease state, and a physical examination.

The physical appearance of an inflamed eye is classified by a variety of methods. One method uses the terms *anterior* as well as *intermediate* and *posterior forms of uveitis*. Uveitis involving the middle portion of the eye depends on which intraocular layer is involved. The terms *choroiditis* and *retinitis* are used when the choroid or retina is involved. *Retinochoroiditis* (ret-i-nō-kō-royd-Ī-tis) or *chorioretinitis* (kō-rē-ō-ret-in-Ī-tis) is used when both layers are affected. Here the first part of the term indicates the most heavily involved eye layer.

Questions

I. Fill in the Blank

Fill in the blank with the appropriate term.

1. What is the term used for most forms of intraocular inflammation?

   _____

2. List the components of the uvea. _____

   _____

3. What is inflammation of the ciliary body called?

   _____

4. What does the term choroiditis mean? _____

5. What are the two terms used to indicate involvement of both the choroid and retina in a clinical condition?

   a. _____
   b. _____

II. Spell Check

Circle each incorrectly spelled term and write it correctly in the space provided.

1. irtis   _____
2. uvae   _____
3. corioretinitis _____
4. vescular   _____
5. iridocyclitis _____
6. choroiditis _____
7. retinochoroiditis _____
8. ciliery   _____

M. Increasing Your Medical Terminology Word Power 3

1. Read the following report.
2. Prepare to answer the questions at the end of the section.
3. Circle all unfamiliar terms with a red pencil.
4. Underline familiar terms with a blue pencil.
5. Use your knowledge of word elements, a medical dictionary, and the key terms to find the meaning of unfamiliar terms.

Tinnitus in Children

Key Terms

audiometry (aw-dē-OM-e-trē)   procedures to test hearing

computerized tomographic scan (computerized axial tomography)   use of x-rays directed through a body plane, with the information obtained being processed by a computer to form a transverse picture of body organs

electroencephalography (ē-lek-trō-en-sef-a-LOG-graf-ē)   procedure used to obtain a record of the electrical activity of the brain

group A, beta-hemolytic streptococci   a bacterial group known to cause sore throats and middle ear infections

magnetic resonance brain scan   a procedure that uses magnetic waves to obtain images of the heart, large blood vessels, brain, and soft body tissues

tic   involuntary muscular contractions (spasms) involving the face, head, neck, or shoulder muscles

tinnitus (tin-Ī-tus)   ringing sound in the ear

tympanometry (tim-pa-NOM-e-trē)   a procedure used to evaluate the functioning of the eardrum and detect middle-ear disorders

I NTRODUCTION

Tinnitus is any sound sensation perceived by the individual to have its origin inside the head, unrelated to external mechanoacoustic or electric signals or, loosely translated, "ear noise." The disorder is subdivided into *subjective tinnitus*, which is apparent only to the individual, and *objective tinnitus*, which can also be heard by others.

C ASE HISTORY

The patient, a seven-year-old girl, had nasal congestions and sore throat unaccompanied by fever, cough, facial pain, headache, rash, or gastrointestinal signs and symptoms. Pharyngeal cultures were negative for group A, beta-hemolytic streptococci. The patient was treated for her signs and symptoms. She returned twelve days later, reporting that her respiratory-tract infection cleared up, but new symptoms developed. The patient noted "clicking" in both ears, with a more pronounced sound in the left ear. Her mother also heard the sound when near her. There were no facial tics, difficulty with talking or swallowing, or neurologic signs.

The clicking irritated the patient as she tried to fall asleep, but she and her mother were unsure whether it persisted during sleep.

On examination, the patient was cooperative, verbal, and in no distress. The tympanic membranes, nose, and pharynx were normal. A snapping sound, similar to flicking the edges of fingernails could be heard near the patient's ear with a stethoscope. The timing of the clicking sometimes was faster and sometimes slower than the pulse. Tympanometry and audiometry were normal.

One month later the patient's symptoms and examination findings remained unchanged. She and her parents requested therapy and consented to further examinations. Computer tomographic (CT) scans of the brain, with and without contrast agents, and electroencephalography were normal.

The young patient's condition remained unchanged for six months. Her overall health was normal. The suggestion for a magnetic resonance brain scan was refused. The family moved and was lost for a follow-up study.

Questions

I.   Fill in the Blank

Fill in the blank with the appropriate term.

1. What is the medical term used for the condition of "ear noise"?

    _____

2. Besides nasal congestion, did the patient have any other signs or symptoms during the first examination? _____

3. Did the patient experience "clicking" in one or both ears?
_____

4. Were the tympanic membranes, nose, and pharynx normal on physical examination of the patient? _____

5. Was the timing of the clicking faster or slower than the patient's pulse? _____

6. List the diagnostic procedures used to determine the cause of the patient's tinnitus. _____, _____,
_____, _____

II.   Spell Check

Circle each incorrectly spelled term and write it correctly in the space provided.

1. tinitus   _____
2. timpanometry _____
3. stethoscope   _____
4. tic   _____
5. audiometry   _____
6. tomografic   _____

Term Search Challenge

Locate 16 terms in the puzzle.

1. Write the specific term next to its definition. Then find that term in the puzzle diagram and circle it.
2. Terms may be read from left to right, backward, up, down, or diagonally.
3. If a term appears more than once, circle it only once. (A term or abbreviation may be found inside others.)
4. Check your answers.

Clues:

1. the area of the eye behind the cornea and in front of the lens that contains the aqueous humor _____ (two words)
2. the photosensitive receptor cells responsible for color vision
_____
3. the lining of the eyelids _____
4. the tough, white, outer coat of the eyeball _____
5. the cranial nerve that carries impulses from the retina to the brain nerve
_____
6. the dark opening of the eye through which light rays pass
_____
7. two combining forms for cornea are _____
8. combining form for retina _____
9. two combining forms for tear(s) are _____,
_____
10. combining form for eyelid _____
11. the term for poor vision due to old age _____
12. the snail-shaped spirally wound tube in the inner ear _____
13. term for bacterial infection of the middle ear _____ media
14. the projecting part or flap of the ear _____

Term Search Puzzle

```
C  O  N  E  S  P  R  E  S  B  Y  O  P  I  A
O  A  C  U  C  O  N  J  U  N  C  T  I  V  A
J  U  F  U  V  E  C  E  N  T  R  A  L  I  S
T  R  O  R  R  S  T  H  A  U  R  I  C  L  E
U  O  I  E  S  N  D  P  I  O  L  O  T  Y  Z
S  C  L  S  C  E  E  A  L  A  C  R  I  M  O
A  C  S  C  L  E  R  A  T  S  U  W  X  P  Y
N  O  P  P  T  K  Y  G  R  S  U  M  N  R  R
T  R  O  U  O  E  C  O  C  H  L  E  A  E  C
E  N  P  P  L  R  O  T  L  C  U  S  I  S  A
R  E  T  I  N  A  T  O  T  I  T  I  S  B  D
I  A  I  L  E  T  O  N  O  M  E  T  R  Y  T
O  I  C  U  N  O  S  S  I  C  L  E  S  I  O
R  R  E  T  I  N  O  C  A  T  A  R  A  C  T
C  H  A  M  B  E  R  B  L  E  P  H  A  R  O
```

Pharmacology

"In my hunt for the secret of life, I started my research in histology. Unsatisfied by the information it could give me about life, I turned to physiology. Finding physiology too complex, I took up pharmacology."

—Albert Szent-Gyorgyi

INFORMATIONAL CHALLENGE

A. Pharmacology, Subdivisions, Drug Names, Standards, and Information Sources

I.   Fill in the Blank

Fill in the blank with the appropriate term.

1. The individual licensed to prepare and dispense drugs is known as a(n) _____.
2. The study of toxic substances and their effects on the body is known as _____.
3. The term used for the treatment of infectious diseases and cancers by chemicals with specific effects is known as _____.
4. A substance that neutralizes the harmful effect of a drug is called a(n) _____.

II.   Matching 1: Pharmacology Subdivisions

Match the term to its meaning. (The same meaning may be used more than once.) Insert the appropriate letter in the space next to the question number.

Choices:

_____ 1. molecular pharmacology
_____ 2. pharmacokinetics
_____ 3. toxicology
_____ 4. pharmaceutical chemistry
_____ 5. pharmacodynamics

a. the chemistry of drugs, their composition, actions, formation, and analysis

b. the study of drug action at subcellular levels

c. includes the study of transport, distribution, action, and elimination of a drug

d. associated with finding antidotes

e. the general study of drugs and their effects on living tissues

III.   Matching 2: Drug Names and References

Match the term to its meaning. (The same meaning may be used more than once.) Insert the appropriate letter in the space next to the question number.

Choices:

_____ **1.** proprietary name
_____ **2.** pharmacopeia
_____ **3.** brand name
_____ **4.** generic name
_____ **5.** chemical name
_____ **6.** official name
_____ **7.** *Physician's Desk Reference*

a. a collection of drug information
b. term used to identify a drug for legal and specific purposes
c. term used to identify a drug manufactured by a drug company
d. indicates atomic and molecular structure of a drug
e. listing of drug products sponsored by drug companies
f. provides information about drugs and their clinical use

IV.   Spell Check

Circle each incorrectly spelled term and write it correctly in the space provided.

1. pharmacopieia   _____
2. pharmocy   _____
3. pharmacology   _____
4. pharmcodynamics   _____
5. formulary   _____
6. generric   _____

B. Drug Preparations, Routes of Drug Administration, and the Apothecaries' System

I.   Fill in the Blank

Fill in the blank with the appropriate term.

1. List five examples of solid forms of drugs. _____,
_____, _____,
_____, _____

2. List five examples of semisolid forms of drugs.
_____, _____,
_____, _____,
_____

3. List five examples of liquid forms of drugs. _____,
_____, _____,
_____, _____

4. What is the smallest unit of weight in the apothecaries' system?
_____

5. What is the smallest unit of volume in the apothecaries' system?
_____

II.   Matching 1: Sites for Drug Administration

Match the term to its meaning. (The same meaning may be used more than once.)
Insert the appropriate letter in the space next to the question number.

Choices:

_____ **1.** buccal   **a.** eyelid
_____ **2.** sublingual   **b.** mouth
_____ **3.** conjunctiva   **c.** in a joint space
_____ **4.** intra-arterial   **d.** under the tongue
_____ **5.** intra-articular   **e.** pleural cavity
_____ **6.** intrathecal   **f.** artery
_____ **7.** intrapleural   **g.** skin
_____ **8.** intradermal   **h.** cerebrospinal fluid
_____ **9.** subcutaneous   **i.** below top skin layers

III.   Matching 2: Abbreviations Used with the Forms of Drugs

Match the term to its meaning. (The same meaning may be used more than once.)
Insert the appropriate letter in the space next to the question number.

Choices:

_____ **1.** elix   **a.** extract
_____ **2.** tab   **b.** tincture
_____ **3.** ext   **c.** oil
_____ **4.** ol   **d.** elixir
_____ **5.** tr   **e.** tablet
_____ **6.** sol   **f.** ointment
_____ **7.** ung   **g.** solution
_____ **8.** fld   **h.** fluid
_____ **9.** caps   **i.** capsule

IV.   Matching 3: Administration Routes and Sites

Match the term to its meaning. (The same meaning may be used more than once.)
Insert the appropriate letter in the space next to the question number.

Choices:

_____ **1.** intravenous   **a.** IM
_____ **2.** intramuscular   **b.** Po
_____ **3.** right eye   **c.** IV
_____ **4.** left eye   **d.** OD
_____ **5.** by mouth   **e.** OU
_____ **6.** in each eye   **f.** Subq
_____ **7.** subcutaneously   **g.** OS

V.   Matching 4: Abbreviations for Amounts

Match the term to its meaning. (The same meaning may be used more than once.)
Insert the appropriate letter in the space next to the question number.

Choices:

_____	**1.** gm or Gm	**a.**	grain
_____	**2.** U	**b.**	drop
_____	**3.** ss	**c.**	microgram
_____	**4.** gr	**d.**	gram
_____	**5.** mg	**e.**	unit
_____	**6.** gtt	**f.**	milligram
_____	**7.** mcg	**g.**	one-half
_____	**8.** o	**h.**	ounce
_____	**9.** oz	**i.**	pint
_____	**10.** M	**j.**	minim

VI.   Matching 5: Time Schedules

Match the term to its meaning. (The same meaning may be used more than once.) Insert the appropriate letter in the space next to the question number.

Choices:

_____	**1.** twice per day	**a.**	od/qd
_____	**2.** every hour	**b.**	t.i.d.
_____	**3.** every day	**c.**	b.i.d.
_____	**4.** immediately	**d.**	Omn hr
_____	**5.** once if necessary	**e.**	Stat
_____	**6.** three times/day	**f.**	Sos
_____	**7.** as much as required	**g.**	Q3h
_____	**8.** four times/day	**h.**	Qs
_____	**9.** after meals	**i.**	Q.i.d.
_____	**10.** every three hours	**j.**	Pm
_____	**11.** when required	**k.**	pc

VII.   Spell Check

Circle each incorrectly spelled term and write it correctly in the space provided.

1. losenges   _____

2. capsules   _____

3. tinkture   _____

4. minnum   _____

5. supositoreies   _____

6. ointment   _____

7. suspension   _____

8. apathecaries'   _____

C. Word Elements Associated with Pharmacology

I.   Fill in the Blank

Fill in the blank with the appropriate term.

1. List two combining forms used for "drug." _____,

_____

2. Give two word roots used for "poison." _____,

_____

3. Give the suffix used to indicate "stopping" or "controlling."

_____

4. Give the suffix pertaining to "killing." _____

5. List two prefixes used to indicate "against." _____,

_____

II.   Matching 1: Word Roots and/or Combining Forms Related to Pharmacology

Match the term to its meaning. (The same meaning may be used more than once.)
Insert the appropriate letter in the space next to the question number.

Choices:

_____ **1.** erg   **a.** work
_____ **2.** pyr/e   **b.** treatment
_____ **3.** alges   **c.** mixture
_____ **4.** narc/o   **d.** individual
_____ **5.** esthesi/o   **e.** feeling
_____ **6.** hypn/o   **f.** numbers
_____ **7.** iatr/o   **g.** sensitivity to pain
                                h. sleep
                                i. fever

III.   Matching 2: Suffixes Associated with Pharmacology

Match the term to its meaning. (The same meaning may be used more than once.)
Insert the appropriate letter in the space next to the question number.

Choices:

_____ **1.** mimic, copy   **a.** phylaxis
_____ **2.** destroy   **b.** mimetic
_____ **3.** stopping   **c.** -cidal
_____ **4.** pertaining to killing **d.** -lytic
_____ **5.** protection   **e.** -static

IV.   Spell Check

Circle each incorrectly spelled term and write it correctly in the space provided.

1. itrogenic   _____
2. narcotik   _____
3. prophilaxis   _____
4. sympathomimetic   _____
5. anelgesic   _____
6. parental   _____
7. antibiotic   _____
8. antihelmenthic   _____

V.   Word Analysis: Word Elements Associated with Pharmacology

Table 27-10 lists a number of terms with their pronunciations and definitions.

TABLE 27-10   WORD ANALYSIS: WORD ELEMENTS ASSOCIATED WITH PHARMACOLOGY

Term and Pronunciation	Definition or Brief Description
adrenergic (ad-ren-ER-jik)	pertaining to working like adrenaline; refers to drug- or nerve-associated adrenaline (epinephrine) actions
analgesic (an-al-JĒ-sik)	pertaining to a drug that relieves pain
antihelminthic (an-tī-hel-MIN-thik)	pertaining to against worms
antimycotic (an-tī-mī-KŌ-tik)	pertaining to against fungi
bactericidal (bak-tēr-ē-SĪ-dal)	pertaining to killing or destroying bacteria
chemotherapy (kē-mō-THER-a-pē)	the treatment of disease with chemicals
dermal (DER-mal)	pertaining to the skin
hemolytic (hē-mō-LIT-ik)	blood destroying
hypnogenic (hip-nō-JEN-ik)	producing sleep
iatrogenic (ī-at-rō-JEN-ik)	pertaining to a reaction produced by treatment
narcotic (nar-KOT-ik)	pertaining to producing numbness or sleep
parenteral (par-EN-ter-al)	pertaining to other than involving the intestines
pharmacotherapy (far-ma-kō-THER-a-pē)	use of drugs for treatment
prophylaxis (prō-fi-LAK-sis)	prevention
pyretic (pī-RET-ik)	pertaining to fever
sympathomimetic (sim-pa-thō-mim-ET-ik)	initiating or copying effects resulting from sympathetic-nervous system stimulation
toxemia (toks-Ē-mē-a)	condition of poison in the blood
toxicologist (toks-i-KOL-ō-jist)	specialist in the field of toxicology

---

1. Analyze each term.
2. Circle all prefixes, combining forms, word roots, and suffixes and label them **p, cf, wr**, and **s**, respectively.
3. Check your answers (shown in Table 27-11).

D. Drug Effects, Action, and Interactions and Drug Families

I.   Fill in the Blank

Fill in the blank with the appropriate term.

1. An illness developing from the actual treatment is referred to as being

   _____.

2. A decreased body response to single or repeated exposure to a drug is called _____.

3. The development of signs and symptoms of an illness when a drug is withdrawn is referred to as _____.

4. When a potentiation situation occurs through the combined use of drugs, the effect is _____ than either drug could cause individually.

5. List three ways in which drugs may be grouped or classified.

   a. _____
   b. _____
   c. _____

6. List six categories of drug interactions in addition to adverse reactions.

   a. _____
   b. _____
   c. _____
   d. _____
   e. _____
   f. _____

II.   Matching: Drugs and Their Actions

Match the term to its meaning. (The same meaning may be used more than once.) Insert the appropriate letter in the space next to the question number.

Choices:

_____ 1. alkylating agents
_____ 2. antimetabolites
_____ 3. streptokinase
_____ 4. topical hemostatics
_____ 5. anticoagulants
_____ 6. heparin
_____ 7. tissue plasminogen activator
_____ 8. mercaptopurine

a. reduce blood loss at surfaces
b. damage to DNA
c. interfere with DNA synthesis
d. used to prevent emboli formation
e. purine or pyrimidine analogues
f. stimulate natural process of dissolving blood clots
g. prevent increases in blood-clot size
h. prevents clotting of blood used for transfusions

III.   Spell Check

Circle the incorrectly spelled term and write it correctly in the space provided.

1. ideosyncratic _____
2. anaphilaxis _____
3. allergic _____
4. cumulative _____
5. alklating _____
6. anticoagulant _____
7. alkylating _____
8. proteinaceous _____
9. tolerance _____
10. antieoplatic _____
11. analoques _____
12. dependance _____

E. Antimicrobials

I.   Fill in the Blank

Fill in the blank with the appropriate term.

   1. A drug that causes the death of bacteria is referred to as being

   _____.

   2. A drug that inhibits or stops bacterial growth without killing is referred to as being _____.

   3. Antibiotics that are active against several different bacteria are called _____ antibiotics.

   4. The resulting antibiotic effect when the use of one drug interferes with the activity of another is called _____.

   5. Combined drugs producing an effect greater than when each drug is given separately is an example of _____ effect.

II.   Matching: Anti-Microbial and Anti-Inflammatory Agents and Antipyretics

Match the term to its meaning. (The same meaning may be used more than once.) Insert the appropriate letter in the space next to the question number.

Choices:

_____ **1.** antimycotic	**a.** used against ringworm
_____ **2.** antimycobacterial drug	**b.** amphotericin B
_____ **3.** antimalarial drug	**c.** quinine
_____ **4.** antiprotozoan drug	**d.** metronidazole
_____ **5.** used for systemic fungal infections	**e.** nystatin
	f. AZT
_____ **6.** antiviral drug	**g.** isoniazid
_____ **7.** antihelminthics	**h.** used against worms
_____ **8.** insecticides	**i.** used against lice and mites
_____ **9.** used against fevers	**j.** scabies
_____ **10.** anti-inflammatory agent	**k.** acetylsalicylic acid
	l. antipyretics

III.   Spell Check

Circle each incorrectly spelled term and write it correctly in the space provided.

   1. synirgistic   _____
   2. antibiotic   _____
   3. aditive   _____
   4. isoniazid   _____
   5. astringant   _____
   6. flucytosine   _____
   7. metronidazole   _____
   8. quinin   _____
   9. asetaminophen   _____
   10. acetylsalicyclic _____

F. Drugs for Body Systems

I.   Matching 1: Cardiovascular Drugs

Match the term to its meaning. (The same meaning may be used more than once.) Insert the appropriate letter in the space next to the question number.

Choices:

_____ 1. chronotropic
_____ 2. ionotropic
_____ 3. dromotropic
_____ 4. anti-lipemics
_____ 5. diuretic
_____ 6. digitalis
_____ 7. antiarrhythmics
_____ 8. vasodilators
_____ 9. vasoconstrictors

a. affects cardiac muscle contraction
b. affects cardiac tissue conductivity
c. affects rate of heart tissue contraction
d. reduce body lipoprotein levels
e. used to correct abnormal heart-contraction patterns
f. relieves angina pectoris
g. increases urine secretion
h. lower blood pressure by relaxation of smooth muscles in blood vessels
i. cause constriction of blood vessels

II.   Matching 2: Drugs Affecting GI Tract

Match the term to its meaning. (The same meaning may be used more than once.)
Insert the appropriate letter in the space next to the question number.

Choices:

_____ 1. promote breakdown of food
_____ 2. neutralize hydrochloric acid
_____ 3. reduce discomfort caused by excess gas
_____ 4. reduce nausea
_____ 5. stop diarrhea
_____ 6. induce vomiting
_____ 7. stimulate fecal elimination

a. antiemetics
b. emetics
c. digestants
d. antacids
e. antiflatulents
f. antidiarrheal
g. laxative

III.   Matching 3: Drugs for the Respiratory System

Match the term to its meaning. (The same meaning may be used more than once.)
Insert the appropriate letter in the space next to the question number.

Choices:

_____ 1. bronchodilator
_____ 2. methlyxanthines
_____ 3. expectorants
_____ 4. sympathomimetics
_____ 5. antitussives
_____ 6. antihistamines
_____ 7. decongestants

a. stimulates autonomic nervous system
b. reduces thickness of mucus
c. expands bronchi
d. Robitussin
e. improves air flow by reducing bronchospasm
f. brings relief from coughs
g. relieves nasal stuffiness
h. blocks action of histamines

IV.   Matching 4: CNS Drugs

Match the term to its meaning. (The same meaning may be used more than once.)
Insert the appropriate letter in the space next to the question number.

Choices:

_____ 1. stimulant
_____ 2. anticholinergics

a. narcotic and nonnarcotic pain relievers

_____ **3.** depressant
_____ **4.** sedatives
_____ **5.** analgesics
_____ **6.** hypnotics
_____ **7.** anesthetics
_____ **8.** tranquilizers
_____ **9.** beta-blockers
_____ **10.** sympatholytics

b. induces relaxation without necessarily producing sleep
c. speeds up vital processes
d. has effects opposite of the parasympathomimetics
e. depresses CNS activity
f. induces relaxation and produces sleep
g. control anxiety
h. causes loss of sensation throughout the body
i. block action of epinephrine

V.   Matching 5: Endocrine Drugs

Match the term to its meaning. (The same meaning may be used more than once.) Insert the appropriate letter in the space next to the question number.

Choices:

_____ **1.** androgen
_____ **2.** tamoxifen
_____ **3.** insulin
_____ **4.** glucocorticoids
_____ **5.** progesterones
_____ **6.** thyroid hormone
_____ **7.** mineral corticoids
_____ **8.** Humulin

a. replacement hormone therapy for Addison's disease
b. anti-estrogen
c. reduces blood sugar to normal levels
d. promotes normal sexual function
e. prevent and treat cretinism
f. treatment for hormone-sensitive cancers
g. treatment for inflammatory diseases involving liver and blood vessels
h. treatment of various female-reproductive-system disorders
i. recombinant-DNA product

VI.   Spell Check

Circle each incorrectly spelled term and write it correctly in the space provided.

1. glycoside   _____
2. digitales   _____
3. antiarhythmicks   _____
4. hyperlipimia   _____
5. antidiarheal   _____
6. antiflatulant   _____
7. antiusives   _____
8. sympathomimetics _____
9. barbiturates   _____
10. anulgesics   _____

G. Vitamins

I.   Fill in the Blank

Fill in the blank with the appropriate term.

1. List four fat-soluble vitamins. _____,

_____, _____,

_____

2. List the water-soluble vitamins. _____ ,
_____

II. Matching 1: Vitamin Function

Match the term to its meaning. (The same meaning may be used more than once.)
Insert the appropriate letter in the space next to the question number.

Choices:

_____ **1.** thiamine	**a.** essential for normal function of the retina (eye)
_____ **2.** vitamin B$_6$	
_____ **3.** vitamin A	**b.** essential for normal nerve function
_____ **4.** folacin	**c.** essential for formation of cholesterol
_____ **5.** niacin	**d.** essential for DNA synthesis
_____ **6.** vitamin D	**e.** serves an important role in the metabolism of amino acids
_____ **7.** vitamin C	
_____ **8.** vitamin B$_{12}$	**f.** promotes absorption of iron
_____ **9.** vitamin E	**g.** necessary for proper metabolism of calcium and phosphorus
_____ **10.** vitamin K	
_____ **11.** biotin	**h.** may reduce or slow effects of air pollution and cellular aging
	i. essential for the formation of prothrombin and other clotting proteins
	j. essential for fatty acid formation

III. Matching 2: Alternate Vitamin Names

Match the term to its meaning. (The same meaning may be used more than once.)
Insert the appropriate letter in the space next to the question number.

Choices:

_____ **1.** thiamine	**a.** vitamin A
_____ **2.** retinol	**b.** vitamin B$_1$
_____ **3.** riboflavin	**c.** niacin
_____ **4.** nicotinic acid	**d.** vitamin B$_2$
_____ **5.** ascorbic acid	**e.** B$_{12}$
_____ **6.** cyanocobalamin	**f.** folic acid
_____ **7.** folacin	**g.** vitamin C
_____ **8.** pyridoxine	**h.** cholecalciferol
_____ **9.** vitamin D	**i.** vitamin B$_6$
_____ **10.** tocopherol	**j.** vitamin K
_____ **11.** menadione	**k.** vitamin E

IV. Matching 3: Vitamin-Deficiency Diseases

Match the term to its meaning. (The same meaning may be used more than once.)
Insert the appropriate letter in the space next to the question number.

Choices:

_____ **1.** night blindness	**a.** thiamine
_____ **2.** pellagra	**b.** vitamin B$_{12}$
_____ **3.** beriberi	**c.** vitamin C
_____ **4.** scurvy	**d.** riboflavin
_____ **5.** pernicious anemia	**e.** vitamin A

_____ **6.** rickets   **f.** niacin
_____ **7.** osteomalacia   **g.** vitamin D

V.   Spell Check

Circle each incorrectly spelled term and write it correctly in the space provided.

1. tiamine   _____
2. niasin   _____
3. pernicious   _____
4. xeroofthalmia   _____
5. pyridoxine   _____
6. ascorbic   _____

H. Medical Vocabulary Building

I.   Matching

Match the term to its meaning. (The same meaning may be used more than once.) Insert the appropriate letter in the space next to the question number.

Choices:

_____ **1.** cathartic
_____ **2.** cardiotonic
_____ **3.** beta-blocker
_____ **4.** antidote
_____ **5.** contraindications
_____ **6.** transport

a. drug that promotes the efficiency and force of the heart
b. drug that relieves constipation
c. a substance that counteracts an unwanted drug effect
d. a drug that blocks the action of epinephrine at sites on heart muscle cell receptors
e. a factor in a patient's condition that prevents the use of a particular treatment
f. movement of a substance across a cell's plasma membrane

II.   Spell Check

Circle each incorrectly spelled term and write it correctly in the space provided.

1. kathartik   _____
2. cardiotonic   _____
3. antianjinal   _____
4. betta-blocker _____
5. antinaseant   _____
6. antidot   _____

I. Increasing Your Medical Terminology Word Power 1

1. Read the following report.
2. Prepare to answer the questions at the end of the section.
3. Circle all unfamiliar terms with a red pencil.
4. Underline familiar terms with a blue pencil.
5. Use your knowledge of word elements, a medical dictionary, and the key terms to find the meaning of unfamiliar terms.

Selected Parts of a Drug Insert Containing Prescribing Information

Key Terms

asthenia (as-THĒ-ne-a)   lack or loss of strength

dyspepsia (dis-PEP-se-a)   painful digestion

lethargy (LETH-ar-jē)   sluggishness

paresthesia (par-es-THĒ-ze-a)   sensation of numbness, prickling, or tingling

Read the following sections adapted from a drug package insert for content and specific details.

B RIEF SUMMARY

Contraindications: known hypersensitivity to the drug, sinus bradycardia, heart block, cardiogenic shock, and overt cardiac failure.

 Adverse reactions: adverse events reported in U.S.-controlled studies include bradycardia, edema, headache, dizziness, fatigue, lethargy, insomnia, nervousness, bizarre dreams, depression, impotence, dyspnea, pharyngitis, rhinitis, upper respiratory infection, dyspepsia, nausea, diarrhea, chest pain, arthralgia, and rash.

 In European-controlled clinical trials the following adverse reactions were noticed: bradycardia, palpitation, edema, cold extremities, headache, dizziness, fatigue, asthenia, insomnia, paresthesia, nausea, dyspepsia, diarrhea, chest pain, joint pain, and myalgia.

Questions

I. Fill in the Blank

Indicate under which of the following conditions a patient should continue to take the medication for which adverse reactions were specified in the package insert.

  1. The patient experiences lethargy, insomnia, strange dreams, and nervousness during the day: _____

  2. The patient experiences dyspnea, pharyngitis, and arthralgia: _____

  3. The patient does not experience rhinitis, bradycardia, or edema: _____

  4. The drug should not be taken by individuals with sinus bradycardia or cardiac shock: _____

II. Matching 1: Adverse Reactions Found in the United States

Match the term to its meaning. (The same meaning may be used more than once.) Insert the appropriate letter in the space next to the question number.

           Choices:

_____ **1.** pain in a joint	**a.** bradycardia
_____ **2.** localized swelling	**b.** edema
_____ **3.** sensation of numbness and tingling	**c.** lethargy
	d. insomnia
_____ **4.** painful or labored breathing	**e.** paresthesia
	f. dyspnea

_____ **5.** sore throat   **g.** pharyngitis
_____ **6.** inability to sleep   **h.** rhinitis
_____ **7.** nasal inflammation   **i.** dyspepsia
_____ **8.** abnormal sensitivity   **j.** arthralgia
_____ **9.** slow heart beat   **k.** hypersensitivity
_____ **10.** painful digestion
_____ **11.** sluggishness

III.   Matching 2: Results of European Clinical Trials

Match the term to its meaning. (The same meaning may be used more than once.)
Insert the appropriate letter in the space next to the question number.

                                                      Choices:

_____ **1.** feeling of spinning   **a.** palpitation
_____ **2.** loss of strength   **b.** asthenia
_____ **3.** feeling usually before   **c.** paresthesia
            vomiting   **d.** myalgia
_____ **4.** frequency of fluid bowel   **e.** dizziness
            movements   **f.** nausea
_____ **5.** muscle pain   **g.** diarrhea
_____ **6.** feeling of tiredness   **h.** fatigue
_____ **7.** tingling, prickling feeling
_____ **8.** rapid or violent
            throbbing

IV.   Spell Check

Circle each incorrectly spelled term and write it correctly in the space provided.

        1. lethergy   _____
        2. insonnia   _____
        3. pharyngitis   _____
        4. palpiation   _____
        5. paresthesia   _____
        6. dizzyness   _____

J. Increasing Your Medical Terminology Word Power 2

1. Read the following report.
2. Prepare to answer the questions at the end of the section.
3. Circle all unfamiliar terms with a red pencil.
4. Underline familiar terms with a blue pencil.
5. Use your knowledge of word elements, a medical dictionary, and the
     key terms to find the meaning of unfamiliar terms.

Taxol, An Effective Anticancer Agent

Key Terms

bronchospasm (BRONG-kō-spazm)   abnormal narrowing of the bronchi caused
by contraction of surrounding muscles (peribronchial)

cytotoxic (sī-tō-TOKS-ik)   destructive to cells

hematopoietic (hē-ma-tō-poy-ET-ik)   red blood cell development and production

histamine (HIS-ta-mēn) a chemical produced from the amino acid histidine; functions include increasing gastric secretion, dilation of capillaries, and constriction of bronchial smooth muscle

hypersensitivity (hī-per-sen-si-TIV-i-tē) in this presentation, refers to an allergic reaction to a drug

hypotension (hī-pō-TEN-shun) decrease of blood pressure below normal

microtubule (mī-krō-TU-būl) an elongated hollow or tubular structure found in cells; important functions include maintaining cellular rigidity, forming mitotic spindle during cell division, and transporting various substances in different cellular areas

mucositis (mū-kō-SĪ-tis) mucous membrane inflammation

neutropenia (nū-trō-PĒ-nē-a) abnormally small number of neutrophils in the blood

palliative (PAL-ē-a-tiv) refers to relieving symptoms without curing

paresthesia (par-es-THĒ-zē-a) sensation of numbness, prickling, or tingling

refractory (rē-FRAK-tō-re) resistant or stubborn

urticaria (ur-ti-KĀ-rē-a) a vascular condition in which skin eruptions develop accompanied by extreme itching; hives

I NTRODUCTION

The *taxanes* (TAK-sāns) are an important new class of anticancer agents that produce their cytotoxic effects through an unusual mechanism. *Taxol* (TAKS-ōl), the first taxane tested in clinical trials, is active against a broad range of cancers that are generally considered to be refractory to conventional chemotherapy. This finding has led to the regulatory approval of Taxol in many countries for use in the palliative therapy of patients with ovarian and breast cancer resistant to chemotherapy.

Taxol was discovered as part of a National Cancer Institute program in which extracts of thousands of plants were screened for anticancer activity. In 1963, a crude extract from the bark of the Pacific yew (yū), a scarce and slow-growing evergreen found in the old-growth forests of the Pacific Northwest, was found to have cytotoxic activity against many tumors.

M ECHANISM OF ACTION

Cells containing numerous microtubules, which are long, hollow tubular structures consisting of great numbers of protein subunits known as *tubulins* (TŪ-bū-lins). Microtubules have a principal function in the forming of the mitotic spindle during cell division. They are also involved in many vital cellular functions such as maintenance of cell shape and intracellular transport of substances important to cell activity. Taxol works by stimulating the formation of dysfunctional microtubules, thereby causing a disruption of cell division and other vital intracellular processes. The end result is cell death.

T HE QUESTION OF TOXICITY

In the early phases of clinical testing, a number of obstacles were encountered that threatened the prospects for Taxol's further development, including hypersensitivity reactions, neutropenia, neurotoxicity, and certain drug-related gastrointestinal effects. Most patients exhibiting hypersensitivity experienced dyspnea with bronchospasm, urticaria, and hypotension. Protective measures, which included the premedication with corticosteroids and histamine, proved to be effective in preventing initial hypersensitivity and recurrences.

Neutropenia is the principal toxic effect of Taxol. Its action was not found to be cumulative and only rarely was thrombocytopenia and anemia experienced by patients.

Taxol also induces some neuropathy that is characterized by symptoms such as numbness and paresthesia. Severe neurotoxicity is rarely encountered at normal doses of the drug.

Drug-related gastrointestinal effects of Taxol use such as vomiting and diarrhea are infrequent. High doses of the drug may cause mucositis, especially in patients with leukemia.

$\mathcal{F}$UTURE DIRECTIONS

The encouraging results obtained with Taxol have required a long-term solution to the drug-supply problem. Until recently, the supply of Taxol came only from Pacific yew tree bark, but in the future it will be derived increasingly from other tree parts, as well as from semisynthetic materials, and plant-tissue cultures.

The novel mechanism of anticancer action of Taxol and related chemicals has stimulated interest in further development and the use of natural products in oncologic therapy.

Questions

I.   Matching

Match the term to its meaning. (The same meaning may be used more than once.) Insert the appropriate letter in the space next to the question number.

Choices:

_____ 1. bronchospasm
_____ 2. cytotoxic
_____ 3. hematopoietic
_____ 4. hypotension
_____ 5. neutropenia
_____ 6. palliative
_____ 7. paresthesia
_____ 8. refractory

a. destruction to cells
b. red blood cell development and production
c. abnormal narrowing of bronchi caused by surrounding muscles
d. decrease in blood pressure below normal
e. resistant
f. numbness, or tingling sensations
g. relieving symptoms without curing
h. abnormally low numbers of neutrophils in blood

II.   Spell Check

Circle each incorrectly spelled term and write it correctly in the space provided.

1. broncspasm   _____
2. microtubuole   _____
3. hipertension   _____
4. paristhesia   _____
5. sitotoxic   _____

6. urticaria   _____

7. palliative   _____

8. hematopoietic _____

K. *Increasing Your Medical Terminology Word Power 3*

    1. Read the following report.

    2. Prepare to answer the questions at the end of the section.

    3. Circle all unfamiliar terms with a red pencil.

    4. Underline familiar terms with a blue pencil.

    5. Use your knowledge of word elements, a medical dictionary, and the key terms to find the meaning of unfamiliar terms.

New Drug Delivery Vehicles

Key Terms

angina (an-JĪ-na) a condition characterized by severe pain and constriction about the heart, usually spreading to the left shoulder and down the left arm; caused by an insufficient blood supply to the heart

compliance (kom-PLĪ-ans) cooperative performance in relation to using or following a prescribed therapy or use of certain medications

hypertension (hī-per-TEN-shun) a condition in which the patient has a higher than normal blood pressure

microinfusion (mī-krō-in-FŪ-zhun) refers to introducing small amounts of a liquid into the body through a vein for therapeutic purposes

permeability (per-mē-a-BIL-i-tē) capability of passage of fluids or other substance into solution

transdermal (tranz-DER-mal) refers to a medicine delivery system applied to the skin

1 NTRODUCTION

With numerous biotechnology drugs on the market and many more likely to be launched over the next decade, barriers to drug delivery have to be addressed. Today's researchers face the dual challenge of finding safer and more effective delivery systems for new drugs. Better formulations and advanced drug delivery systems can provide enabling technology and patient compliance not only with drugs currently in use but with those to be provided in the near future.

    There are many delivery approaches to drug delivery, including injectable, oral, transdermal, nasal, and microinfusion. Researchers are attempting to overcome the pain and inconvenience experienced by patients during traditional delivery approaches while devising systems that can make drugs act at specific times and body sites for maximum results.

O RAL DELIVERY

A substantial portion of drugs taken orally in pill or liquid form is lost to digestive processes and removed by the liver, and what remains can irritate the intestinal tract. Barriers to oral delivery of drugs include metabolic breakdown of the medication, elimination, and regional permeability.

$\mathcal{T}$RANSDERMAL DELIVERY

Transdermal delivery of proteins and related materials avoids gastrointestinal degradation. Transdermal patches slowly deliver drugs through the skin from a reservoir of the drug located within the patch, and usually carry small-molecule drugs that can diffuse through the skin. This approach is being used to treat conditions such as hypertension and angina. Other patches have been designed to deliver pharmaceuticals to motion-sickness sufferers and individuals needing estrogen replacement.

$\mathcal{T}$RANSCUTANEOUS DELIVERY

Transcutaneous patches are being considered as an effective and painless approach to immunization and a stimulant for immune responses. These patches deliver drugs to *epidermal Langerhans* (LANG-er-hanz) *cells*. These cells compose about 25 percent of the epidermis and provide an effective barrier to microorganisms.

$\mathcal{N}$EEDLE-FREE DELIVERY

New devices to replace intramuscular injections also are under development. One approach involves forcing a liquid medication at high speed through a tiny instrument held against the skin. The force creates an ultra-fine stream of fluid that penetrates the skin, delivering medication in a fraction of a second. This approach, once perfected, can deliver injectable medications comfortably, accurately, and quickly without the use of a needle. The system can deliver both intramuscular and subcutaneous injectable drugs. In addition, because needles are not involved, the system provides health-care workers with an unparalleled level of protection against accidental needle-stick injuries.

$\mathcal{A}$EROSOLS

Pulmonary delivery of medications and other materials through the use of aerosols to the systemic circulation can achieve excellent availability for treatment because of the large surface area of the respiratory system, the thinness of the air–blood barrier, and the relative absence of inactivating enzymes. Inhalers, which are the best-known examples using an aerosol approach, are limited in effectiveness. However, improvements are being made with a better understanding of the factors influencing aerosol deposition in the lungs.

$\mathcal{F}$UTURE OUTLOOK

Large numbers of protein and related drugs for the prevention and treatment of a large number of diseases and disorders are continually being developed. However, satisfactory ways with which to accurately deliver them have not kept up. What is needed is a way to place effective drugs into the bloodstreams of patients so that the drugs go directly to where they are needed and only there, and do exactly what they are intended to do, and only that. Biotechnology has not reached this point yet.

Questions

I.   Fill in the Blank

Fill in the blank with the appropriate term.

1. List five drug delivery vehicles.

   a. _____
   b. _____
   c. _____
   d. _____
   e. _____

2. A patch that slowly delivers drugs through the skin from a reservoir within the patch is _____.

3. A patch that delivers drugs to epidermal Langerhans cells is

   _____.

4. List two barriers to the oral delivery of medications.

   a. _____
   b. _____

II.   Spell Check

Circle each incorrectly spelled term and write it correctly in the space provided.

1. hypertenson   _____
2. microinfuzun   _____
3. permeebility   _____
4. anjina   _____
5. complience   _____
6. airosol   _____
7. transcutanous _____
8. Langerhans   _____

Term Search Challenge

Locate 12 terms in the puzzle.

1. Write the specific term next to its definition. Then find that term in the puzzle diagram and circle it.
2. Terms may be read from left to right, backward, up, down, or diagonally.
3. If a term appears more than once, circle it only once. (A term or abbreviation may be found inside others.)
4. Check your answers.

Clues:

1. Study of drugs, including their origin and effect on the body

   _____

2. Use of drugs for treatment of infectious diseases and cancer

   _____

3. Study of harmful chemicals and their effects on the body

   _____

4. Substance given to neutralize undesirable or unwanted effects of drugs

   _____

5. Material that promotes vomiting _____

6. Gastrointestinal drug that neutralizes an acid condition
   _____

7. Commercial or trade names for a drug _____

8. Legal, noncommercial name for a drug _____

9. Drug that produces sleep _____

10. Two combining forms for a drug _____ and
    _____

11. Suffix pertaining to killing _____

Term Search Puzzle

```
P  H  A  R  M  A  C  O  L  O  G  Y  P  C  A
S  H  P  H  A  R  M  A  C  O  T  T  H  O  N
Y  P  A  R  E  H  T  O  M  E  H  C  Y  N  T
G  S  A  R  A  B  X  I  S  Y  Y  A  L  V  A
O  A  T  L  M  L  R  P  R  U  T  A  U  C
L  T  N  A  G  A  H  P  N  H  X  L  I
O  N  P  T  T  E  C  E  N  Y  O  A  I  S  D
C  P  R  U  I  I  S  I  S  D  T  R  S  A  C
I  T  R  P  H  D  C  I  S  L  I  T  S  N  I
X  A  T  U  Y  L  O  T  O  T  C  I  T  T  D
O  T  A  R  R  A  S  T  A  T  I  C  I  R  A
T  I  C  A  T  I  C  E  E  L  A  S  T  P  L
T  A  R  R  H  Y  T  H  I  C  X  I  S  L  O
G  E  G  E  N  E  R  I  C  G  C  H  E  M  O
T  N  A  L  U  G  A  O  C  E  M  E  T  I  C
```

CHAPTER 28

Radiology, Radiotherapy, and Nuclear Medicine

"Insults and injuries to the human have always challenged the ingenuity of individuals and groups to devise means and forms toward their prevention, control, and treatment."

—David Landy

INFORMATIONAL CHALLENGE

A. Specialty Areas, Radiological Personnel, Diagnostic Procedures and Techniques, Patient Positioning, and Contrast Media

I. Fill in the Blank

Fill in the blank with the appropriate term.

1. A physician who specializes in the practice of diagnostic radiology is called a *radio* _____.
2. A physician trained in the use of diagnostic nuclear medical procedures is a(n) _____ physician.
3. A physician specializing in the treatment of disease with radiation is a *radio*_____.
4. Supportive health-care professionals working with physicians in the specialty areas of radiotherapy, nuclear medicine, and radiology are known as _____ technologists.
5. A substance used to make a body structure, fluid, or other material of importance obvious is referred to as a _____ medium.

II. Matching 1: Processes and Substances Associated with Radiology, Nuclear Medicine, and Radiation Therapy

Match the term to its meaning. (The same meaning may be used more than once.) Insert the appropriate letter in the space next to the question number.

_____ 1. x-rays
_____ 2. gamma rays
_____ 3. ionization
_____ 4. ions
_____ 5. half-life
_____ 6. translucent
_____ 7. barium sulfate
_____ 8. radiopaque
_____ 9. air, carbon dioxide, and nitrous oxide
_____ 10. iodine

Choices:

    a. process by which neutral particles become charged

    b. time required for radioactive substrate to lose half of its radioactivity

    c. charged particles

    d. invisible waves of energy produced by an energy source such as a cathode ray tube

    e. waves of energy, similar to x-rays, that are used in nuclear medicine

    f. gases used as contrast media for the examination of organs such as the brain and spinal cord

    g. a substance that permits passage of most x-rays

    h. a metallic powder used for the examination of the GI tract

    i. a substance that absorbs most x-rays to which it is exposed

    j. an example of a radiopaque material used in obtaining x-ray images of blood vessels and certain body organs

III.   Matching 2: Positioning Terms Used in Diagnostic and Related Radiologic Procedures

Match the term to its meaning. (The same meaning may be used more than once.) Insert the appropriate letter in the space next to the question number.

Choices:

_____ **1.** eversion

_____ **2.** recumbent

_____ **3.** extension

_____ **4.** prone

_____ **5.** flexion

_____ **6.** inversion

_____ **7.** PA view

_____ **8.** abduction

_____ **9.** oblique view

_____ **10.** supine

_____ **11.** adduction

_____ **12.** lateral decubitus

a. x-ray tube is placed at an angle from the perpendicular plane

b. lying on the abdomen (belly)

c. turning outward

d. lying down in either a prone or supine position

e. lying on the back

f. individual is standing with the back to an x-ray machine and the film to the chest

g. turning inward

h. bending a part of the body

i. moving the body toward the midline

j. moving part of the body away from the midline

k. straightening a flexed body part

l. lying on the side with the x-ray beam positioned horizontally

IV.   Spell Check

Circle each incorrectly spelled term and write it correctly in the space provided.

    1. rontgenology _____

    2. radioopaque _____

    3. ionization _____

    4. abducktion _____

5. irons   _____

6. radionuclide   _____

7. betta   _____

8. gama   _____

9. radiografer   _____

10. envirsion   _____

B. Contrast Media and Techniques

I.   Fill in the Blank

Fill in the blank with the appropriate term.

1. List three diagnostic radiologic techniques that require the use of a contrast medium.

a. _____

b. _____

c. _____

2. List recent diagnostic radiologic techniques that may or may not require the use of a contrast medium.

a. _____

b. _____

c. _____

3. What does the abbreviation for the radiologic technique CAT mean?

C = _____ , A = _____ , T = _____

4. What do the abbreviations used for the radiologic technique NMR and MRI mean?

N = _____ , M = _____ , R = _____

M = _____ , R = _____ , I = _____

5. What is the record produced by ultrasonography called?

_____

II.   Matching 1: Diagnostic X-Ray Techniques Requiring Contrast Medium, Part 1

Match the term to its meaning. (The same meaning may be used more than once.) Insert the appropriate letter in the space next to the question number.

Choices:

_____ **1.** angiocardiogram

_____ **2.** venogram

_____ **3.** intravenous cholangiogram

_____ **4.** upper GI series

_____ **5.** bronchogram

_____ **6.** sialogram

_____ **7.** arteriogram

_____ **8.** hysterosalpingogram

a. uses barium sulfate to outline the area from the esophagus through the duodenum

b. used to obtain a record of the salivary ducts

c. used to detect any blockage of the uterine (Fallopian) tubes

d. used to obtain an x-ray image of the renal pelvis and urinary tract

_____ **9.** intravenous pyelogram
_____ **10.** myelogram

e. provides an image of the blood vessels and heart
f. used to obtain an x-ray of the bronchial tubes
g. may be used to detect any blockage of the bile ducts
h. used to obtain an x-ray of an artery
i. provides an x-ray image of veins
j. may be used to detect a bone pressing on the spinal cord

III.   Matching 2: Diagnostic X-Ray Techniques Requiring Contrast Medium, Part 2

Match the term to its meaning. (The same meaning may be used more than once.) Insert the appropriate letter in the space next to the question number.

_____ **1.** used to detect gallstones in the common bile duct
_____ **2.** used to obtain views of a joint
_____ **3.** used to identify tumors of the spinal cord
_____ **4.** provides x-ray records of the renal pelvis and urinary tract
_____ **5.** involves the use of two x-rays, one without contrast medium, and the removal of blocking view by a computer
_____ **6.** provides x-ray record of lymphatic vessels
_____ **7.** the use of air for an x-ray examination of the brain and spinal cord
_____ **8.** used to obtain x-rays of brain ventricles with the injection of air

Choices:

a. myelogram
b. digital subtraction angiography
c. cholecystogram
d. arthrogram

e. encephalogram
f. lymphangiogram
g. retrograde pyelogram
h. ventriculogram

IV.   Matching 3: Radiologic Diagnostic Procedures Usually Not Involving Contrast Media

Match the term to its meaning. (The same meaning may be used more than once.) Insert the appropriate letter in the space next to the question number.

Choices:

_____ **1.** nuclear magnetic resonance
_____ **2.** laminagraphy
_____ **3.** tomography
_____ **4.** position-emission tomography
_____ **5.** ultrasonography
_____ **6.** xeroradiography

a. the use of a series of x-rays focusing on an organ at different levels
b. positions create a cross-sectional image of radioactivity distribution
c. an x-ray is first made on a charged plate and then reproduced on copy paper
d. the use of a magnetic field and radio waves to form body images
e. the use of high-frequency sound waves bouncing off body tissue to obtain records of body organs

V.   Spell Check

Circle each incorrectly spelled term and write it correctly in the space provided.

  1. flouressence   _____
  2. kolecystogram   _____
  3. hysterosalpingogram   _____
  4. pneumoencefalogram   _____
  5. cholangiogram   _____
  6. mylogram   _____
  7. angiography   _____
  8. bronchogram   _____

VI.   Vision Quiz: Radiologic Techniques

Figure 28-8 shows the results of a brain examination that does not require a contrast medium or x-rays to produce a cross-sectional image. Identify and write the name of the technique in the space provided.

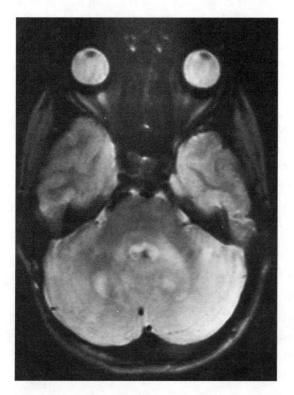

FIGURE 28-8   Vision Quiz. Radiologic Techniques.

_____

C. Nuclear Medicine

I.   Fill in the Blank

Fill in the blank with the appropriate term.

  1. The time required for a radioactive substance to lose half of its radioactivity is referred to as its _____.

2. List the three types of radioactivity associated with radionuclides.

a. _____

b. _____

c. _____

3. An organ susceptible to the effects of radiation is referred to as being *radio*_____.

4. What do the letters in **rad** mean?

r_____, a_____, d_____

5. List four possible undesirable side effects of radiotherapy.

a. _____

b. _____

c. _____

d. _____

II.   Matching 1: Diagnostic Imaging Procedures, Techniques, and Materials

Match the term to its meaning. (The same meaning may be used more than once.) Insert the appropriate letter in the space next to the question number.

_____ **1.** IV injection of technetium-99m to label phosphates in the body skeleton

_____ **2.** IV injection of a radioactive substance to produce a cross-sectional image of biochemical processes in the body

_____ **3.** IV injection of technetium-99m pertechnate to detect tumors in the CNS

_____ **4.** IV injection of ^{99m}Tc human serum albumin

_____ **5.** applicable to the study of brain chemistry

_____ **6.** oral ingestion of radioactive iodine

_____ **7.** IV injection of radioactive iodine

_____ **8.** following radionuclide distribution to obtain a body image

_____ **9.** can be used to determine thyroid gland size and shape

_____ **10.** IV injection of ^{99m}Tc and sulfur colloid

Choices:

a. scanning   **e.** brain scan

b. thyroid scan   **f.** heart scan

c. bone scan   **g.** iodine uptake

d. positron-emission   **h.** liver scan
tomography

III.   Matching 2: Radiation Therapy Terminology

Match the term to its meaning. (The same meaning may be used more than once.) Insert the appropriate letter in the space next to the question number.

                                                  Choices:

_____ **1.** killing effect   **a.** palliative

_____ **2.** susceptible to radiation   **b.** intercavitary

_____ **3.** placed or lying between   **c.** brachytherapy

_____ **4.** relieves symptoms but   **d.** lethal
does not cure

                                          e. interstitial

_____ **5.** placed within a cavity   **f.** teletherapy

_____ **6.** placement of radioactive   **g.** radiosensitive
materials at site of a tumor

_____ **7.** treatment from a distance

IV.   Spell Check

Circle each incorrectly spelled term and write it correctly in the space provided.

1. radionulide   _____

2. sintillation   _____

3. phamasutical   _____

4. perfusion   _____

5. alopechsia   _____

6. technetium   _____

7. pertechnatate   _____

8. interstitial   _____

9. brachytheraoy   _____

10. myelosuppression   _____

D. Word Elements Associated with Radiology, Nuclear Medicine, and Radiation Therapy

I.   Matching: Word Elements Associated with Radiologic Procedures and Techniques

Match the term to its meaning. (The same meaning may be used more than once.)
Insert the appropriate letter in the space next to the question number.

Choices:

_____ **1.** radi/o   **a.** x-rays

_____ **2.** tele/o   **b.** same

_____ **3.** ion   **c.** distant

_____ **4.** xer/o   **d.** rays

_____ **5.** ech/o   **e.** to wander

_____ **6.** roentgen   **f.** sound

_____ **7.** tom/o   **g.** dry

_____ **8.** iso-   **h.** luminous

_____ **9.** fluor/o   **i.** to cut

_____ **10.** son/o   **j.** short

_____ **11.** brachy

II.   Spell Check

Circle each incorrectly spelled term and write it correctly in the space provided.

1. ultrasenography   _____

2. radiographer   _____

3. ionezation   _____

4. echocardiographer   _____

5. flouroscope   _____

6. zeroradiography   _____

III.   Word Analysis: Word Elements Associated with Radiology, Nuclear Medicine, and Radiation Therapy

Table 28-8 lists a number of terms with their pronunciations and definitions.

TABLE 28-8   WORD ANALYSIS: WORD ELEMENTS ASSOCIATED WITH RADIOLOGY, NUCLEAR MEDICINE, AND RADIATION THERAPY

Term and Pronunciation	Brief Explanation
brachytherapy (brak-ē-THER-a-pē)	a form of radiation therapy applied a short distance from a tumor
echoencephalogram (ek-ō-en-SEF-a-lō-gram)	a record of the ultrasonic echoes of the brain
fluoroscope (FLOO-rō-skōp)	instrument used to see a fluorescent image produced by x-rays on a fluorescent screen
ionogenic (ī-on-ō-JEN-ik)	any substance that can be ionized (becomes an ion)
radiography (rā-de-OG-ra-fē)	process of making x-ray images
roentgenogram (RENT-gen-ō-gram)	film record produced by x-rays
sonography (sō-NOG-ra-fē)	process of recording an image of an organ or tissue
tomography (tō-MOG-ra-fē)	diagnostic technique using x-rays to obtain images of tissue or an organ at difficult levels or planes
ultrasonography (ul-tra-son-OG-ra-fē)	procedure using sound to produce an image of an organ or tissue
xeroradiography (zē'-rō-rā-dē-OG-ra-fē)	process of making an x-ray image on a specially coated plate that is then photographed on copy or special paper

1. Analyze each term.
2. Circle all combining forms, word roots, prefixes, and suffixes and label them **cf, wr, p**, and **s**, respectively.
3. Check your answers (shown in Table 28-9).

E. Medical Vocabulary Building

I.   Matching

Match the term to its meaning. (The same meaning may be used more than once.) Insert the appropriate letter in the space provided next to the question number.

_____ **1.** alopecia   _____ **3.** artifact
_____ **2.** ampere   _____ **4.** ionization

_____	**5.**	cassette	_____	**9.**	shield
_____	**6.**	cyclotron	_____	**10.**	tagging
_____	**7.**	decontamination	_____	**11.**	volt
_____	**8.**	half-life	_____	**12.**	watt

Choices:

a. the process of tracing a radioactive isotope involved in a metabolic reaction

b. a protective structure used to prevent or reduce the passage of radioactive particles

c. the unit of pressure for the flow of electricity

d. the unit of electrical power

e. the process of freeing an object of some contaminating substance

f. the time required for half of the radioactivity of a substance to be reduced by radioactive decay

g. a megavoltage machine used in external radiation therapy

h. pertaining to hair loss

i. the unit of strength of electricity

j. an artificially produced structure

k. the process of irradiating an atom

l. a lightproof holder for film

II.   Spell Check

Circle each incorrectly spelled term and write it correctly in the space provided.

1. wat   _____

2. ampire   _____

3. cycletron   _____

4. megavoltege _____

5. alopesia   _____

6. artifact   _____

7. decontanination _____

8. taging   _____

F. Abbreviations Used in Diagnostic Radiology, Nuclear Medicine, and Radiation Therapy

I.   Fill in the Blank

Fill in the blank with the appropriate term.

1. List six symbols of radioactive chemicals used in radiological and related specialties.

a. _____

b. _____

c. _____

d. _____

e. _____

f. _____

2. Give the meanings of the following abbreviations: CT, PECT:

C = _____ , T = _____

P = _____ , E = _____ , C = _____ , T = _____

3. List two units of radiation measurement.

    a. _____

    b. _____

II.   Matching

Match the term to its meaning. (The same meaning may be used more than once.)
Insert the appropriate letter in the space next to the question number.

Choices:

_____ **1.** CXR

_____ **2.** IVC

_____ **3.** MRI

_____ **4.** IVP

_____ **5.** RP

_____ **6.** DI

_____ **7.** NMR

_____ **8.** ERCP

_____ **9.** SPECT

_____ **10.** PTHC

a. nuclear magnetic resonance

b. intravenous cholangiogram

c. intravenous pyelogram

d. chest x-ray

e. magnetic resonance imaging

f. diagnostic imaging

g. single-photon-emission computed tomography

h. retrograde pyelogram

i. endoscopic retrograde cholangiopancreatography

j. percutaneous transhepatic cholangiography

III.   Spell Check

Circle each incorrectly spelled term and write it correctly in the space provided.

1. simbol   _____

2. intirventional   _____

3. milliampere   _____

4. retrograde   _____

5. millikurie   _____

6. techneteum   _____

IV.   Abbreviation Meanings

Give the meaning of the following abbreviations. Write the responses in the spaces
provided next to the abbreviations.

1. DI _____

2. ERCP _____

3. MRI _____

4. PET _____

G. Increasing Your Medical Terminology Word Power 1

1. Read the following report.

2. Prepare to answer the questions at the end of the section.

3. Circle all unfamiliar terms with a red pencil.

4. Underline familiar terms with a blue pencil.

5. Use your knowledge of word elements, a medical dictionary, and the key terms to find the meaning of unfamiliar terms.

Pleomorphic Adenoma

Key Terms

adenoma (ad-e-NŌ-ma)   an abnormal growth of glandular tissue

benign (bē-NĪN)   opposite of malignant or cancerous

en bloc (en BLOK)   in surgery, refers to removal as a whole or as a lump

foci (FŌ-sī)   locations or sites

hemicranial (hem-ē-KRĀ-nē-al)   pertaining to one side of the head

hypervascularity (hī'-per-vas-kū-LAR-e-tē)   pertaining to an extensive concentration of blood vessels

intradiploic (in-tra-dip-LŌ-ik)   pertaining to spongy tissue between two layers of a compact bone of the skull

parotidectomy (pa-rot-i-DEK-tō-mē)   surgical removal of the parotid gland

pleomorphic (plē-ō-MOR-fik)   having many shapes

resection (rē-SEK-shun)   partial excision of a bone or other structure

C ASE REPORT

A thirty-year-old male presented with an enlarging scalp mass over a period of four months and left-sided hemicranial headaches for the past three months. Fourteen years prior to admission, he had a left superficial parotidectomy for a benign pleomorphic adenoma measuring 2.5 cm.

Skull radiographs and a CT scan showed a large intradiploic mass. A radioisotope bone scan revealed a central area of decreased uptake surrounded by a rim of increased uptake of the radioactive material. No additional abnormal foci were noted in the rest of the skeleton.

An MRI study of the neck and skull base showed no evidence of a recurrent parotid tumor. En bloc surgical resection was performed. Histological and ultrastructural examination confirmed the diagnosis of a benign pleomorphic tumor.

D ISCUSSION

Pleomorphic adenomas of the salivary glands are benign neoplasms characterized by slow growth and may remain unchanged in size for many years. They occur most commonly in the parotid gland and account for the majority of parotid neoplasms. They appear slightly more often in women, with the peak age being between thirty and fifty years.

Questions

I.   Matching

Match the term to its meaning. (The same meaning may be used more than once.) Insert the appropriate letter in the space provided next to the question number.

Choices:

_____ 1. new growth

_____ 2. opposite of cancerous

_____ 3. removal as a whole

_____ 4. on one side of the head

_____ 5. an abnormal growth of glandular tissue

_____ 6. excessive concentration of blood vessels

_____ 7. location

_____ 8. pertains to spongy tissue between two layers of compact bone of the skull

_____ 9. removal of the parotid gland

_____ 10. having many shapes

_____ 11. partial removal of a structure

a. *en bloc*

b. hypervascularity

c. foci

d. neoplasm

e. adenoma

f. parotidectomy

g. intradiploic

h. benign

i. hemicranial

j. pleomorphic

k. resection

II.   Spell Check

Circle each incorrectly spelled term and write it correctly in the space provided.

1. adinoma   _____
2. hemecranial   _____
3. intradiploik   _____
4. reesection   _____
5. benine   _____
6. hipervascularite _____
7. parotidectomy   _____
8. neoplazm   _____

H. Increasing Your Medical Terminology Word Power 2

1. Read the following report.
2. Prepare to answer the questions at the end of the section.
3. Circle all unfamiliar terms with a red pencil.
4. Underline familiar terms with a blue pencil.
5. Use your knowledge of word elements, a medical dictionary, and the key terms to find the meaning of unfamiliar terms.

Bone Injury from Electrical Current

Key Terms

debridement (dā-brēd-MON)   removal of foreign material and dead or damaged tissue

fixation   holding or fastening position

myoglobinuria (mī-ō-glō-bin-Ū-rē-a)   the presence in urine of a form of hemoglobin found in muscle; usually occurs after muscular injury or activity

reduction   pertaining to restoration to normal position, as a fractured bone or hernia

sequestra (sē-KWES-tra)   fragments of damaged bone that have become separated from surrounding tissue

triaged (trē-AZHD)   pertaining to grouping of the sick or injured during emergency situations to determine priority needs for efficient use of health-care personnel, equipment, and facilities

volar (VŌ-ler)   relating to the palm of the hand or the sole of the foot

1 NTRODUCTION

The damage to bone from electrical current may be direct or indirect. Bone, having the greatest electrical resistance of any tissue, generates the greatest heat when conducting an electrical current. Although its structure provides some protection against heat damage, the result may be necrosis of bone, producing sequestra.

C ASE REPORT

A forty-two-year-old male delivering a load of stone to a construction site suffered an electrical injury when the bed of his dump truck hit a high-tension line while unloading. The patient was standing next to the truck at the time of contact and fell to the ground. He lost consciousness briefly, then awoke, and crawled away from the truck. Rescue workers found the patient awake and alert. He was initially triaged at a nearby hospital and then transferred to a burn center, where he was found to have a 3-cm-full thickness burn (entrance wound) on the volar surface of his left forearm and superficial exit wounds on the plantar surfaces of both feet.

Three days following the injury he was taken to the operating room for debridement of his entrance wound. Throughout his hospitalization the patient complained of groin pain, which was felt to be muscle strain. Fracture was not suspected, and radiographs were not obtained. Due to the persistence of this pain, a pelvic radiograph was obtained four days after injury; it revealed bilateral displaced femoral neck fractures.

The patient was promptly taken to the operating room and underwent bilateral reduction and internal fixation with screws. The postoperative course was uneventful, and the patient was discharged to his home nine days after injury.

Questions

I.   Fill in the Blank

Fill in the blank with the appropriate term.

1. Where was the entrance wound located on the patient?

_____

2. Where were the exit wounds located on the patient?

_____

3. Did the patient experience any cardiac or neurologic injuries?

_____

4. What types of fractures did the radiograph reveal?

_____

II.   Spell Check

Circle each incorrectly spelled term and write it correctly in the space provided.

1. voler   _____

2. plantar   _____

    3. sequestra   _____

    4. femorel   _____

    5. superficiel   _____

    6. mioglobinuria   _____

I. Increasing Your Medical Terminology Word Power 3

    1. Read the following report.

    2. Prepare to answer the questions at the end of the section.

    3. Circle all unfamiliar terms with a red pencil.

    4. Underline familiar terms with a blue pencil.

    5. Use your knowledge of word elements, a medical dictionary, and the key terms to find the meaning of unfamiliar terms.

Advances in Nuclear Medicine Instrumentation

Key Terms

aerobic (er-Ō-bik)   pertaining to the presence of oxygen

analogue (AN-a-log)   pertaining to chemical use of the term; a compound that is structurally similar to another

colorectal (kō-lō-REK-tal)   pertaining to the colon and rectum

dissection (dī-SEK-shun)   cutting parts for purposes of separation and/or study

glycolysis (glī-KŌL-i-sis)   pertaining to a series of metabolic reactions in which sugar is broken down; involves water

isotope (Ī-sō-tōp)   one of a series of chemical elements that have nearly identical chemical properties but differ in their atomic weights and electric charge

lymphoma (lim-FŌ-ma)   a general term for the growth of new tissue in the lymphatic system

melanoma (mel'-a-NŌ-ma)   a pigmented mole or tumor that may or may not be cancerous

positron (POZ-i-tron)   an atomic vehicle having the same mass as a negative electron, but having a positive charge

1 NTRODUCTION

A number of technological developments within the past 12 or more years have had positive effects on almost all medical specialties. Within the imaging specialties, advances in computer processing capabilities have allowed more efficient collecting and processing of extremely large volumes of imaging data. Nuclear medicine has long been associated with physiologic imaging and the use of the radiotracer principle. A deeper understanding of the complex relationship between physiology, biochemistry, and genetics, along with technological improvements in instrumentation, has allowed better imaging of physiologic processes. This is also true at the molecular level, which the nuclear medicine community sometimes refers to as *molecular nuclear medicine*. Unlike most studies in radiology, nuclear medicine studies generally depend on the use of radiotracers or radiolabeled pharmaceuticals that are imaged externally.

*P*OSITRON EMISSION TOMOGRAPHY (PET)

Positron emission tomography (PET) rapidly has become an integral part of clinical medicine. This method relies on imaging of radiolabeled tracers that emit positrons. The most common positron-emitting isotope approved for clinical use is the glucose analogue fluorodeoxyglucose F 18 (FDG). PET imaging has long been used in research, but it was not until the U.S. Food and Drug Administration (FDA) and the former U.S. Health Care Financing Administration (HCFA) approved reimbursement for certain indications that PET became an accepted clinical imaging method.

The first approved indication for PET imaging was established in 1998 by HCFA and Medicare. Both agencies agreed that PET imaging is invaluable and cost-effective in the diagnosis of non-small-cell lung cancer (NSCLC) and in the evaluation of indeterminate single pulmonary nodules that are found on occasion during other imaging studies.

PET imaging with FDG relies on the demonstration of an increased rate of aerobic glycolysis by cancer cells. With the use of a glucose analogue, tumor uptake generally is associated with increased metabolic activity. Such changes are well documented for NSCLC, lymphoma, colorectal adenocarcinoma, and malignant melanoma.

Several types of dedicated and nondedicated PET systems are in use; dedicated systems have a more expensive design that enables them to detect positron-emitting agents with a much higher sensitivity and efficiency. Nondedicated systems are usually a modified form of single-photon-emission computed tomography (SPECT) cameras and additional components.

*R*ADIOISOTOPE LYMPHATIC MAPPING

Lymphoscintigraphy (lim'-fō-sin-TIG-gra-fē) is the imaging of lymphatic channels after the injection of radioactive material. Lymphatic mapping is based on the sentinel node concept, which is that the first lymph node to receive lymphatic drainage from a tumor location will be tumor-positive if there has been any lymphatic spread. If the sentinel lymph node is tumor-free, the patient is spared unnecessary lymph node dissection.

Lymphatic mapping has been performed with a variety of radiopharmaceuticals. The only FDA-approved agent is technetium-99m (^{99m}Tc) sulfur colloid preparation. Between 400 and 600 μC of this agent is diluted in 2–4 ml of isotonic sodium chloride and injected into a selected area. There are four main sites of injection: peritumoral, subdermal, intradermal, and intratumoral.

*C*ONCLUDING COMMENTS

The appropriate use of the advanced nuclear medicine technologies requires a team approach to patient care. With more accurate staging of disease processes such as lung cancer, expensive surgical interventions can be avoided and better treatment options used.

Questions

I.   Fill in the Blank

Fill in the blank with the appropriate term.

1. Write the meaning of the following abbreviations in the spaces provided.

    a. PET _____

    b. FDA _____

    c. HCFA _____

    d. FDG _____

    e. NSCLC _____

    f. SPECT _____

2. What is the only FDA-approved agent for lymphatic mapping?

    _____

3. List the four sites of injection used in lymphatic mapping.

    a. _____

    b. _____

    c. _____

    d. _____

II.   Spell Check

Circle each incorrectly spelled term and write it correctly in the space provided.

1. glicolysis   _____

2. nucler   _____

3. cholorectel   _____

4. analoque   _____

5. lymphoma   _____

6. magnetic   _____

Term Search Challenge

Locate 22 terms in the puzzle.

1. Write the specific term next to its definition. Then find that term in the puzzle diagram and circle it.
2. Terms may be read from left to right, backward, up, down, or diagonally.
3. If a term appears more than once, circle it only once. (A term or abbreviation may be found inside others.)
4. Check your answers.

Clues:

1. The study of x-rays _____
2. Medical specialty that involves the use of radioactive substances in disease diagnosis and treatment _____
3. Physician specializing in diagnostic radiology _____
4. Three types of radioactive particles and rays _____, _____, _____.
5. The x-ray procedure in which a fluorescent screen is used instead of a photographic plate _____

6. Abbreviation for chest x-ray _____
7. Combining form for sound _____
8. Combining form for x-rays _____
9. Combining form for rays or radioactivity _____
10. Diagnostic procedure in which a series of picture or views are taken at different depths of an organ _____
11. Diagnostic procedure in which positrons create a cross-sectional image of the metabolism of the body: positron- _____ tomograph
12. Substance that releases high-energy particles or rays as it breaks down _____
13. Term for body position with the face down _____
14. Two abbreviations for computed tomography _____ _____
15. Record of internal body parts produced by ultrasonic _____gram or _____gram
16. Metallic powder mixed in water and used for examination of the upper and lower gastrointestinal tract _____ sulfate
17. Term for electrically charged particles _____
18. Badge worn by individuals working with x-rays _____

Term Search Puzzle

```
B  A  G  U  L  T  R  A  S  O  T  E  N     N
X  E  L  A  X  R  A  Y  O  F  I  L  M  C  U
E  S  T  P  M  G  O  T  N  R  P  O  L  H  C
R  F  T  A  H  M  I  O  O  S  I  R  C  O  L
O  L  T  S  T  A  A  M  O  V  M  A  A  C  E
M  E  M  I  S  S  I  O  N  N  M  D  T  T  A
A  X  B  F  T  S  I  G  O  L  O  I  D  A  R
M  I  A  L  F  I  N  R  T  P  R  O  N  E  O
M  O  R  O  M  A  G  A  S  T  N  N  O  I  E
O  N  I  U  E  S  U  P  I  N  E  U  N  O  N
C  T  U  R  L  E  N  H  Y  A  T  C  U  N  T
X  C  M  E  S  C  P  Y  E  L  U  L  C  S  G
R  A  D  I  O  A  R  T  H  R  O  I  N  O  E
F  L  U  O  R  O  S  C  O  P  Y  D  N  T  N
R  A  D  I  O  L  O  G  Y  I  O  E  C  H  O
```

Pearson Education, Inc.

**YOU SHOULD CAREFULLY READ THE TERMS AND CONDITIONS BEFORE USING THE CD-ROM PACKAGE.
USING THIS CD-ROM PACKAGE INDICATES YOUR ACCEPTANCE OF THESE TERMS AND CONDITIONS.**

Pearson Education, Inc. provides this program and licenses its use. You assume responsibility for the selection of the program to achieve your intended results, and for the installation, use, and results obtained from the program. This license extends only to use of the program in the United States or countries in which the program is marketed by authorized distributors.

LICENSE GRANT

You hereby accept a nonexclusive, nontransferable, permanent license to install and use the program ON A SINGLE COMPUTER at any given time. You may copy the program solely for backup or archival purposes in support of your use of the program on the single computer. You may not modify, translate, disassemble, decompile, or reverse engineer the program, in whole or in part.

TERM

The License is effective until terminated. Pearson Education, Inc. reserves the right to terminate this License automatically if any provision of the License is violated. You may terminate the License at any time. To terminate this License, you must return the program, including documentation, along with a written warranty stating that all copies in your possession have been returned or destroyed.

LIMITED WARRANTY

THE PROGRAM IS PROVIDED "AS IS" WITHOUT WARRANTY OF ANY KIND, EITHER EXPRESSED OR IMPLIED, INCLUDING, BUT NOT LIMITED TO, THE IMPLIED WARRANTIES OR MERCHANTABILITY AND FITNESS FOR A PARTICULAR PURPOSE. THE ENTIRE RISK AS TO THE QUALITY AND PERFORMANCE OF THE PROGRAM IS WITH YOU. SHOULD THE PROGRAM PROVE DEFECTIVE, YOU (AND NOT PRENTICE-HALL, INC. OR ANY AUTHORIZED DEALER) ASSUME THE ENTIRE COST OF ALL NECESSARY SERVICING, REPAIR, OR CORRECTION. NO ORAL OR WRITTEN INFORMATION OR ADVICE GIVEN BY PRENTICE-HALL, INC., ITS DEALERS, DISTRIBUTORS, OR AGENTS SHALL CREATE A WARRANTY OR INCREASE THE SCOPE OF THIS WARRANTY.

SOME STATES DO NOT ALLOW THE EXCLUSION OF IMPLIED WARRANTIES, SO THE ABOVE EXCLUSION MAY NOT APPLY TO YOU. THIS WARRANTY GIVES YOU SPECIFIC LEGAL RIGHTS AND YOU MAY ALSO HAVE OTHER LEGAL RIGHTS THAT VARY FROM STATE TO STATE.

Pearson Education, Inc. does not warrant that the functions contained in the program will meet your requirements or that the operation of the program will be uninterrupted or error-free.

However, Pearson Education, Inc. warrants the diskette(s) or CD-ROM(s) on which the program is furnished to be free from defects in material and workmanship under normal use for a period of ninety (90) days from the date of delivery to you as evidenced by a copy of your receipt.

The program should not be relied on as the sole basis to solve a problem whose incorrect solution could result in injury to person or property. If the program is employed in such a manner, it is at the user's own risk and Pearson Education, Inc. explicitly disclaims all liability for such misuse.

LIMITATION OF REMEDIES

Pearson Education, Inc.'s entire liability and your exclusive remedy shall be:

1. the replacement of any diskette(s) or CD-ROM(s) not meeting Pearson Education, Inc.'s "LIMITED WARRANTY" and that is returned to Pearson Education, or

2. if Pearson Education is unable to deliver a replacement diskette(s) or CD-ROM(s) that is free of defects in materials or workmanship, you may terminate this agreement by returning the program.

IN NO EVENT WILL PRENTICE-HALL, INC. BE LIABLE TO YOU FOR ANY DAMAGES, INCLUDING ANY LOST PROFITS, LOST SAVINGS, OR OTHER INCIDENTAL OR CONSEQUENTIAL DAMAGES ARISING OUT OF THE USE OR INABILITY TO USE SUCH PROGRAM EVEN IF PRENTICE-HALL, INC. OR AN AUTHORIZED DISTRIBUTOR HAS BEEN ADVISED OF THE POSSIBILITY OF SUCH DAMAGES, OR FOR ANY CLAIM BY ANY OTHER PARTY.

SOME STATES DO NOT ALLOW FOR THE LIMITATION OR EXCLUSION OF LIABILITY FOR INCIDENTAL OR CONSEQUENTIAL DAMAGES, SO THE ABOVE LIMITATION OR EXCLUSION MAY NOT APPLY TO YOU.

GENERAL

You may not sublicense, assign, or transfer the license of the program. Any attempt to sublicense, assign or transfer any of the rights, duties, or obligations hereunder is void.

This Agreement will be governed by the laws of the State of New York.

Should you have any questions concerning this Agreement, you may contact Pearson Education, Inc. by writing to:
Director of New Media
Higher Education Division
Pearson Education, Inc.
One Lake Street
Upper Saddle River, NJ 07458

Should you have any questions concerning technical support, you may write to:

**New Media Production
Higher Education Division
Pearson Education, Inc.
One Lake Street
Upper Saddle River, NJ 07458
1-800-677-6337 Monday–Friday, between 8:00 a.m. and 5:00 p.m. CST.**

You can also get support by filling out the web form located at http://247.pearsoned.com/mediaform

YOU ACKNOWLEDGE THAT YOU HAVE READ THIS AGREEMENT, UNDERSTAND IT, AND AGREE TO BE BOUND BY ITS TERMS AND CONDITIONS. YOU FURTHER AGREE THAT IT IS THE COMPLETE AND EXCLUSIVE STATEMENT OF THE AGREEMENT BETWEEN US THAT SUPERSEDES ANY PROPOSAL OR PRIOR AGREEMENT, ORAL OR WRITTEN, AND ANY OTHER COMMUNICATIONS BETWEEN US RELATING TO THE SUBJECT MATTER OF THIS AGREEMENT.